HEPARIN:
Structure, Cellular Functions, and Clinical Applications

Academic Press Rapid Manuscript Reproduction

The Symposium was generously supported by the College of Medicine, the Department of Physiology, the College of Graduate Studies and Research, and the University of Saskatchewan, Saskatoon

Abbott Laboratories Limited, Montreal, Quebec
Canada Packers Limited, Toronto, Ontario
Ciba-Geigy Canada Ltd., Dorval, Quebec
Cohelfred Laboratories, Inc., Illinois
Inolex Corporation, Illinois
Organon, Inc., West Hill, Ontario
Oscar Mayer & Co., Wisconsin
Riker Laboratories, Inc., California
Upjohn International, Inc., Michigan

Canadian Heart Foundation
Canadian Hemophilia Society
Saskatchewan Heart Foundation

City of Saskatoon
Province of Saskatchewan

HEPARIN: Structure, Cellular Functions, and Clinical Applications

Edited by

Norman M. McDuffie

Department of Physiology
College of Medicine
University of Saskatchewan
Saskatoon, Saskatchewan, Canada

ACADEMIC PRESS **New York San Francisco London** **1979**
A Subsidiary of Harcourt Brace Jovanovich, Publishers

ACADEMIC PRESS, INC.
111 Fifth Avenue, New York, New York 10003

United Kingdom Edition published by
ACADEMIC PRESS, INC. (LONDON) LTD.
24/28 Oval Road, London NW1 7DX

Library of Congress Cataloging in Publication Data

International Symposium on Heparin, Saskatoon, Sask., 1977.
Heparin, structure, cellular functions, and clinical applications.

1. Heparin—Congresses. I. McDuffie, Norman M.
QP702.H4157 1977 612′.115 78-31254
ISBN 0-12-484850-8

PRINTED IN THE UNITED STATES OF AMERICA

79 80 81 82 9 8 7 6 5 4 3 2 1

CONTENTS

STRUCTURE

STRUCTURE AND PHARMACODYNAMICS

CELLULAR FUNCTION

CONTRIBUTORS AND PARTICIPANTS

Numbers in parentheses indicate pages on which authors' contributions begin.

D. R. AMIES, 200 Scott Building, Moose Jaw, Saskatchewan, Canada, S6H 0C1

N. G. ARDLIE, P. O. Box 4, Canberra, A.C.T. 2600 Australia

M. ARMANIOUS, Department of Physiology, College of Medicine, University of Saskatchewan, Saskatoon, Saskatchewan, Canada, S7N 0W0

K. F. AUSTEN (67), Harvard Medical School and Robert B. Brigham Hospital, Boston, Massachusetts 02215

W. E. BARNETT, Riker Research Building, 218-1, 3M Company, St. Paul, Minnesota 55016

E. A. BECK (189), Hämatologisches Zentrallabor, Inselspital, CH-3010 Bern, Switzerland

J. P. BENTLEY, University of Oregon Medical School, Portland, Oregon 97201

H. BERTRAND (299), Institut Choay, 46 Avenue Theophile Gautier, 75782 Paris-Cedex 16, France

P. BIANCHINI (99), Laboratori Ricerche Opocrin S.r.l. Via Pacinotti 3 - Corlo(MO) Italia

E. J. BOYER, The Upjohn Co., 7171 Portage Road, Kalamazoo, Michigan 49001

R. T. CARD, Department of Medicine, College of Medicine, University of Saskatchewan, Saskatoon, Saskatchewan, Canada, S7N 0W0

I. A. CARR, Department of Pathology, College of Medicine, University of Saskatchewan, Saskatoon, Saskatchewan, Canada, S7N 0W0

J. CARR, Department of Physiology, College of Medicine, University of Saskatchewan, Saskatoon, Saskatchewan, Canada, S7N 0W0

H. CHIU (323), Department of Pathology, McMaster University Medical Center, 1200 Main Street West, Hamilton, Ontario, Canada, L8S 4J9

L. L. COLEMAN, The Upjohn Co., 7000 Portage Road, Kalamazoo, Michigan 49002

D. M. COHEN (39), Departmento Bioquimica e Farmacologia, Escola Paulista de Medicina, Rua Botucatu 865, Caixa Postal 20372, São Paulo, Brazil 01000

H. E. CONRAD, Department of Biochemistry, University of Illinois, Urbana, Illinois 61801

N. W. COWIE (79), Department of Physiology, College of Medicine, University of Saskatchewan, Saskatoon, Saskatchewan, Canada, S7N 0W0

E. COYNE, Cohelfred Laboratories Inc., Chicago, Illinois 60618

T. A. CUNNINGHAM, Department of Pathology, College of Medicine, University of Saskatchewan, Saskatoon, Saskatchewan, Canada, S7N 0W0

H. L. DAVIS (191), The University of Nebraska Medical Center, Department of Surgery, Omaha, Nebraska 68105

N. L. DAVIS (191), The University of Nebraska Medical Center, Department of Surgery, Omaha, Nebraska 68015

C. P. DIETRICH (39), Departmento Bioquimica e Farmacologia, Escola Paulista de Medicina, Rua Botucatu 865, Caixa Postal 20372, São Paulo, Brazil 01000

K. A. DONNELLY, Department of Biochemistry, University of Utah, Salt Lake City, Utah 84113

R. G. DONOVAN, Canada Packers Limited, 2211 St. Claire Avenue West, Toronto, Ontario, Canada, M6N 1K4

J. EDSTROM, Department of Physiology, College of Medicine, University of Saskatchewan, Saskatoon, Saskatchewan, Canada, S7N 0W0

S. FEDEROFF, Department of Anatomy, College of Medicine, University of Saskatchewan, Saskatoon, Saskatchewan, Canada, S7N 0W0

L. M. FISHER, Department of Clinical Pathology, Medical College of Virginia, Richmond, Virginia 23298

W. C. FROST, Organon Canada Limited, 565 Coronation Drive, West Hill, Ontario, Canada, M1E 4S2

H. GASTPAR (347), Faculty of Medicine, University of Munich, Pettenkoferstr. 8a D8000 Munich 2, West Germany

S. G. GHANI, Pharmaceutical Evaluation Division, Place Vanier, Tower B, 355 River Road, Vanier, Ontario, Canada, K1A 1B8

R. GOODMAN, Department of Physiology, College of Medicine, University of Saskatchewan, Saskatoon, Saskatchewan, Canada, S7N 0W0

P. GORIN, Prairie Regional Laboratory, National Research Council, Saskatoon, Saskatchewan, Canada, S7N 0W9

C. HALL, Department of Anatomy, College of Medicine, University of Saskatchewan, Saskatoon, Saskatchewan, Canada, S7N 0W0

H. HASTIE, Department of Physiology, College of Medicine, University of Saskatchewan, Saskatoon, Saskatchewan, Canada, S7N 0W0

J. HAYES, Department of Physiology, College of Medicine, University of Saskatchewan, Saskatoon, Saskatchewan, Canada, S7N 0W0

L. M. HIEBERT (289), Department of Physiology, College of Medicine, University of Saskatchewan, Saskatoon, Saskatchewan, Canada, S7N 0W0

R. D. HIGGINBOTHAM, Department of Microbiology, University of Louisville, Health Science Center, Louisville, Kentucky 40203

R. HILL, Department of Physiology, College of Medicine, University of Saskatchewan, Saskatoon, Saskatchewan, Canada, S7N 0W0

J. HIRSH (323), Department of Pathology, McMaster University Medical Center, 1200 Main Street West, Hamilton, Ontario, Canada, L8S 4J9

A. A. HORNER (51), Department of Physiology, University of Toronto, Toronto, Ontario, Canada, M5S 1A8

P. HOVINGH (3), Veterans Administration Hospital, Salt Lake City, Utah 84113

R. E. HURST, Center for Developmental and Learning Disorders, University of Alabama in Birmingham, University Station, Birmingham, Alabama 35294

R. HUTCHINSON, Department of Physiology, College of Medicine, University of Saskatchewan, Saskatoon, Saskatchewan, Canada, S7N 0W0

D. IRVINE, Psychiatric Research, College of Medicine, University of Saskatchewan, Saskatoon, Saskatchewan, Canada, S7N 0W0

L. B. JAQUES (373), Department of Physiology, College of Medicine, University of Saskatchewan, Saskatoon, Saskatchewan, Canada, S7N 0W0

M. J. JERIA, Department of Anatomy, College of Medicine, University of Saskatchewan, Saskatoon, Saskatchewan, Canada, S7N 0W0

B. JOHNSON, Bushell Park, Saskatchewan, Canada, S0H 0N0

B. H. J. JUURLINK, Department of Anatomy, College of Medicine, University of Saskatchewan, Saskatoon, Saskatchewan, Canada, S7N 0W0

V. V. KAKKAR, Thrombosis Research Unit, Department of Surgery, King's College Hospital Medical School, University of London, Denmark Hill, London, UK SE5 8RX

L. W. KAVANAGH (333), #107, 217 Third Avenue North, Saskatoon, Saskatchewan, Canada, S7K 2H7

A. KHER Pharmuka, 35 a 41, Quai du Moulin de Cage, 92231, Gennevilliers, France

T. Y. KOH, Canada Packers Ltd., 2211 St. Clair Avenue West, Toronto, Ontario, Canada, M6N 1K4

R. KOOB, Department of Physiology, College of Medicine, University of Saskatchewan, Saskatoon, Saskatchewan, Canada, S7N 0W0

T. KOVATS, Chemical and Pharmaceutical Works of Gedeon Richter, H-1475 Budapest 10. Pf.27. Hungary

P. M. KRAEMER (211), Cellular and Molecular Biology Group, University of California, Los Alamos Scientific Laboratory, P.O. Box 1663, Los Alamos, New Mexico 87545

T. KRUKOFF, Department of Anatomy, College of Medicine, University of Saskatchewan, Saskatoon, Saskatchewan, Canada, S7N 0W0

M. KYLE, Nursing, College of Medicine, University of Saskatchewan, Saskatoon, Saskatchewan, Canada, S7N 0W0

O. G. LANE, Victoria Union Hospital, Bag 300, Prince Albert, Saskatchewan, Canada, S6V 5T4

Y. LAPIDOT, Department of Biological Chemistry, The Hebrew University of Jerusalem, Jerusalem, Israel

S. E. LASKER (143), Department of Medicine, New York Medical College, Flower and Fifth Avenue Hospitals, New York, New York 10029

W. W. LAUTT, Department of Physiology, College of Medicine, University of Saskatchewan, Saskatoon, Saskatchewan, Canada, S7N 0W0

U. LINDAHL (167), Department of Medical Chemistry, Royal Veterinary College, Biomedicum, Box 575, B-75123 Uppsala, Sweden

A. LINKER (3), Veterans Administration Hospital, Salt Lake City, Utah 84113

W. L. LOW, Box 310, Invermay, Saskatchewan, Canada, S0A 1M0

W. S. LYNN, BC-3711, Duke University Medical Center, Durham, North Carolina

J. G. McCORMICK, The Bowman Gray School of Medicine of Wake Forest University, Winston-Salem, North Carolina 27103

H. McDUFFIE, Division of Medical Genetics, Department of Pediatrics, Ellis Hall, University Hospital, Saskatoon, Saskatchewan, Canada, S7N 0W8

N. M. McDUFFIE (79), Department of Physiology, College of Medicine, University of Saskatchewan, Saskatoon, Saskatchewan, Canada, S7N 0W0

K. McDUFFIE, Department of Physiology, College of Medicine, University of Saskatchewan, Saskatoon, Saskatchewan, Canada, S7N 0W0

B. McLENNAN, Department of Biochemistry, College of Medicine, University of Saskatchewan, Saskatoon, Saskatchewan, Canada, S7N 0W0

J. McMULLEN, Galaxo Laboratories, 1 Dorchester Avenue, Toronto, Ontario, Canada, M8Z 4W1

J. MADLAND-ULMER, Department of Physiology, College of Medicine, University of Saskatchewan, Saskatoon, Saskatchewan, Canada, S7N 0W0

J. MAHADOO (181, 333), Department of Physiology, College of Medicine, University of Saskatchewan, Saskatoon, Saskatchewan, Canada, S7N 0W0

J. MARDIGUIAN, Department Biologie-Pharmuka, 35 a 41, Quai de Cage, 92231 Gennevilliers, France

R. K. MARGOLIS (227), Department of Pharmacology, State University of New York Downstate Medical Center, Brooklyn, New York 11203

R. U. MARGOLIS (227), Department of Pharmacology, N.Y.U. Medical Center, School of Medicine, New York, New York 10016

I. S. MENDELSON, Alvin Buckwold Center, Department of Pediatrics, University Hospital, Saskatoon, Saskatchewan, Canada, S7N 0W8

J. E. MERRIMAN, 7518 S. Evanston Avenue, Tulsa, Oklahoma 74136

K. MEYER, Belfer Graduate School of Science, New York, New York 10033

Y. M. MICHELACCI (39), Departmento Bioquimica e Farmacologia, Escola Paulista de Medicina, Rua Botucatu 865, Caixa Postal 20372, São Paulo, Brazil 01000

G. J. MILLAR, Department of Physiology, College of Medicine, University of Saskatchewan, Saskatoon, Saskatchewan, Canada, S7N 0W0

V. G. MOSS, Oscar Mayer & Co., Research Department, P.O. Box 7188, Madison, Wisconsin 53707

H. B. NADER (39), Departmento Bioquimica e Farmacologia, Escola Paulista de Medicina, Rua Botucatu 865, Caixa Postal 20372, São Paulo, Brazil 01000

R. S. NAGI, Department of Anatomy, College of Medicine, University of Saskatchewan, Saskatoon, Saskatchewan, Canada, S7N 0W0

N. NAKAMURA, Engineering Biophysics, University of Alabama, University Station, Birmingham, Alabama 35294

V. OSTERTAG, Department of Physiology, College of Medicine, University of Saskatchewan, Saskatoon, Saskatchewan, Canada, S7N 0W0

F. T. OTERUELO, Department of Anatomy, College of Medicine, University of Saskatchewan, Saskatoon, Saskatchewan, Canada, S7N 0W0

J. PADAWER (251), Department of Anatomy, Albert Einstein College of Medicine, New York, New York 10461

J. L. PEREZ-REQUEJO, Banco De Sangre De Carabo BO-Avda. Luis Pérez Carreño Qta. Wanda Cristina Urb. Guaparo Valencia Edo. Carabobo Venezuela

A. S. PERLIN (25), Department of Chemistry, Otto Mass Chemistry Bldg., McGill University, Montreal, Quebec, Canada, H3C 3G1

J. W. PHILLIS, Department of Physiology, College of Medicine, University of Saskatchewan, Saskatoon, Saskatchewan, Canada, S7N 0W0

M. W. PIEPKORN, Department of Pathology, School of Medicine, RC-72, University of Washington, Seattle, Washington 98195

W. F. PROUTY, Inolex Corporation, Park Forest South, Illinois 60466

C. RABY (299), Institut Choay, 46 Avenue Theophile Gautier, 75782 Paris-Cedex 16, France

B. ROBERTSON, Organon Canada Ltd., 565 Coronation Drive, West Hill, Ontario, Canada, M1E 4S2

B. ROBSON, Department of Physiology, College of Medicine, University of Saskatchewan, Saskatoon, Saskatchewan, Canada, S7N 0W0

R. D. ROSENBERG Sidney Farber Cancer Center, Harvard Medical School, Boston, Massachusetts 02215

B. S. R. SASTRY, Department of Physiology, College of Medicine, University of Saskatchewan, Saskatoon, Saskatchewan, Canada, S7N 0W0

C. SCHAFER, Department of Nuclear Medicine, St. Barnabas Hospital, New York City, New York 10457

S. SHERRY, Department of Medicine, Temple University, School of Medicine, Philadelphia, Pennsylvania 19140

J. E. SILBERT (67), Veterans Administration Hospital, Outpatient Clinic, Boston, Massachusetts 02108

A. SILVERGLADE, 19901 Nordhoff Street, Northridge, California 91324

P. K. SINGAL, Department of Physiology, College of Medicine, University of Saskatchewan, Saskatoon, Saskatchewan, Canada, S7N 0W0

D. SINGER, College of Dentistry, University of Saskatchewan, Saskatoon, Saskatchewan, Canada, S7N 0W0

L. SPOLTER, Cell Biochemistry Research, Veterans Administration Hospital, Sepulveda, California 91342

B. STANLEY, Department of Physiology, College of Medicine, University of Saskatchewan, Saskatoon, Saskatchewan, Canada, S7N 0W0

S. STECKLER, Department of Physiology, College of Medicine, University of Saskatchewan, Saskatoon, Saskatchewan, Canada, S7N 0W0

T. K. SUE (159), Department of Physiology, College of Medicine, University of Saskatchewan, Saskatoon, Saskatchewan, Canada, S7N 0W0

G. B. SUTHERLAND, Department of Physiology, College of Medicine, University of Saskatchewan, Saskatoon, Saskatchewan, Canada, S7N 0W0

Y. TANAKA, Department of Chemistry, Premedical Course, Kurume University School of Medicine, 1635 Mii-Machi, Kurume, 830, Japan

D. W. TYLER, College of Dentistry, University of Saskatchewan, Saskatoon, Saskatchewan, Canada, S7N 0W0

M. UDDIN, College of Dentistry, University of Saskatchewan, Saskatoon, Saskatchewan, Canada, S7N 0W0

B. UVNÄS (243), Department of Pharmacology, Karolinska Institutet, FACK S-10401, Stockholm, Sweden

W. G. VAN AKEN (323), Department of Pathology, McMaster University Medical Center, 1200 Main Street West, Hamilton, Ontario, Canada, L8S 4J9

G. VAN DEDEM, Diosynth BV., P.O. Box 20, Oss, Holland

E. G. VARIEL, Institut Choay, 46 Avenue Theophile Gautier, 75782 Paris-Cedex 16, France

G. VIELLE, 1782 Belfoux IFR, Switzerland

B. WEISSMAN, Department of Biological Chemistry, University of Illinois at Medical Centre, Chicago, Illinois 60612

S. S. WEST, Department of Engineering Biophysics, University Alabama Medical Center, Birmingham, Alabama 35233

P. WEISSGERBER (347), Faculty of Medicine, University of Munich, Pettenkoferstr. 8a D8000 Munich 2, West Germany

S. WICE, Department of Physiology, College of Medicine, University of Saskatchewan, Saskatoon, Saskatchewan, Canada, S7N 0W0

T. WICKES, Cohelfred Laboratories, Inc., Chicago, Illinois 60618

A. WOLLIN, Unite de Recherches Gastrointestinales, Centre Hospitalier Universitaire, Sherbrooke, Quebec, Canada, J1H 5N4

C. J. WRIGHT, Department of Surgery, College of Medicine, University of Saskatchewan, Saskatoon, Saskatchewan, Canada, S7N 0W0

E. YOUNG (51), Department of Physiology, University of Toronto, Toronto, Ontario, Canada M5S 1A8

R. W. YURT (67), Harvard Medical School and Robert B. Brigham Hospital, Boston Massachusetts 02215

FOREWORD

It is an honor, indeed, for me to have this opportunity to say a few words at the opening of this important international symposium on heparin.

One cannot overestimate the importance of the substance or substances referred to generically as heparin, for few agents have had a more profound influence on the development of medicine and surgery. Not only has heparin been the leader in antithrombotic therapy ever since its introduction some 40 years ago initiated a new field of therapeutics, but it also has made possible dramatic advances in cardiac surgery, vascular surgery, acute and chronic hemodialysis, and a variety of other medical and surgical procedures. Furthermore, were it not for heparin, many experimental studies in animals and on blood, which have been and continue to be fundamental for important clinical developments, never could have been carried out. Thus, while few, if any, have ever suggested that heparin be included in any survival kit, it would be interesting to contemplate the nature of medicine or medical practice today without its presence. Such considerations, along with the fact that ever since its introduction heparin has continued to enjoy a sustained growth, both in volume of use and variety of applications, provide sufficient reason that new knowledge, both of a basic and applied nature, be reviewed at appropriate intervals. This is such a time, particularly since a number of important advances have occurred recently.

The site for this symposium is a most fitting one. It takes place in a country where heparin was first introduced for clinical use, and where pioneering work on this compound has continued uninterrupted for some two score years; and it takes place in an institution whose Department of Physiology has been a world leader in heparin research by virtue of its many significant advances to our knowledge. But, perhaps most importantly, it offers the many scientists who have come near and far to attend this meeting the opportunity to honor a senior and elder statesman at the University of Saskatchewan who has devoted his entire research career to the investigation of these unique macromolecules, and whose studies on this subject are so well recognized internationally that a word association between heparin and L. B. Jaques has developed spontaneously.

As frequently happens with imortant medical breakthroughs, serendipity played a major role in Jay McLean's discovery of heparin. Howell had asked him to investigate tissue sources of thromboplastin other than brain, and had suggested he try to extract such a material from the heart and the liver. The heart material turned out to be less potent than the controversial brain extract but the liver preparation actually prevented clotting rather than accelerating it. The rest is history!

I have no intention to review the heparin story. Its early phase is well covered in previous publications by McLean and such other famous heparin pioneers as Erik Jorpes, Charles Best, and Gordon Murray, and a complete classified bibliography of all heparin publications through July 1958 is available. And as for the period since then, no purpose would be served by my doing this, particulaly since Professor Jaques will be addressing us later on "Forty Years of Heparin Research: Past and Future."

This symposium is not designed to cover all aspects of our knowledge of heparin; such an undertaking would be much too formidable for a three-day meeting. Rather the organizers, under the wise leadership of Dr. McDuffie, have chosen certain topics of current interest for major consideration. These include the structure of heparin and related compounds, its interactions in carrying out its functional activity, the cellular role of heparin, and selected aspects of clinical application.

Before concluding these introductory remarks, I would like to say a few words about the man being honored by this symposium and for whom the published proceedings undoubtedly will be dedicated. As many of you know, almost two decades went by, following the initial discovery of heparin in 1916, before purified preparations of this substance were made available for clinical investigation in man and this occurred almost simultaneously and independently in Canada and Sweden. It is indeed fortunate for us that, just at the time that Connaught Laboratories made such preparations available to Dr. Gordon Murray for patient studies, Louis Barker Jaques, who had been born in Toronto some 22 years earlier, decided to pursue a Masters Degree in Physiology at the University of Toronto and was assigned to assist Murray in his studies. This collaboration between a brilliant academic surgeon and a dedicated and determined student, so reminiscent of the Banting and Best association some ten years earlier, soon resulted in the first demonstration of the clinical usefulness of heparin, namely, in vascular surgery. From this early trail-blazing work, Jaques has maintained a commitment and devotion to heparin research which is unique; he is the only one of the early pioneers who has maintained a total interest in this agent. This interest now spans four decades and includes 128 publications of original research work on this substance.

Among Jaques' firsts are the demonstration of the use of heparin in preventing thrombosis, the use of pharmacodynamic studies for establishing dosage, identification of differences in heparins among various mammalian species, variability of activity among commercial preparations, methods for the determination of heparin such as protamine titration, metachromatic staining, and clotting times, demonstration of the platelet aggregating effect of commercial heparin preparations, heparin's reaction with toluidine blue, identification of iduronic acid as a major component of heparin, and the identification of circulating heparin in canine anaphylaxis. Thus Jaques' career has spanned not only the entire active period of investigation of this substance, but his own studies have covered the entire spectrum of heparin investigation: its chemistry, physiology, pharmacology, and therapeutics. And in the tradition of the "complete" scientist, he has adopted, adapted, and created techniques to solve problems rather than seeking problems to be solved by a specific technique.

The first 12 years of Jaques' research career were spent in the Department of Physiology at the University of Toronto, but in 1946 at the age of 35, he was summoned to the University of Saskatchewan as Professor and Head of their Department of Physiology, a position he held for the next 25 years. In 1971 he relinquished this responsibility, and since then has served as Director of the Department's Haemostasis-Thrombosis Research Unit. His importance to the University has been recognized in many ways; one evidence of this has been his appointment in 1972 as the first W. S. Lindsay Professor of this University's College of Medicine.

While his research accomplishments and the leadership he has given to the heparin field speak for themselves, all of us have admired this man for his personal qualities as well. He has taught us all that one need not be flashy to be impressive—all one has to do is to have the facts. And where heparin is concerned, Louis Barker Jaques has more than anyone else in this world today. All of us here salute you Professor Jaques and wish you many more years of wise counsel, leadership, and productive research.

SOL SHERRY

Department of Medicine
Temple University

PREFACE

The International Symposium on Heparin was held at Saskatoon, July 6–8, 1977. The purposes of the symposium were multiple. Foremost among them was the opportunity to honor a persistent and gifted scientist who had unflaggingly devoted over 40 years to heparin research. Although Louis Barker Jaques' contributions are legion, the timing of the symposium was perhaps equally dictated by the novel findings emanating from research centers in Boston, Uppsala, São Paulo, Toronto, Montreal, London, and Saskatoon. The mid-1970's produced a surge in application of new techniques to the age-old problems of heterogeneity and polydispersity of the mucopolysaccharides. Results of these studies suggested better understanding of the complex molecules termed heparin could be obtained. With this objective in mind, the symposium was organized to bring together experts from diverse disciplines that related to the heparin problem. Individuals were encouraged to discuss at length older and newer concepts pertaining to the heparin molecule, its pharmacology, physiology, and clinical application.

The response was most gratifying. The interaction between the participants was extraordinary, and I commend to the reader the edited discussion sections of the book.

The final word at the symposium was left to Professor Jaques whose commentary on the field and the conference closes the book. I am indebted to all participants and particularly those individuals who worked diligently toward the completion of the book.

STRUCTURE

ENZYMATIC DEGRADATION OF HEPARIN AS A TOOL FOR STRUCTURAL ANALYSIS

Alfred Linker and Peter Hovingh

Veterans Administration Hospital
and
Departments of Biological Chemistry and Pathology
University of Utah College of Medicine

Heparin fractions obtained originally from a variety of biological sources were degraded by Flavobacterial heparinase, and the products obtained were analyzed for structural details. In addition periodate oxidation and nitrous acid degradation were used on the polysaccharides as well as on their enzymatic breakdown products to gain further information about the distribution of uronic acid units and about sulfate substitution. Based on these data an arrangement of lower sulfated regions in an otherwise higher sulfated polymer has been proposed.

I. INTRODUCTION

Heparin was first isolated about sixty years ago and its general physical, chemical, and biological properties have been known for a long time. It is, therefore, quite surprising that despite continuing interest and extensive research effort some major questions about this polysaccharide still remain unanswered.

Over many years, Dr. Jaques has consistently and relentlessly reminded all of us who would be only too willing to rest on our laurels that the two most important questions one can ask about a biologically active material have remained elusive. These are: what is heparin and what is its true biological activity?

Recent very interesting work by Rosenberg and coworkers (1) and Lindahl and coworkers (2,3) dealing with "active" heparin has shown that only one half, or even considerably less, of what is considered to be heparin interacts strongly with antithrombin. This makes the unanswered questions even more significant.

ISBN 0-12-484850-8

The main interest of our laboratory has been directed toward the elucidation of the structural details of the polysaccharide chains and their relation to the activities of the polymer in biological systems. Our approach to this problem has involved the use of specific degradative enzymes as well as chemical methods when suitable. One of the more obvious problems in structural studies is the rather ill-defined nature of the polysaccharide itself. Heparins from different sources vary in uronic acid composition and sulfate content (4,5) and closely related glycosaminoglycans such as heparan sulfate confuse the issue further. In addition even a single heparin preparation contains a variable collection of individual chains as shown clearly by electrophoretic studies (6) and also by the work on "active" heparin mentioned above. Table I shows representative analyses of heparin samples from different sources which we have used. A heparan sulfate fraction is included for comparison. Though the samples vary particularly in acetyl content and the proportion of glucuronic acid, they can all be considered to be heparin by chemical definition as well as by their anticoagulant activities, which are known to be in the same range (4,5). This includes the whale heparin, while the heparan sulfate fraction (we have chosen one with the highest sulfate content available) though very similar, does not actually overlap with the heparin as pointed out by us previously (7).

The composition, degree of sulfation, and major linkage types of heparin seem by now well established. Though it is only fairly recently that the presence of sulfated iduronic acid as a major component (8) and the presence of α-L-iduronidic and β-D-glucuronidic linkages as the major uronidic bonds has been demonstrated (9,10). What remains to be shown if one wants to understand biological or pharmacological activity is the detailed arrangement of the sulfate groups, the L-iduronic and the D-glucuronic acid units, and perhaps the N-acetyl groups in the polymer chains.

Valuable information on this has been obtained by chemical methods (11,12), but precise details are still unknown.

II. EXPERIMENTAL

Analytical and chemical methods have been described by us previously (7,13,14). Periodate oxidation and Smith degradation were carried out as described by Painter *et al.* (15) and Baker *et al.* (16). Crude and purified heparinase was prepared as described previously, and products of enzymic degradation were isolated on Sephadex and ion exchange columns (17,18,19). The specificity of the purified *Flavobacterium* heparinase had been tested on a variety of naturally occurring

TABLE I Analyses of Standard Heparins

Source	Optical Rotation	% Uronic Acid (Carbazole)	% Glucuronic Acid [a]	% Hexosamine (Ehrlichs)	% Hexosamine (Indole)	% Acetyl	% Sulfate	Molecular Weight
NBC 2825 Beef Liver[b]	+51	40	45	21	26	1.8	31	11000
Upjohn 3858W Beef Mucosa[c]	+41	40	-	22	25	1.4	31	11300
Sigma 79B-1610 Pig Mucosa[d]	+48	41	-	22	26	1.6	32	9500
Upjohn ZX317 Beef Lung[c]	+43	38	30	20	27	0.4	34	10300
w-heparin[e]		34	64	18	20	2.5	25	
Heparan Sulfate[f]	+65	46	70	30	27	3.7	17	11600

[a] As % of total uronic acid. The rest is L-iduronic acid.
[b] Commercial sample from Nutritional Biochemical Co.
[c] We want to thank the Upjohn Co. for these samples.
[d] Commercial sample from Sigma Co.
[e] We want to thank Dr. Zensaku Yosizawa for this whale heparin.
[f] Heparan sulfate 1.4 NaCl fraction.

and modified substrates (13,19). The enzyme requires the presence of α-linked N-sulfated D-glucosamine and sulfated L-iduronic acid (D-glucuronic acid?) for activity. Size specificity is uncertain but there are indications that it acts more rapidly on larger fragments. It will not act if the amino groups are N-acetylated or if the sulfate group is missing on the uronic acid. The 6-sulfate on the glucosamine does not seem to be essential.

III. RESULTS

We had previously shown that crude heparinase degrades heparin to monosaccharides (18), while the purified enzyme degrades it to a mixture of oligosaccharides by an eliminase type mechanism (20). We have extended this work since then and have compared heparins from different sources.

Figure 1 shows the oligosaccharide mixture obtained by the action of purified heparinase on different heparin samples. In all cases, except whale heparin, the major product is a trisulfated disaccharide containing an α-, β unsaturated uronic acid. This compound has been well characterized by us (13) and Perlin *et al.* (9). Its structural significance is limited to the fact that this disaccharide must come from an area of the polymer chain containing a continuous series of repeating units containing disulfated hexosamine and sulfated uronic acid. As can be seen, the relative amounts of di- and oligosaccharides obtained vary with the source of the heparin used. Whale heparin is degraded very poorly. The tetra and higher oligosaccharides, which appear not to be degraded further significantly even with additional enzyme, represent areas which are structurally different from those degradable to disaccharide. They represent, therefore, a clue to structural variation. Their analyses are shown in Table II. The absorbance due to the unsaturated uronic acid on the non-reducing end, and other data (20), show that one deals indeed with a tetrasaccharide. The glucuronic acid content reflects that of the parent heparin but is increased. However, the presence of substantial amounts of iduronic acid in all samples shows that one must be dealing with at least two different tetrasaccharides in each fraction as only the internal uronic acid has remained intact after enzyme degradation (see Fig. 8). The sulfate content is somewhat low for a fully sulfated (i.e., 6 sulfate groups) tetrasaccharide, but the available methods would not readily distinguish between 5 or 6 sulfate groups. It should be noted that there is very little N-acetyl present. We were unable to resolve the tetrasaccharide mixture into individual components by any method we tried.

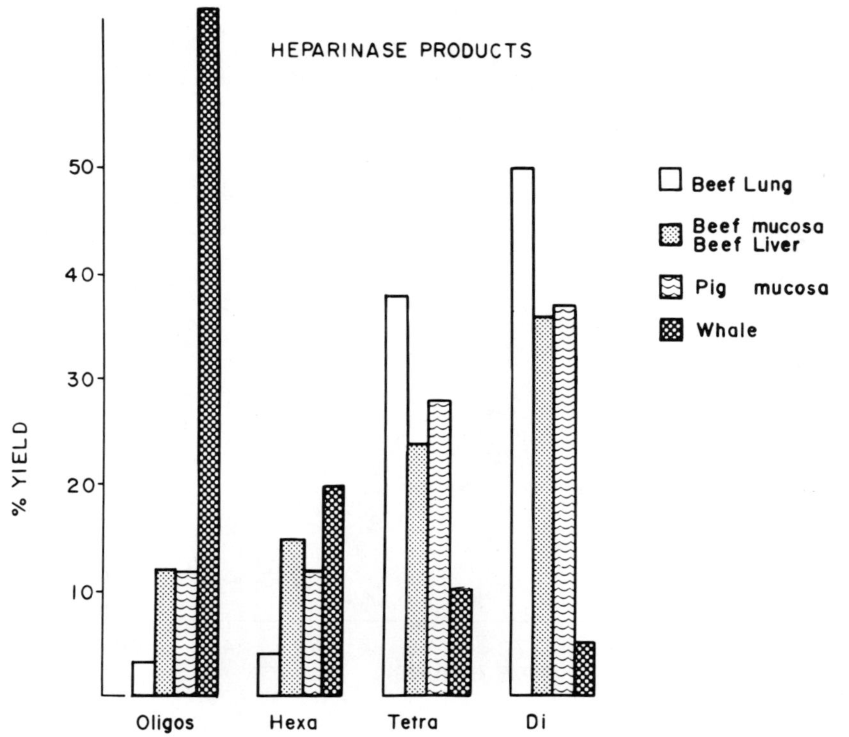

Fig. 1. Products obtained by the action of purified heparinase on heparins from different sources. Oligos, stands for oligosaccharides; Hexa, for hexasaccharides; Tetra, for tetrasaccharides; and Di, for disaccharide.

The data obtained were quite significant in a comparative sense but did not give very much information about structural details. Therefore, as the tetrasaccharides contained substantial amounts of glucuronic acid and as it is this uronic acid in heparin which appears to be degraded by periodate (8), we felt that it might be interesting to investigate periodate degradation again in conjunction with our enzyme results. This method had previously given interesting, but difficult to interpret, data.

A. Periodate Degradation

Beef liver heparin was treated with periodate and consumption measured. Fig. 2 shows the rate of reaction and the loss of uronic acid as measured by the carbazole reaction.

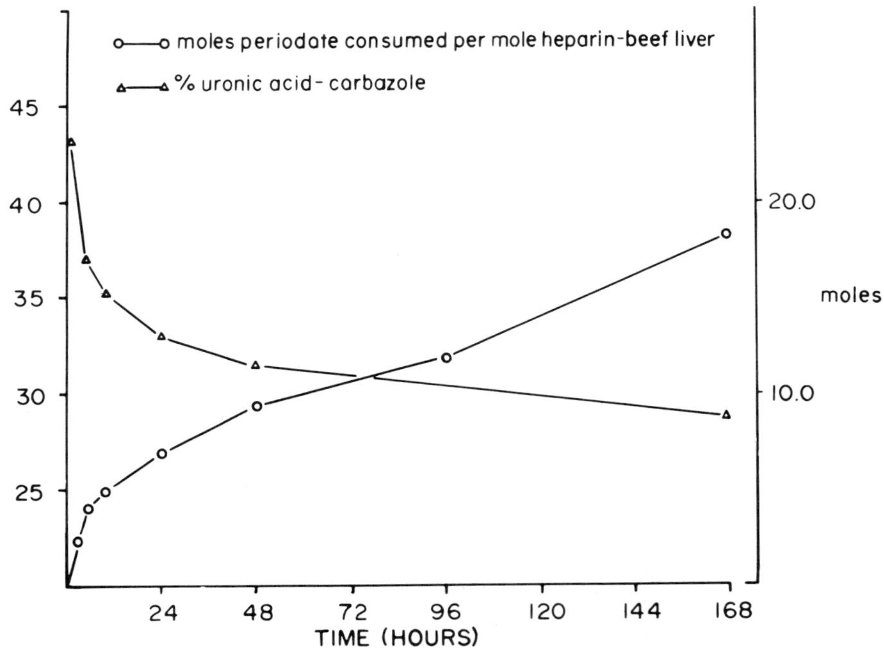

Fig. 2. Periodate treatment of beef liver heparin. The rate of periodate consumption and decrease of uronic acid content as measured by the carbazole reaction are shown.

Other heparin samples used less periodate per mole of polysaccharide with lung heparin using least (1.6 moles per mole heparin). In addition, several heparins were treated by Smith degradation and chromatographed on columns of Sephadex G-50. It can be seen in Fig. 3 that the products obtained are quite heterogeneous in size with some of the chains remaining relatively intact, while others are extensively degraded. The degree of degradation appears to be inverse to that of the heparinase, with lung heparin (most extensively degraded by the enzyme) being degraded least by periodate. The major products of the lung material appear to have a molecular weight of approximately half that of the original polymer. This indicates that most of the chains are oxidized near their center. The other heparins are degraded more extensively, which is reasonable considering that they contain more glucuronic acid. On the other hand, they are degraded less than the lung material by the heparinase which requires sulfated uronic acid. In addition, it is apparent

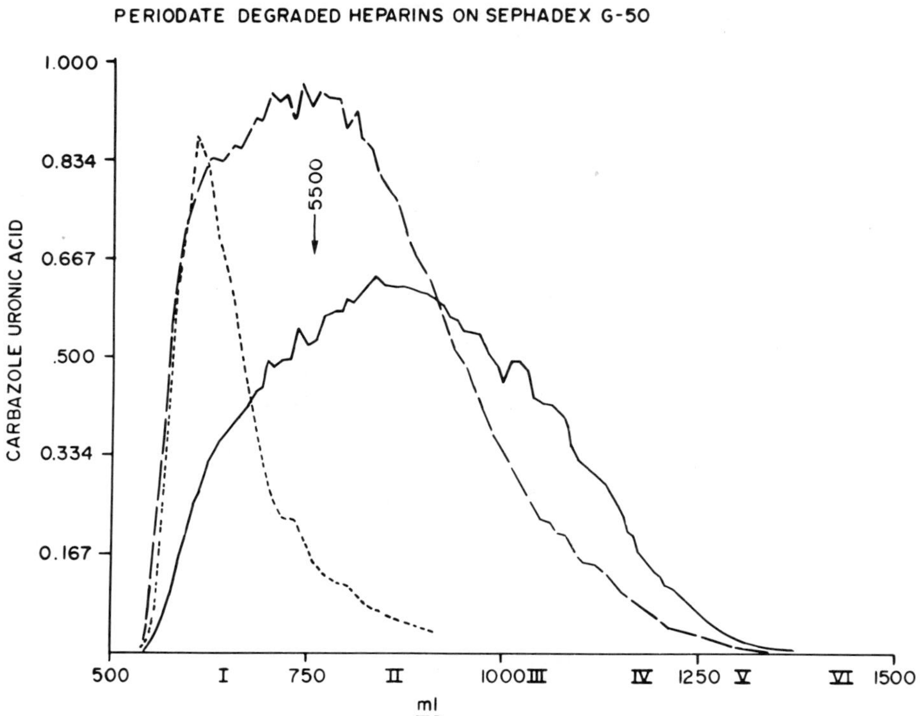

Fig. 3. Chromatography on Sephadex G-50 columns of Smith degraded heparins. Short dashes show undegraded control; long dashes show degraded beef lung heparin; solid line shows products from beef mucosa, beef liver, and pig mucosa. 5,500 indicates the elution peak of a standard with this molecular weight.

that the glucuronic acid units are distributed throughout the chains with most of them in the interior portions of the polymer. This agrees with data reported by Cifonelli *et al.* (4).

Periodate treated heparin could be degraded readily by heparinase, however, the yield of disaccharide was only about 50% and that of tetrasaccharide 70% of untreated material. The rest appeared in the oligosaccharide fraction. Table II (bottom line) shows the analyses for tetrasaccharide isolated from periodate treated and heparinase degraded beef liver heparin. As can be seen, this fraction contains little or no glucuronic acid.

Commerical lung and liver heparin, which are known to contain very little serine, were first reduced with sodium

TABLE II Analysis of Unsaturated Tetrasaccharides From Various Heparins

Source	Optical Rotation	Absorbance per mg at 232 nm	% Uronic Acid (Carbazole)	% Glucuronic[b] Acid	% Hexosamine (Indole)	% Hexosamine (Ehrlichs)	% Acetyl	% Sulfate
Beef Liver	+23	4.4	46	58	17	22	0.5	33
Beef Lung - Commercial	+17	4.3	43	35	18	17	0.0	34
Pig Mucosa	+23	4.6	44	62	21	21	0.6	35
PR Beef Liver[a]	+15	3.6	32	?	16	16	0.3	32

[a] Obtained from heparin that was first treated with periodate, followed by borohydride reduction, and then degraded with heparinase.

[b] As % of total uronic acid. The rest is L-iduronic acid.

borotritide and then submitted to Smith degradation. The products were chromatographed on Sephadex G-50 and the results are shown in Fig. 4. Relatively little label can be seen to appear in the very low molecular weight range indicating that the susceptible D-glucuronic acid units are generally not located near the reducing end of the polymer chains.

B. Enzymatic Degradation of "Active" and "Inactive" Heparin

We were fortunate in obtaining samples of "active" (about 300 units per mg) and "inactive" (about 20 units per mg) mucosal heparin from Dr. Lindahl. These samples which show little chemical difference were degraded with heparinase and the products chromatographed on Sephadex G-25[a]. As can be seen in Fig. 5 the inactive fraction shows a pattern similar to unfractionated material while the active fraction shows less disaccharide, very much less tetrasaccharide, and much more oligosaccharides. This difference in breakdown products was certainly very significant but difficult to interpret as we were not certain of the detailed structure of the tetrasaccharide mixture. Therefore, we carried out the following experiments to obtain more structural information about the tetrasaccharides.

C. Structure of Tetrasacchardies

As mentioned above, the tetra and higher oligosaccharides are not further degraded by purified heparinase. They are, however, acted on by the crude enzyme. The products are the same monosaccharides as those obtained from heparin itself, that is an α-keto acid, and monosulfated and disulfated glucosamine (18). Due to the alteration of the uronic acid and the presence of rather ill-defined sulfatases very little information about structure can be derived from these products.

If the tetrasaccharides indeed lack sulfate groups on some of the uronic acid they should be susceptible to periodate degradation. They were, therefore, treated with periodate and reisolated after desalting on Sephadex G-10. Analyses before and after periodate are shown in Table III.

---

[a] *A. Linker, M. Höök, and U. Lindahl, unpublished observation.*

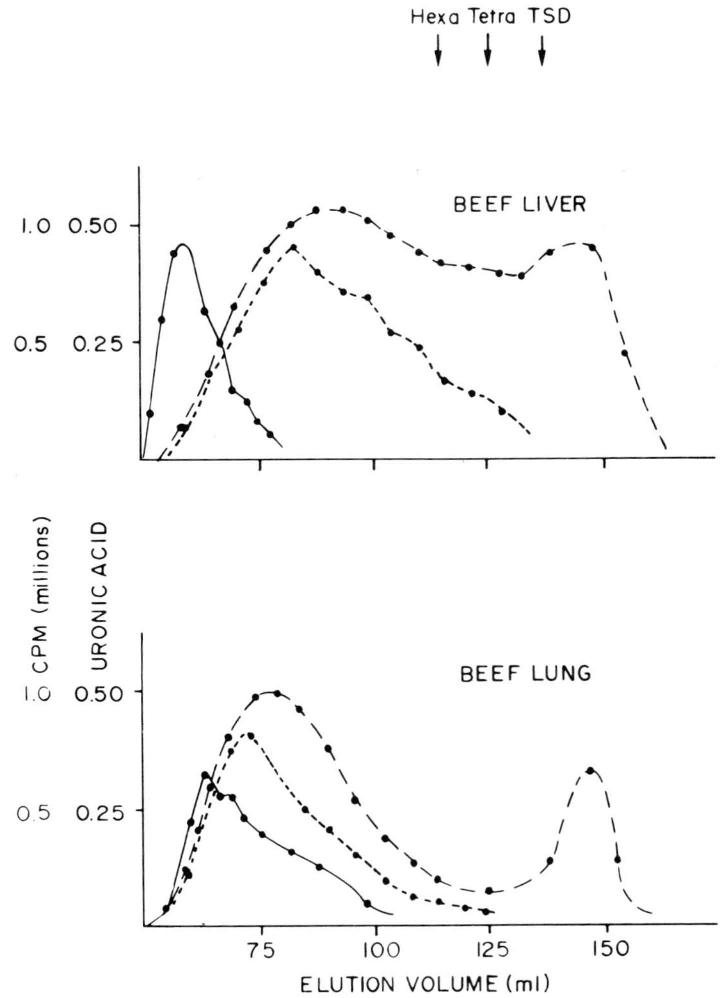

Fig. 4. Chromatography on Sephadex G-50 columns of sodium borotritide reduced and Smith degraded heparins. Both radioactive label and uronic acid content were used to follow the elution. Hexa, indicates where hexasaccharide standard is eluted; Tetra, where tetrasaccharide standard is eluted; TSD, where trisulfated disaccharide standard is eluted. Long dashes indicate label; short dashes uronic acid; the solid line shows undegraded control.

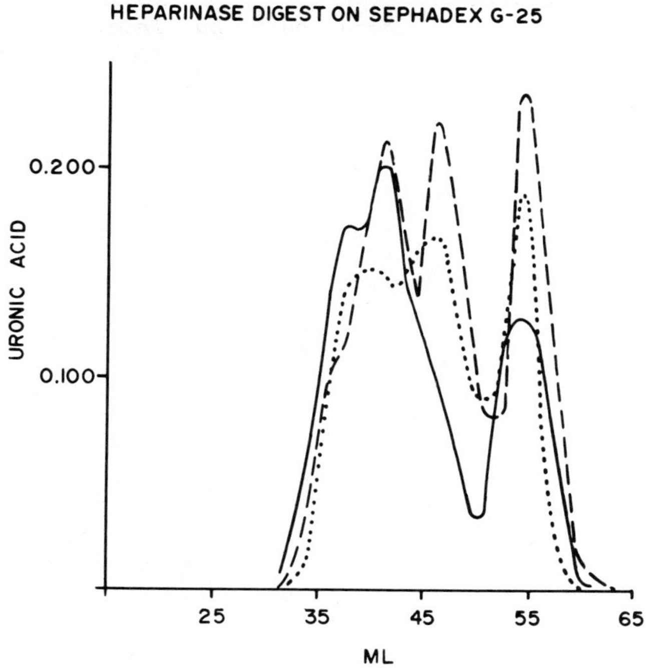

Fig. 5. Degradation of "active" and "inactive" heparin fractions by purified heparinase. Products were chromatographed on Sephadex G-25 columns. Elution was followed by the carbazole reaction for uronic acid. The dashed line shows the products of pig mucosal heparin; the dotted line the products of the "inactive" fraction obtained by antithrombin affinity chromatography; the solid line shows the products of the "active" fraction. The peak at about 54 ml is the point of elution of disaccharide; the peak at about 46 ml that of tetrasaccharide; the peak at 40 ml that of hexasaccharide; and the shoulder at about 36 ml that of higher molecular weight oligosaccharides.

TABLE III Analysis of Tetrasaccharides After Treatment with Periodate[a]

Source	*Absorbance per mg at 232 nm*	*% Uronic Acid by Carbazole*	*% Hexosamine by Indole Reaction*	*% Sulfate*
Beef Lung	*5.0 (4.1)*	*25 (32)*	*28 (27)*	*35 (31)*
Beef Liver	*5.0 (4.1)*	*21 (32)*	*22 (27)*	*31 (30)*
PR Beef Liver	*4.4 (4.0)*	*25 (25)*	*25 (26)*	*33 (30)*

[a]*Values in parenthesis are those of the tetrasaccharide samples before periodate treatment.*

The only significant change noticeable is a loss in uronic acid content as measured by the carbazole reaction. This loss is greater for the beef liver derived compound than for lung, which is in agreement with the higher glucuronic acid content of the former. The tetrasaccharide obtained from previously periodate treated heparin shows no change in analysis. As changes in color reactions cannot be interpreted too precisely the periodate treated tetrasaccharides were hydrolyzed with 0.1 *M* HCl at 25° for three days and then chromatographed on Sephadex G-25. The results are shown in Fig. 6. The elution pattern indicates that the tetrasaccharide from periodate treated heparin was not further degraded, while the lung compounds were degraded to an extent of about 25% with 75% remaining intact, and the liver compounds showed about 40% degradation.

D. Nitrous Acid Degradation of Tetrasaccharides

Tetrasaccharides from beef mucosa were degraded by the low pH method of Shively and Conrad (21) and the resulting disaccharides fractionated on columns of DEAE-Sephadex A-25. They were then desalted on Sephadex G-10. The more highly sulfated disaccharide, which also showed u.v. absorption, was eluted by 0.8 *M* NaCl and was desalted readily, while we could not separate the lower sulfated material eluted with 0.4 *M* NaCl from the salt. Analyses for the desalted disaccharide are compared with those of other disaccharides prepared by nitrous acid degradation in Table IV.

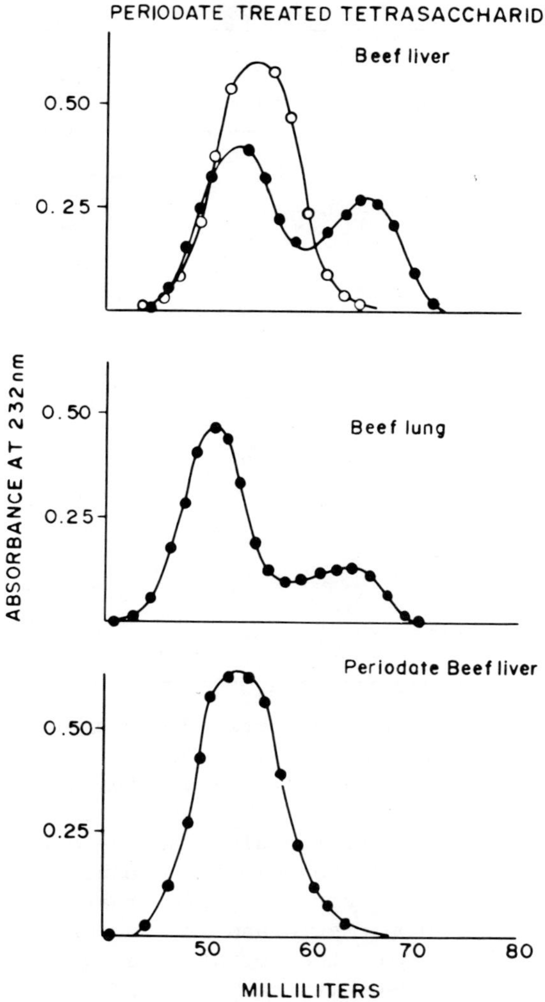

Fig. 6. Chromatography on Sephadex G-25 columns of periodate degraded tetrasaccharides (see text). The elution was followed by absorbance at 232 nm as the unsaturated, sulfated uronic acid at the nonreducing end is not affected by periodate. Open circles indicate the elution peak of untreated tetrasaccharides; solid circles indicate the elution pattern of the periodate treated material.

TABLE IV Analysis of Disaccharides Obtained From Treatment with Nitrous Acid

Source	*Heparin*	*Tetrasaccharide*	*Trisulfated[a] Disaccharide*
Ultraviolet Absorbance per mg at 232 nm	*0*	*8.6*	*9.0*
% Uronic Acid (Carbazole)	*14*	*27*	*24*
% Uronic Acid (Orcinol)	*47*	*14*	*11*
% Sulfate	*28*	*28*	*25*
% Hexosamine (Ehrlichs)	*1.8*	*2.3*	*0.4*
% Hexosamine (Indole)[b]	*26*	*20*	*5*

[a] *This is the unsaturated trisulfated disaccharide obtained by heparinase action (see text).*
[b] *What is measured here is actually 2,5 anhydromannose.*

It should be noted that the disaccharide obtained from the tetrasaccharide shows an ultraviolet absorbance identical to that of the heparinase product indicating that it contains only α,β unsaturated uronic acid and is, therefore, derived from the nonreducing end of the tetrasaccharide. The sulfate and indole reactions agree with that of the well characterized anhydromannose containing disaccharide from heparin (8,22). The carbazole reactions differ due to the unsaturation. The low value for the indole reactions of the nitrous acid treated trisulfated disaccharide is not explained but may be due to the fact that this compound does not yield anhydromannose but another derivative (23). The data show that the nonreducing portion of the tetrasaccharides consist of trisulfated disaccharide.

In order to obtain information about the disaccharide portion at the reducing end of the tetrasaccharides, the following experiments were carried out. Beef liver tetrasaccharides were first treated by Smith degradation to remove the glucuronic acid containing material. The remaining tetrasaccharides were then reduced with sodium borotritide and degraded with nitrous acid. Chromatography on Sephadex G-25 columns indicated that disaccharides had been formed with no tetrasaccharide remaining. After elution from the Sephadex columns, the disaccharides were placed on an analytical DEAE Sephadex column and eluted with solutions of NaCl of increasing molarity. The disulfated derivative of the unsaturated trisulfated disaccharide from the nonreducing end (therefore not labeled with tritium) was eluted with 0.6 to 1.0 *M* NaCl, as shown by its ultraviolet absorbance. Labeled material was eluted also at the same position indicating the presence of an equally sulfated disaccharide (fraction C) from the reducing end of the original tetrasaccharide. In addition, labeled material was eluted at 0.2 to 0.4 *M* NaCl indicating the presence of disaccharide with lower sulfate content (fraction B). The disaccharides eluted from the column were then desalted and checked by electrophoresis on paper. N-acetylglucosamine, monosulfated disaccharide from chondroitin sulfate C, and the disulfated anhydromannitol containing disaccharide from heparin (obtained directly by nitrous acid degradation and reduction) were used as standards. As can be seen in Fig. 7, fraction B migrates at the same rate as the chondroitin sulfate disaccharide, i.e., it is monosulfated while fraction C migrates mainly like the disulfated disaccharide derived from heparin.

This data indicates that the beef liver tetrasaccharides after periodate treatment consist of two compounds, one a tetrasaccharide containing a disulfated disaccharide at the reducing end, the other with a trisulfated disaccharide at the reducing end. Both have trisulfated disaccharides at the nonreducing end. Preliminary data based on sulfatase action indicate that the sulfate group on the monosulfated disaccharide (fraction B) is located on the anhydromannitol unit and that, therefore, the uronic acid has no sulfate. As the glucuronic acid containing tetrasaccharide had been removed previously by periodate, this means that a nonsulfated L-iduronic acid is present in one of the tetrasaccharides (about 1/3 of the total iduronic acid) (see Fig. 8). It is not clear why this nonsulfated iduronic acid moiety was not oxidized by periodate. The same reactions were carried out for beef lung and pig mucosal tetrasaccharides. The final data based on periodate degradation and on the yield of tritium labeled disaccharides indicate that approximately half of the internal uronic acids of the tetrasaccharides are nonsulfated; the other half are sulfated. Fig. 8 shows only tetrasaccharides lacking sulfate on the internal uronic acid;

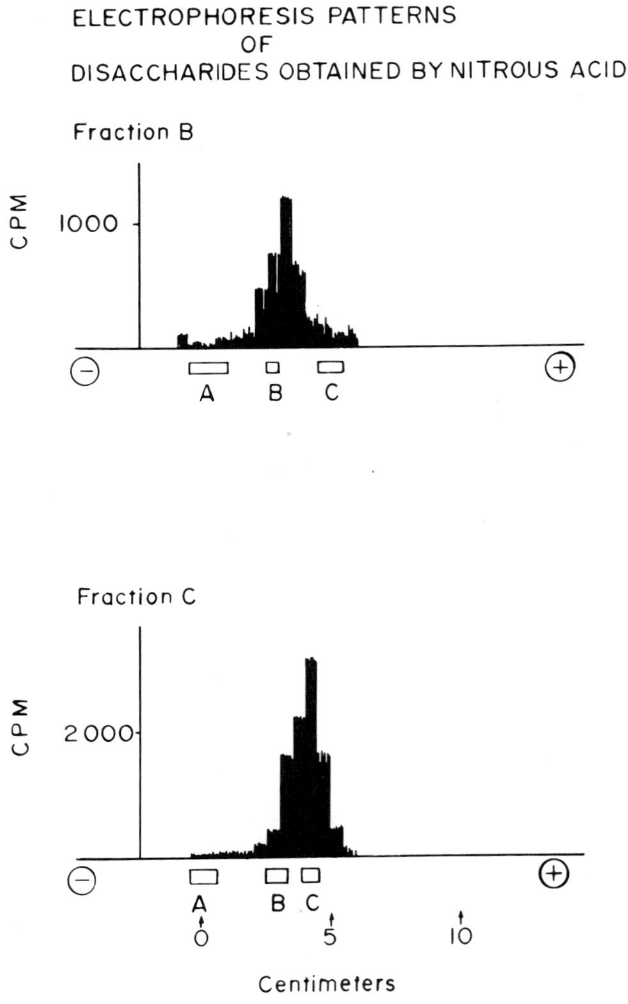

Fig. 7. Electrophoresis patterns of tritium labeled disaccharide fractions obtained by nitrous acid degradation of beef liver tetrasaccharides. The migration position of standards is indicated: A, N-acetylglucosamines; B, monosulfated disaccharide from chondroitin 6-sulfate; C, disulfated anhydromannitol containing disaccharide obtained from heparin. The two runs shown cannot be superimposed.

HEPARIN TETRASACCHARIDES

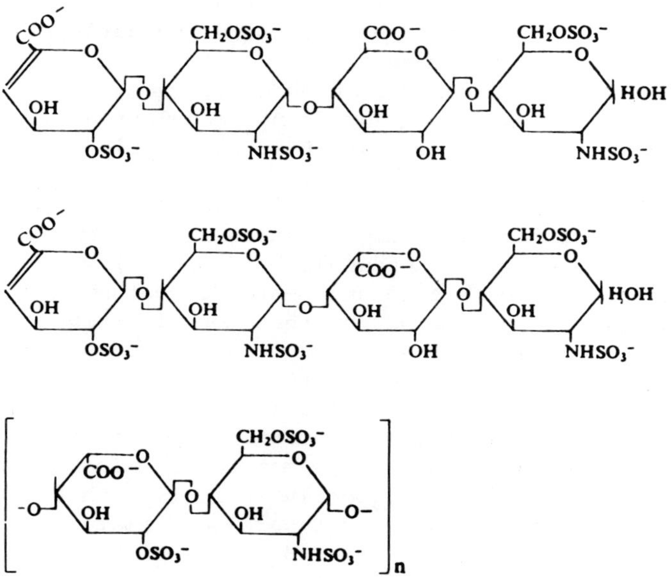

Fig. 8. Proposed structures of tetrasaccharides obtained by purified heparinase degradation of heparin. The unsaturation at the nonreducing end is due to the eliminase type of mechanism by which the enzyme acts. A fully sulfated repeating disaccharide unit is shown on the bottom. A third possible tetrasaccharide, which is not shown, would have an additional sulfate group on the 2 position of the iduronic acid.

the fully sulfated compound would have a sulfate group also on the 2 position of the internal iduronic acid.

IV. DISCUSSION

The biological role of heparin as an anticoagulant and the structural features necessary for this activity have remained unchallenged for a considerable length of time. At this point, however, both have to be called into question. It is well accepted that the N-sulfate group and a high sulfate content in general are necessary for anticoagulant activity. Indeed, other polysaccharides such as dextrans or chitin when highly sulfated by chemical means can serve as anticoagulants, though in most cases they are not as effective as heparin. The liberation of lipoprotein lipase by heparin also seems to be associated with its high charge density. The ideal heparin then would appear to be the fully sulfated (i.e., 3 sulfate groups per repeating unit) polymer. Beef lung heparin most closely approximates this. However, recent evidence on "active" heparin (3), and data presented here, indicate that the absence of sulfate groups in critical positions may be necessary for high activity.

Previous attempts to related anticoagulant activity to sulfate content, D-glucuronic to L-iduronic acid ratios, and N-sulfate vs. N-acetyl content have not led to any clear-cut relation. All the heparins listed in Table I have anticoagulant activities in a fairly narrow range from 130 to 170 units per mg. This includes whale heparin (24) which has quite a high glucuronic acid and N-acetyl content. It has, therefore, become quite apparent that more information about the detailed arrangement of the charged groups is necessary if one wants to relate structure to function.

The data shown in Fig. 1 clearly indicate structural differences between heparins, in particular between lung heparin and the liver and mucosal materials. The whale polysaccharide was degraded very poorly indicating that degradability by heparinase and activity are not related as such. The periodate data (shown in Fig. 3 and 4) give information about the general distribution of glucuronic acid units which are not sulfated in the polymer chains. These same glucuronic acids appear as internal units in some of the tetrasaccharides which are resistant to heparinase. Somewhat less than one half of the tetrasaccharides which contain important clues to the overall structure of the chains appear to have an internal glucuronic acid moiety as shown by the periodate degradation of the tetrasaccharides themselves (see Table III and Figs. 6 and 8). This amounts to only about one third in the lung heparin derived compounds as less total glucuronic acid is present. The data obtained by nitrous acid degradation indicate that in addition about one third of the L-iduronic acid units are not sulfated. Therefore, depending on original source, somewhat better than one half of the tetrasaccharides contain a nonsulfated uronic acid in the internal position of the molecule. The L-iduronic acid even if not sulfated seems resistant to periodate oxidation. This could well be due to its conformation (1C?) in the tetrasaccharide (25). Some of the iduronic units appear to be sulfated and it is not clear why the heparinase was not able to degrade these tetrasaccharides further. Nothing is known about substrate size specificity of this enzyme and this could indeed play a role here. The proposed structures of two of the tetrasaccharides are shown in Fig. 8 along with the disaccharide units. The difficulties in determining structural details were in large part due to the fact that we were dealing with a mixture of 3 tetrasaccharides which we could not resolve. In general, our data are in agreement with those of Silva and Dietrich (26) who reported that a tetrasaccharide, obtained from lung heparin by the same Flavobacterial heparinase used by us, was degraded by their heparitinase II to two disaccharides, one containing three sulfate groups, the other two. These products would indeed be obtained from the tetrasaccharides lacking a sulfate group on the internal uronic acid. However, due to the introduction of unsaturation by the enzyme and the possible presence of sulfatases in the heparitinase, no conclusions about the uronic acid could be deduced, and the degree of sulfation remained somewhat uncertain. We are now investigating the hexasaccharides obtained by heparinase digestion of the various heparins. Preliminary data indicate that they also contain D-glucuronic and L-iduronic acid units which lack sulfate groups. They, therefore, also represent undersulfated areas in the chains. In view of the data presented here, both enzymatic and chemical, a tentative and somewhat general structure of heparins can be proposed. As shown in Fig. 9, all heparins are composed mainly of trisulfated disaccharide repeating units. In addition the chains contain lower sulfated areas. Less of those in lung heparin than in the others. It must also be strongly emphasized that one is not dealing with a single chain type, but that several distributions are possible. For instance the top scheme shown for lung heparin is unlikely, but the other two chains are quite possible. These structures are also quite compatible with those postulated on the basis of chemical data (11,12). The heterogeneity is certainly reinforced by the studies on active heparin mentioned above (1,2) where only some of the chains appear to bind effectively to antithrombin. It should also be quite apparent that the distributions shown or other similar arrangements could account for the biological activities, or lack thereof, of the polymers. Therefore, the data shown in Fig. 5 for breakdown products of "active" vs. "inactive" heparin do represent an important clue. As considerably less disaccharide and tetrasaccharides and more hexa- and oligosaccharides are obtained from the active fraction, it would appear that activity may depend on the exact arrangement of the areas in the chain which are lower in sulfate content. Indeed considering the possible distribution of the charged groups, carboxyl as well as sulfate (see Figs. 8 and 9) it would be easy to arrive at a highly specific arrangement. One must, however, keep in mind that low sulfate content per se cannot be responsible

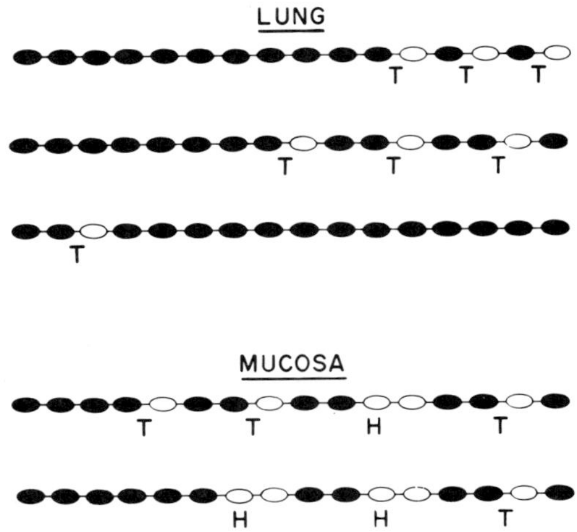

Fig. 9. Schematic structure of heparin chains showing possible arrangements of lower sulfated units. The filled in ellipses represent fully sulfated (i.e., 3 sulfates) disaccharide units; the open ellipses represent disaccharide units which lack sulfate on the uronic acid moiety. The letter T stands for the unit which yields the tetrasaccharide products of heparinase; the letter H for the unit which yields the hexasaccharides.

for anticoagulant action as heparan sulfate which contains similar groupings has little activity. On the other hand, partly synthetic heparinoids which lack L-iduronic acid (or even uronic acid) such as dextran sulfates or chondroitin polysulfate (27) can show good activity. In view of the above and the relatively small proportion of highly active heparin in preparations, one must also ask whether anticoagulant activity is indeed the biological function of heparin or whether it is merely a pharmacological phenomenon? Jaques has raised this point recently in relation to mast cell function (28,29) and indicated a possible role for heparin as an ion exchanger. Silbert *et al.* have isolated native heparin from rat mast cells that appears to have very low anticoagulant activity (30). This of course leaves lipoprotein lipase release as a possible biological role for heparin, and another quite intriguing possibility is activation of chymotrypsin (31), which is also present in mast cells. In conclusion, though much information has been accumulated on a biochemical as well as on a biological and clinical level, it is still quite difficult to define heparin except somewhat arbitrarily by chemical analysis and structure, while the true biological role of this interesting and complex polysaccharide remains elusive at present.

REFERENCES

1. Lam, L.H., Silbert, J.E., and Rosenberg, R.D., Biochem. Biophys. Res. Comm. *69*, 570 (1976).
2. Höök, M., Björk, I., Hopwood, J., and Lindahl, U., FEBS Letters *66*, 90 (1976).
3. Hopwood, J., Höök, M., Linker, A., and Lindahl, U., FEBS Letters *69*, 51 (1976).
4. Cifonelli, J.A., and King, J., Biochim. Biophys. Acta *320*, 331 (1973).
5. Taylor, R.L., Shively, J.E., Conrad, H.E., and Cifonelli, J.A., Biochem. *12*, 3633 (1973).
6. McDuffie, N.M., Dietrich, C.P., and Nader, H.B., Biopol. *14*, 1473 (1975).
7. Linker, A., and Hovingh, P., Carbohyd. Res. *29*, 41 (1973).
8. Lindahl, U., and Axelsson, O., J. Biol. Chem. *246*, 74 (1971).
9. Perlin, A.S., Mackie, D.M., and Dietrich, C.P., Carbohyd. Res. *18*, 185 (1971).
10. Hovingh, P., and Linker, A., Biochem. J. *165*, 287 (1977).
11. Höök, M., Lindahl, U., and Iverius, P.-H., Biochem. J. *137*, 33 (1974).
12. Cifonelli, J.A., and King, J., Connect. Tiss. Res. *3*, 97 (1975).
13. Hovingh, P., and Linker, A., Carbohyd. Res. *37*, 181 (1974).
14. Linker, A., and Hovingh, P., Biochim. Biophys. Acta *385*, 324 (1975).
15. Painter, T., and Larson, B., Acta Chem. Scand. *24*, 813 (1970).
16. Baker, J.R., Rodén, L., and Stoolmiller, A.C., J. Biol. Chem. *247*, 3838 (1972).
17. Linker, A., and Hovingh, P., *in* "Methods in Enzymology" (V. Ginsburg, ed.), Vol. 28, p. 902. Academic Press, New York, 1972.
18. Linker, A., and Hovingh, P., J. Biol. Chem. *240*, 3724 (1965).
19. Hovingh, P., and Linker, A., J. Biol. Chem. *245*, 6170 (1970).
20. Linker, A., and Hovingh, P., Biochem. *11*, 563 (1972).
21. Shively, J.E., and Conrad, H.E., Biochem. *15*, 3932 (1976).
22. Lim, T.W., Leder, I.G., Bach, G., and Neufeld, E.F., Carbohyd. Res. *37*, 103 (1974).

23. Shively, J.E., and Conrad, H.E., Biochem. *15*, 3943 (1976).
24. Yosizawa, Z., Biochem. Biophys. Res. Comm. *16*, 336 (1964).
25. Fransson, L.-Å., Carbohyd. Res. *36*, 339 (1974).
26. Silva, M.E., and Dietrich, C.P., J. Biol. Chem. *250*, 6841 (1975).
27. Voss, H., Sensch, K.H., and Panse, P., Zbl. Bakt. Hyg. *229*, 1 (1974).
28. Jaques, L.B., Gen. Pharmacol. *6*, 235 (1975).
29. Jaques, L.B., Mahadoo, J., and Riley, J.F., The Lancet *I*, 411 (1977).
30. Yurt, R.W., Leid, R.W., Jr., Austen, K.F., and Silbert, J.E., J. Biol. Chem. *252*, 518 (1977).
31. Twining, S.S., and Brecher, A.S., Can. J. Biochem. *55*, 134 (1977).

RECENT STRUCTURAL STUDIES ON HEPARIN

Arthur S. Perlin

McGill University

I. INTRODUCTION

It is a particular pleasure to take part in this symposium, because our studies on the chemistry of heparin were undertaken with the generous collaboration of Professor Louis Jaques.

We set out initially to examine the proton magnetic resonance spectra of heparins accumulated from different sources by Prof. Jaques, looking for possible variations in structure that might be associated with known differences in anticoagulant activity. It soon appeared from these spectra (1,2,3) that there are two general types of heparin--for simplicity they have been called type *A* and type *B*. The most visible distinction between them is a rather strong singlet at ∿2 ppm in one set of spectra (*A*) and its relatively low intensity in the other set (*B*) (Fig. 1). This signal, attributable to an acetamido (CH_3CONH) group, serves to illustrate that *A*-heparins have a notably higher content of 2-acetamido 2-deoxyhexose (N-acetylglucosamine) residues than do those of the *B*-type. Since anticoagulant activities of the two groups of samples, on the average, were found to be comparable (1,2), this compositional difference is not reflected physiologically in the heparin assay. However, that has not precluded the possibility that the two types vary in their effectiveness in some of the numerous other biological functions attributed to heparin.

Preparations from hog mucosa are representative of the *A* type heparin, whereas *B* type is obtained from beef lung. On the basis of the data available, it appears that nmr spectroscopy (^1H or ^{13}C) is a reliable means for distinguishing between samples from these two major commercial sources.

This article summarizes recent structural information about each of the heparin types and focuses on the minor components that permit a distinction between them. It brings together data furnished by several colleagues: B. Casu and G. Gatti (Milan), G.K. Hamer, R. Helleur, and E.C. Mushayakarara (Montreal).

ISBN 0-12-484850-8

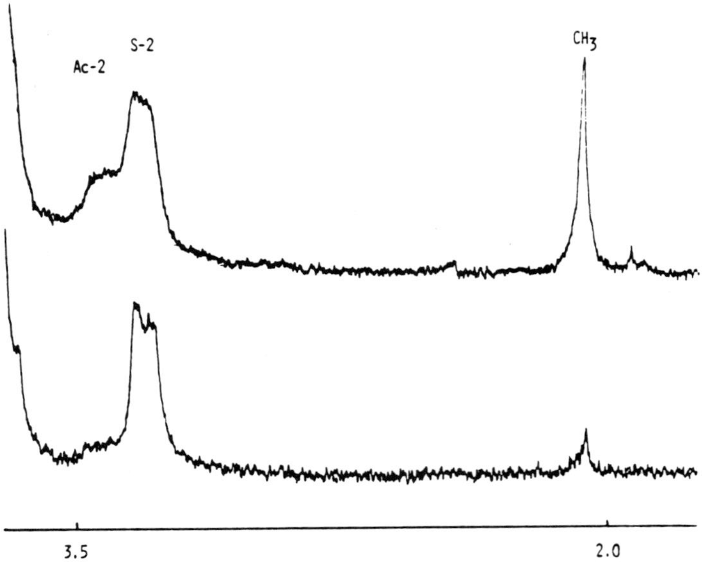

Fig. 1. Partial pmr spectra (220 MHz) (3) of a hog mucosal heparin (A-type) (upper trace) and a beef lung heparin (B-type) in D_2O solution. Ac-2 and CH_3: signals of H-2 and CH_3, respectively, of 2-acetamido-2-deoxyhexose residues; S-2: signal of H-2 of 2-deoxy-2-sulfaminoglucose residues.

II. HEPARIN FROM BEEF LUNG (TYPE B)

Our studies on the structure of *B*-type heparin have dealt mainly with material isolated from beef lung by the Upjohn Company (and provided by that firm in liberal quantity). According to analyses by spectroscopic, chemical, and enzymic methods (1-8), this heparin is constituted preponderantly--perhaps 85-90%--of a repeating sequence represented by *1*, i.e., alternating 1,4-linked residues of α-L-idopyranuronic acid 2-sulfate and 2-deoxy-2-sulfamino-α-D-glucopyranose 6-sulfate.

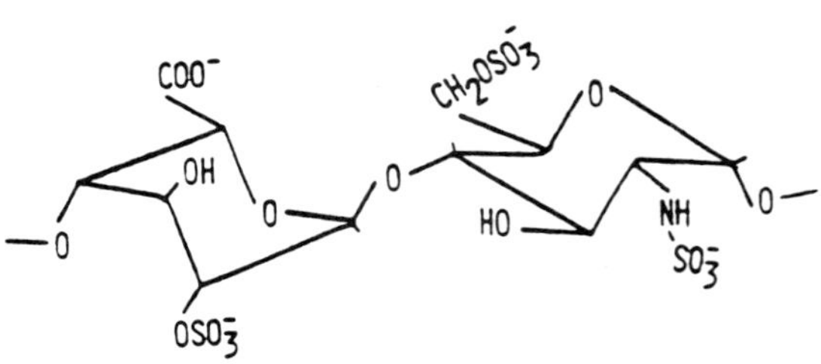

1

Focusing specifically on nmr spectra of this heparin, one can account in substantial detail for structure *1*. For a comprehensive analysis of proton (^{1}H) spectra, high-frequency instruments have been invaluable; i.e., the 220 MHz spectra (3) proved to be a good deal more satisfactory in resolving the various signals present than our initial 100 MHz spectra (1,2). More recent studies at 270 MHz (9), which utilize computer analysis and simulation of the spectra, provide a far superior resolution of signals and furnish definitive data about each of the major proton resonances. According to the 270 MHz data, the pmr spectrum of beef lung consists essentially of 12 proton signals. (Weak resonances (such as that of the acetamido CH_3) that are largely obscured by baseline noise, and may account for 15% of the total spectral intensity, are not included in this treatment.) Not only is this number of signals consistent with sequence *1*, but the chemical shifts and spin-spin coupling patterns observed are wholly in agreement with this structure. The reliability of these data is indicated by the coupling parameters (Table I) obtained for the hexosamine moiety. Since there can be little doubt that its geometry is closely depicted in *1*, it is reassuring that the coupling constants listed for the amino-sugar are precisely those to be expected for the α-*gluco* configuration and Cl (D) conformation shown.

Particularly noteworthy is the fact that the full analysis of coupling constants for the iduronic acid moiety (Table I) readily accommodates the 1C(L) conformation depicted for it in *1*. Although earlier data pointed to this likelihood (3,10), they were far less complete. Therefore, one can affirm with confidence that, in aqueous solution, the α-L-iduronosyl residues of heparin adopt substantially this chair conformation.[a]

The ^{13}C nmr spectrum of beef lung heparin consists of 12 major signals. In the original spectrum examined (6), that of the sodium salt at 25 MHz, several of the signals overlap. This is unusual in ^{13}C spectroscopy--normally, the ability of this technique to account for each of the nonequivalent carbon nuclei in a molecule is its major strength. However, better signal separation is obtained (12) with the barium salt of the polymer (Fig. 2), or its free acid form, and overlap is even more fully alleviated, of course, in ^{13}C spectra of higher frequency (13). The group of 12 carbon nuclei detected in this manner corresponds to a disaccharide repeating structure and, based on analyses (6,13) of the spectra, to the sequence represented by *1*.

---

[a]*This appears to be true also for heparin in the solid state (11).*

Table I Proton-Proton Vicinal Couplings (^3J, Hz) for the 2-deoxy-2-sulfamino-D-glucose and L-iduronic acid Residues of Beef Lung Heparin (9,13)

2-deoxy-2-sulfamino-D-glucose residue		*L-iduronic acid residue*	
$J_{1,2}$	3.6	$J_{1,2}$	3.0
$J_{2,3}$	9.5	$J_{2,3}$	5.5
$J_{3,4}$	9.5	$J_{3,4}$	4.0
$J_{4,5}$	9.4	$J_{4,5}$	3.4
$J_{5,6} \simeq J_{5,6'}$	1.5		

The products formed (14) from beef lung heparin by degradation with nitrous acid (15,16) afford a particularly clear description of the ^{13}C nuclei present in the parent polymer (Fig. 3). Aside from the presence of very weak signals, due to the minor constituents, the spectrum shown in Fig. 3 is indistinguishable from that of the disaccharide *2* isolated

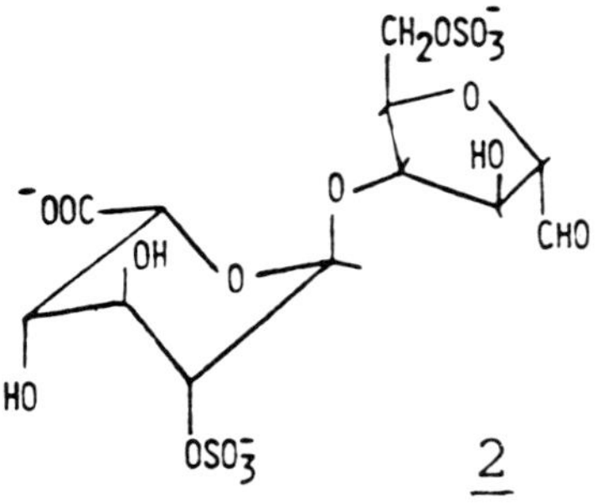

2

chromatographically in 60% yield in an earlier study (6) of these fragmentation products. Disaccharide *2* corresponds, of course, to polymer structure *1*, and since it represents purified material, whereas Fig. 3 depicts the *total* degradation product, it is evident once again that this heparin from beef lung is constituted very largely of a single type of biose sequence *1*.

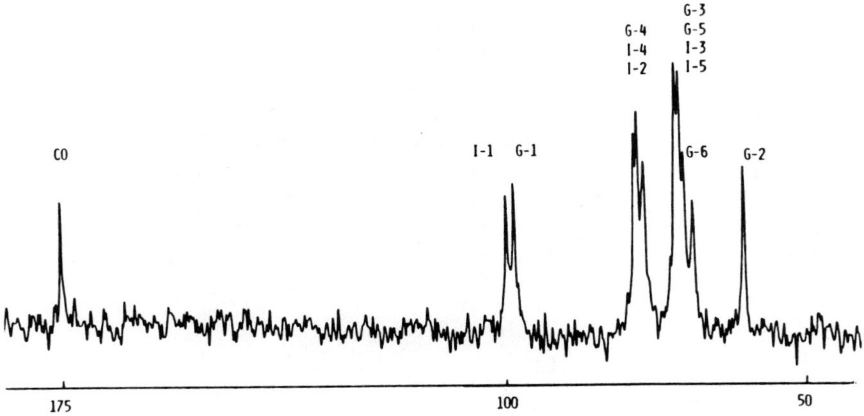

Fig. 2. ^{13}*C nmr spectrum (22.63 (MHz) (12) of beef lung heparin, barium salt in* D_2O*. I: signal due to iduronic acid residures; G: signal due to glucosamine residues; CO: signal due to carboxyl group.*

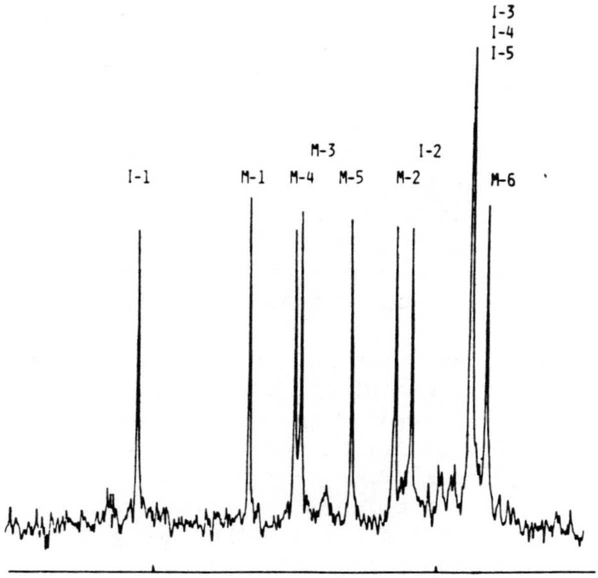

Fig. 3. ^{13}*C nmr spectrum (22.63 (MHz) (14) of the products formed from beef lung heparin by deaminative degradation with nitrous acid (solvent,* D_2O*). I: signal due to iduronic acid residues; M: signal due to anhydromannose residues.*

Other information obtained (14) from these degradation products concerns the minor components (about which more is presented below). One of the disaccharide fractions isolated by gel permeation chromatography was found to include, in addition to *2*, a small proportion of a second compound. According to its ^{13}C spectrum, the latter contains a β-D-glucopyranosyl uronic acid residue (non-O-sulfated), and is formulated (14) as *3*; its β-configuration was confirmed by the C-1, H-1 spacing in its ^{1}H-coupled ^{13}C spectrum (see below). A third disaccharide appears to be an analog of *3*, i.e., one bearing no O-sulfate group on the anhydromannose portion (14).

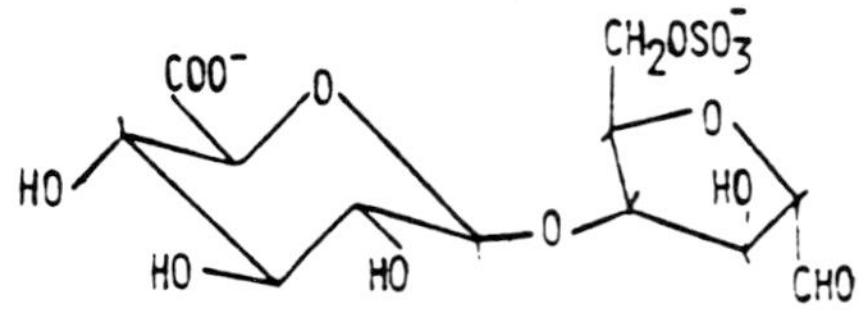

3

III. HEPARIN FROM HOG MUCOSA (TYPE *A*). MINOR CONSTITUENTS OF HEPARINS

Reference has been made above to the acetamido CH_3 signal that characterizes pmr spectra of those heparins called *A*-type. Hog mucosal heparins examined have this characteristic in common. Other minor differences are found in comparing (3) their pmr spectra with that of beef lung heparin, although the origin of some of these weak signals is difficult to interpret.

Better progress has been made in this direction with ^{13}C nmr spectroscopy. For example, a *difference* spectrum has been generated (12) from the data acquired by computer in measuring the ^{13}C Ft spectra of hog mucosal *A* and beef lung *B* heparins. This spectrum (Fig. 4) represents ^{13}C nuclei that are not common to both the *A* and *B* heparins. More precisely, it reflects the fact that *A* has a higher content of certain minor constituent residues than does *B*; as already noted, there are weak signals in both ^{1}H and ^{13}C spectra of beef lung heparin, but minor signals are much more prominent in spectra of type *A* heparin.

Especially noteworthy, is the striking resemblance between this *difference* spectrum and the actual ^{13}C spectrum (Fig. 4) (17) of a major fraction of heparan sulphate from a beef lung source (Upjohn). This fraction is constituted primarily of alternating residues of 2-acetamido-2-deoxy-α-D-glucopyranose and β-D-glucopyranuronic acid, as in *4*, (17) i.e., a structure in accord with much of the evidence now available about heparan sulphate (18-21).

Although one interpretation of these findings is that the type *A* heparin contains a small proportion of heparan sulphate (and type *B*, much less), it is equally possible that they merely reflect the presence of the same kinds of

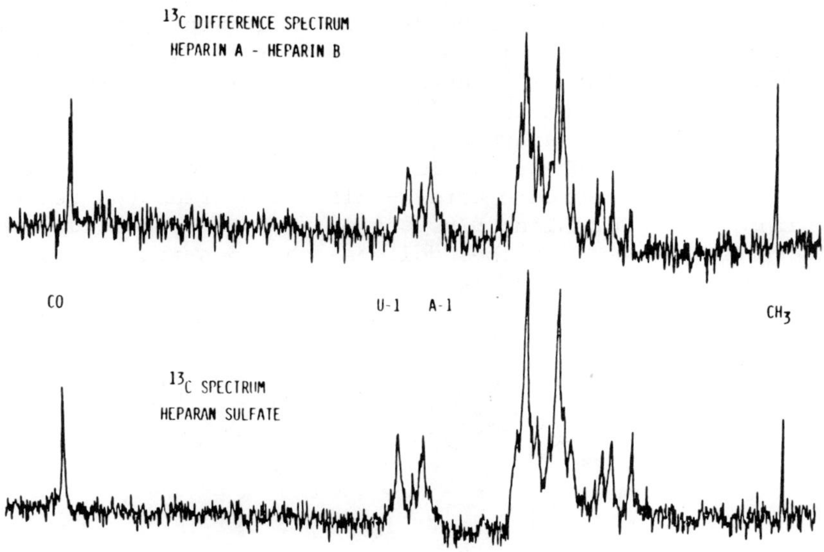

Fig. 4. ^{13}C nmr spectra at 22.63 MHz. Upper trace: represents differences between the ^{13}C spectra of hog mucosal and beef lung heparin in D_2O (12); lower trace: ^{13}C spectrum of a major fraction of heparan sulfate (17). U: signal due to uronic acid residues; A: signal due to aminohexose residues.

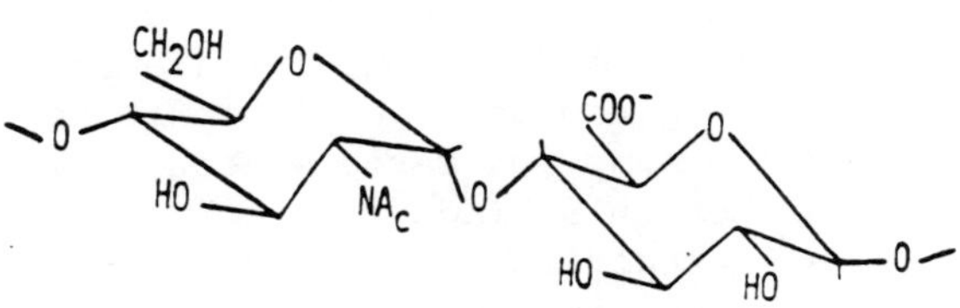

4

constituent residues as present in *4*. Further information about these minor structural features has been obtained (14) by deaminative degradation of hog mucosal heparin.

As with beef lung heparin, the products of treatment with nitrous acid consist preponderantly of disaccharide *2*. This is evidenced by the fact that the major signals of the ^{13}C spectrum of the unfractionated degradation products are the same as in Fig. 3, i.e., they are obviously attributable to *2*. As would be expected, however, signals due to the minor constituents were more prominent in this instance. Gel permeation chromatography of the mixture afforded *2* and, as noted above for the beef lung heparin experiments, a fraction in which *2* was admixed with a minor proportion of disaccharide 3. In addition, two tetrasaccharides were isolated in moderate yield. Based on their ^{13}C and ^{1}H spectra, both were found to contain 2,5-anhydromannose-6-sulfate and 2-acetamido-2-deoxy-α-glucose; the remaining two residues of one tetrasaccharide are α-iduronic acid-2-sulfate, whereas the other contains one such residue *plus* one of β-glucuronic acid. The structures proposed for these oligosaccharides are represented by *5* and *6*, respectively (14).[b]

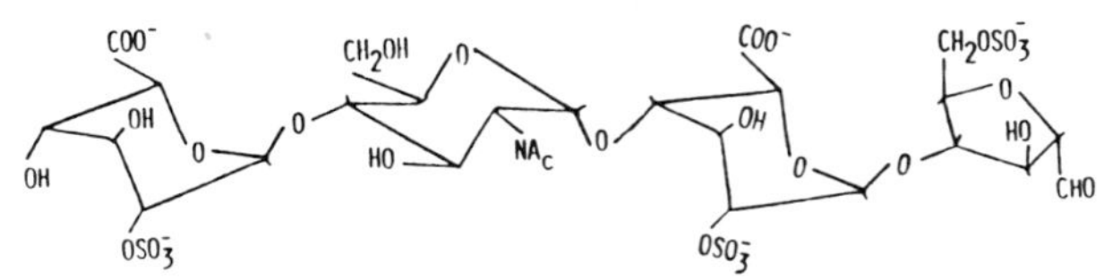

5

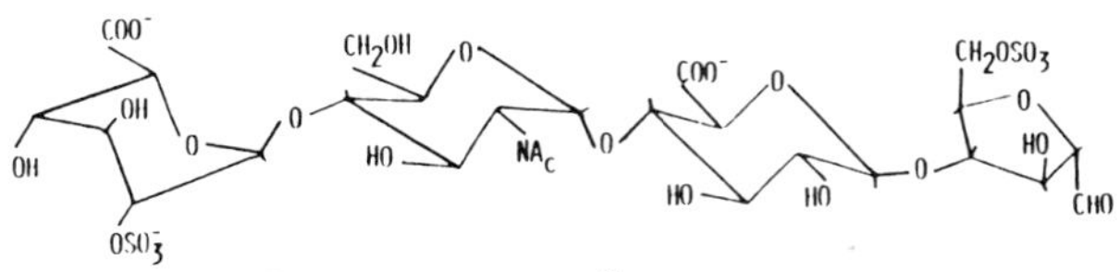

6

Of special note is this evidence from *5* and *6* that *both* 2-acetamido-2-deoxyglucose and 2-deoxy-2-sulfaminoglucose residues, and also *both* glucuronic and iduronic acid residues, are constituents of the *same* polymeric molecules in the heparin sample. Whether this kind of mixed sequence is confined to only a small proporiton of the molecules, or has widespread occurrence, remains to be determined.

---

[b] *These findings are generally consistent with the results of other workers (15,16,22,23), who isolated di- and tetrasaccharides and fragments ranging to octasaccharide and showed enzymatically that β-D-glucuronic acid residues were present in some fragments.*

IV. OBSERVATIONS ON $^{13}C{=}O$ SIGNALS AND ANOMERIC $^{13}C{-}^{1}H$ COUPLING

In the light of the data presented above, it is informative to focus on the carbonyl region of ^{13}C spectra of heparins, i.e., the 175-180 ppm range. Type *A* and *B* heparins should exhibit characteristic differences in this region: for *B*, the only C=0 signal of importance should be that due to the iduronic acid residues, whereas CH_3CONH groups and glucuronic acid residues should add two additional, relatively weaker, C=0 signals to the spectrum. Such distinctions are not apparent with the sodium salts but become evident (12) near the pK_a (24) of the uronide moieties. Hence, in the pH 3.5-4 region, there are three C=0 signals in the spectrum of hog mucosal heparin, and at a lower pH, the uronide signals are shifted well upfield of that due to the acetamido C=0 (Table II). By contrast, only one signal can be detected throughout this pH range in spectra of the beef lung heparin (12).

TABLE II Carbonyl ^{13}C Chemical Shifts (ppm) for Type A and B Heparins (pH dependence)

Type A:	*pH*	*5.7*	*3.5*	*2.0*
		175.8	*175.7*[a]	*175.7*[a]
			175.3[b]	*175.3*[b]
			175.0[c]	*174.0*[c]
Type B:	*pH*	*5.7*	*4.0*	*2.0*
		175.9	*175.6*	*173.7*

[a] *Signal due to CH_3CONH*
[b] *Signal ascribed to COOH of glucuronsyl residue*
[c] *Signal ascribed to COOH of iduronsyl residue; more intense than the other two.*

According to these observations, it should be feasible to determine the relative proportions of acetamidodeoxyglucose, iduronic, and glucuronic acid in heparin samples from the relative intensities of their $^{13}C{=}O$ signals in the pH 2-4 range. Infrared spectroscopy of heparins and other mucopolysaccharides in D_2O and DCl solutions affords (24) a quantitative measure of the ratio of acetamidodeoxyhexose: total uronic acid, although it does not differentiate between isomeric uronic acids.

Another ^{13}C nmr parameter of value is that of coupling between anomeric carbons and protons (^{1}JC-H). All of the ^{13}C spectra described above were recorded with ^{1}H-decoupling, which affords optimum simplicity and sensitivity. Measurements on ^{1}H-coupled spectra, however, provide additional stereochemical information. For example, the anomeric configuration of residues in these polymers can be determined in this way (25). PMR spectroscopy of the products formed by the action of *F. heparinum* on heparin has provided evidence (5) that the L-iduronic acid possesses the α-configuration, and this is confirmed by the 270 MHz proton data (9) cited above, based on the coupling between H-1 and H-2. Coupling between C-1 and H-1 demonstrates this also, because when the C-1--O-1 bond is axial, ^{1}JC-H is about 160 Hz, whereas a value of about 170 Hz is observed when the bond is oriented equatorially (25-27). Consequently, since the C-1, H-1 coupling for the iduronic acid residue of heparin (either type *A* or *B*) is 172 Hz (Table III), the α-L-configuration is indicated. Disaccharide 2 gives the same ^{1}JC-H value as the parent polymer, evidence that the orientation at the anomeric center is the same in both. Similarly, because of its α-D-configuration, the hexosamine component of the heparin gives rise to a ^{1}JC-H value of 170 Hz.

The C-1 signal of the glucuronic acid residue, measured (14) with the deaminative degradation products, is only 160 Hz (Table III), which thus corresponds to a β-configuration, as shown in *3*. This is the value obtained (25) for the β-D-glucuronosyl residues of chondroitins A and C. The same value is observed (17) (Table III) also for C-1 of the glucuronosyl residue of the heparan sulfate fraction described above, so that the β-D-configuration is indicated here, whereas, not unexpectedly, acetamidodeoxyhexose residues of this polymer give ^{1}JC-H of 170 Hz (17), corresponding to the α-D-configuration (as in *4*).

V. SUMMARY

To summarize, these results supplement earlier findings on the structure of heparin. They show that both *A*- and *B*-types are constituted mainly of a disaccharide repeating sequence *1* in which residues of α-L-idopyranuronic acid 2-sulfate (essentially in the 1C(L) conformation) and 2-deoxy2-sulfamino-α-D-glucopyranose 6-sulfate are bound together by 1,4-linkages. Both types of heparin also contain residues of 2-acetamido-2-deoxy-α-D-glucopyranose and β-D-glucopyranuronic acid, which are appended through 1,4 bonds, although heparin *A* is characterized by a content of such residues that is several times that of *B*-type heparin. The location of these minor residues within the polysaccharide chains is not known, but it is clear that they co-occur in at least some of the molecules bonded glycosidically (as in *3*, *5*, and *6*) to residues of the major, sulfated hexosamine and iduronic acid, constituents.

TABLE III Direct-Bond Coupling ($^1J_{C-H}$) Between ^{13}C-1 and ^1H-1, and Anomeric Configuration[a]

	$^1J_{C-H}$ (Hz)	
	α	β
D-Glucopyranuronic acid	*170*	*162*
D-Glucuronic acid residue (chondroitins A and C)		*160-162 (25)*
L-Iduronic acid residue (beef lung heparin)	*172*	
L-Iduronic acid residue (disaccharide 2)	*172 (14)*	
D-Glucuronic acid residue (disaccharide 3)		*160 (14)*
D-Glucuronic acid residue (heparan sulfate fraction)		*160 (17)*
2-Acetamido-2-deoxy-D-glucopyranose	*173*	*160*
2-Acetamido-2-deoxy-D-glucose residue (chondroitins A and C)		*161 (25)*
2-Deoxy-2-sulfamino-D-glucose residue (beef lung heparin)	*170*	
2-Acetamido-2-deoxy-D-glucose residue (heparan sulfate fraction)	*170 (17)*	

[a] *All uronic acids as sodium salts.*

ACKNOWLEDGMENTS

The author expresses his gratitude to B. Casu, G. Gatti, G.K. Hamer, R. Helleur, and E.C. Mushayakara for their generous collaboration in furnishing data for this article.

REFERENCES

1. Jaques, L.B., Kavanagh, L.W., Mazurek, M., and Perlin, A.S., Biochem. Biophys. Res. Commun. *24*, 447 (1966).
2. Perlin, A.S., Mazurek, M., Jaques, L.B., and Kavanagh, L.W., Carbohydr. Res. *7*, 369 (1968).
3. Perlin, A.S., Casu, B., Sanderson, G.R., and Johnson, L.F., Can. J. Chem. *48*, 2260 (1970).
4. Perlin, A.S., and Sanderson, G.R., Carbohydr. Res. *12*, 183 (1970).
5. Dietrich, C.P., Biochem. J. *108*, 647 (1968); Perlin, A.S., Mackie, D.M., and Dietrich, C.P., Carbohydr. Res. *18*, 185 (1971).
6. Perlin, A.S., Ng Ying Kim, N.M.K., Bhattacharjee, S.S., and Johnson, L.F. Can. J. Chem., *50*, 2437 (1972).
7. Perlin, A.S., *in* E.B. Mano (ed.), Proceedings Int. Symp. Macromolecules, Rio de Janeiro, July (1974), p. 337.
8. Perlin, A.S., Fed. Proceedings, *36*, 106 (1977).
9. Gatti, G., Casu, B., and Perlin, A.S., Symposium on Biology of Connective Tissue, Upsala J. Med. Sci. *82*, 131 (1977).
10. Perlin, A.S., Casu, B., Sanderson, G.R., and Tse, J., Carbohydr. Res., *21*, 123 (1972).
11. Atkins, E.D.T., Fed. Proceedings, *36*, 68 (1977).
12. Hamer, G.K., and Perlin, A.S., unpublished results.
13. Gatti, G., and Casu, B., 2nd Joint Conference C.I.C. and A.C.S., Montreal, June (1977). Abstr. Carb. 7.
14. Helleur, R., M.Sc. Thesis, McGill University, Montreal, Sept. (1977).
15. Foster, A.B., Harrison, R., Inch, T.D., Stacey, M., and Webber, J.M., J. Chem. Soc., 2279 (1963).
16. Wolfrom, M.L., and Wang, P.Y., Chem. Commun., 241 (1967).
17. Mushayakarara, E.C., M.Sc. thesis, McGill University, Montreal, Sept. (1977).
18. Linker, A., Hoffman, P., Sampson, P., and Meyer, K., Biochem. Biophys. Acta, *29*, 443 (1958); 43, 366 (1960).
19. Cifonelli, J.A., Carbohydr. Res., *2*, 150 (1966): *9*, 233 (1968).
20. Höök, M., Lindahl, U., and Iverius, P.H., Biochem. J., *137*, 33 (1974).

21. Dietrich, C.P., and Nader, H.B., Biochem. Biophys. Acta. 343, *34* (1974).
22. Lindahl, U., and Axelsson, O., J. Biol. Chem., *246*, 74 (1971).
23. Cifonelli, J.A., and King, J., Carbohydr. Res., *21*, 173 (1972).
24. Casu, B., Scovenna, G., Cifonelli, J.A., and Perlin, A.S., Carbohydr. Res., in press.
25. Hamer, G.K., and Perlin, A.S., Carbohydr. Res., *49*, 37 (1976).
26. Perlin, A.S., and Casu, B., Tetrahedron Lett., 2921 (1969); Schwarcz, J.A., and Perlin, A.S., Can. J. Chem., *50*, 773 (1972).
27. Bock, K., Lundt, J., and Pederson, C., Tetrahedron Lett., 1037 (1972).

STRUCTURE OF SULFATED MUCOPOLYSACCHARIDES FROM NORMAL TISSUES AND FROM PATIENTS WITH MUCOPOLYSACCHARIDOSES[a]

Carl P. Dietrich, Helena B. Nader,
Diana M. Cohen, and Yara M. Michelacci

Escola Paulista de Medicina

A comparative study on the structure of heparin, heparitin sulfates, and chondroitin sulfates from normal tissues and from patients with the Hunter and Hurler syndromes is described. The structural studies were based, among other methods, on the products formed from these compounds by the action of heparinase, heparitinases, chondroitinases, and other enzymes involved in the sequential degradation of these mucopolysaccharides in Flavobacterium heparinum. It is concluded that heparitin sulfate excreted by patients with the Hunter syndrome is a unique and complex structure composed of nine different types of disaccharide units and containing regions akin to heparitin sulfate from normal tissues and regions akin to heparin. It is also concluded that Hurler chondroitin sulfate B is a unique structure which is made almost exclusively of glycosidic linkages susceptible to chondroitinase B, whereas chondroitin sulfate B from normal tissues contain two regions: one susceptible to chondroitinase B and a dodecasaccharide region which is susceptible to chondroitinase AC. The implications of these findings on the possible metabolic errors of the Hunter and Hurler syndromes is discussed.

I. STRUCTURE AND ENZYMATIC DEGRADATION OF HEPARIN AND HEPARITIN SULFATES FROM NORMAL TISSUES

Figure 1 summarizes our findings on the structure of heparin and heparitin sulfates as well as their sequential degradation to monosaccharides by enzymes from *F. heparinum*. This has already been described in detail in several publications from our laboratory (1-10). Briefly, heparin is degraded to a trisulfated disaccharide and a pentasulfated tetrasaccharide by the heparinase. The tetrasaccharide is in turn degraded by a heparitinase (called heparitinase II)since

---

[a]*Aided by grants from FINEP (Financiadora de Estudos e Projetos), FAPESP (Fundacão de Amparo a Pesquisa do Estado de São Paulo), CNPq (Conselho Nacional de Desenvolvimento Cientifico e Tecñologico), and CAPES (Campanha de Aperfeicoamento de Pessoal de Nivel Superior).*

ISBN 0-12-484850-8

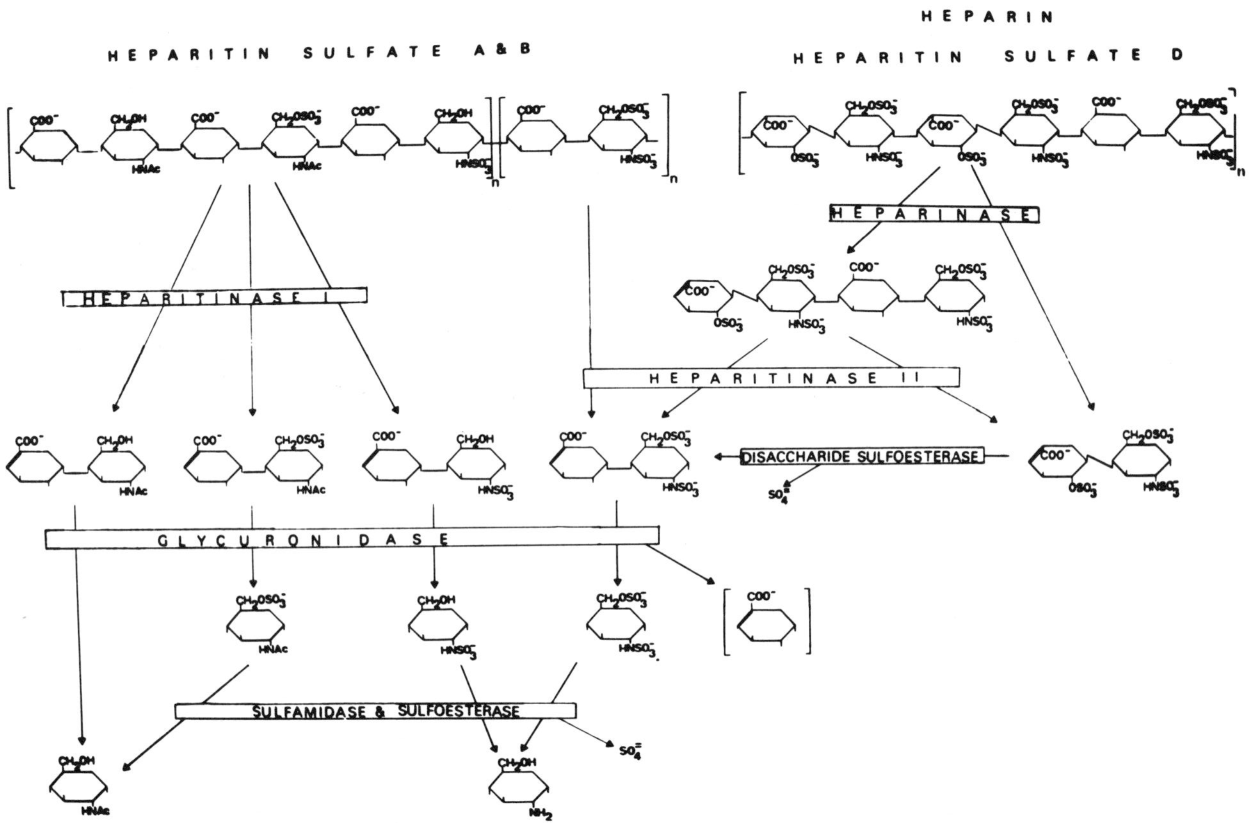

Fig. 1. Structure and sequential degradation of heparin and heparitin sulfates by enzymes from Flavobacterium heparinum.

it also acts upon heparitin sulfate (Fig. 1) to a disulfated disaccharide and trisulfated disaccharide. A disaccharide sulfoesterase removes the sulfate from the uronic acid moiety of the trisulfated disaccharide transforming it into a disulfated disaccharide. Heparitin sulfates A and B[a] are degraded by heparitinase I forming three types of disaccharides, namely, an N-acetylated nonsulfated disaccharide, N-acetylated-6-sulfated disaccharide, and N-sulfated disaccharide, plus an oligosaccharide with an average molecular weight of 6000. The latter is only degraded by heparitinase II forming mainly disulfated disaccharide. The resulting disaccharides from heparitin sulfate and heparin are then degraded by a glycuronidase to monosaccharides and α,β keto acid. The sulfated monosaccharides are then desulfated by a sulfamidase and a sulfoesterase producing glucosamine and N-acetylglucosamine. Several conclusions can be reached regarding the mode of action of the heparinase and heparitinases upon heparin and heparitin sulfates. The specificity of the heparinase seems to be upon αD glucosaminido-iduronic acid linkages, whereas the specificity of heparitinase I is upon αD glucosaminido-glucuronic acid linkages. The specificity of heparitinase II is not fully established. Its action seems to be dependent upon the presence of a sulfate in the 6 position of the glucosamine. The possibility that the difference of specificity of heparitinase I and II would reside in the type of linkage (α 1-3 versus α 1-4) is not ruled out by the present results. Another question that has not been answered in the present studies is the nature of the glycosidic linkages between the uronic acid and hexosamine of the disaccharides. The finding that heparitin sulfate B has a strong positive optical rotation which is around +130 (after extensive purification with removal of protein and chondroitin sulfate B that contaminate these preparations) suggests that the linkages are αD type as shown in Fig. 1. This is corroborated by the finding that these disaccharides are not substrates for a β glycuronidase from *F. heparinum* that acts upon chondroitin sulfate disaccharides (1). Some of these reactions have also been worked out in other laboratories (13-16).

II. STRUCTURE AND ENZYMATIC DEGRADATION OF HEPARITIN SULFATE EXCRETED BY PATIENTS WITH HUNTER SYNDROME

The products formed from Hunter heparitin sulfate compared

---

[a]*We have previously shown that heparitin sulfate from beef lung tissue is a mixture of four sulfated mucopolysaccharides. Heparitin sulfates A and B are susceptible to heparitinases I and II and heparitin sulfates C and D are only degraded by heparinase. For details of their structure and chemical composition see 7, 10, 11, 12.*

with the products formed from heparin and heparitin sulfate from normal tissues (human urine, beef lung) by the action of heparinase and heparitinases are shown in Fig. 2. The disaccharide products formed from both heparitins by action of

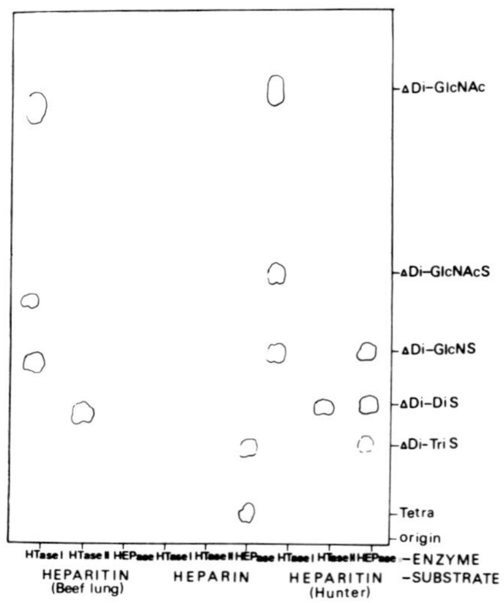

Fig. 2. Disaccharide products formed from heparitin sulfates and heparin by action of heparitinases and heparinase. The substrates as indicated were incubated with the enzymes heparitinase I (HTase I), heparitinase II (HTase II) and heparinase (HEPase) as described in (9) and (10). The incubation mixtures were then chromatographed in isobutyric acid - 1M/NH_3, 5, 3, v/v. The products were identified by silver nitrate reaction and short wave ultra violet light. Δ Di - ... , unsaturated disaccharides. For further details see text.

heparitinases are undistinguishable from each other. Both heparitins formed the four types of disaccharides shown in Fig. 1. Nevertheless these heparitins differ from each other regarding the susceptibility to heparinase. Normal heparitin sulfate is not degraded by heparinase, contrasting with Hunter heparitin which produces disaccharides with chromatographic migrations of di- and monosulfated disaccharide standards. The products are different from the ones produced from heparin which yields only trisulfated disaccharide and tetrasaccharide (Fig. 1). Since the heparitinases I and II susceptible regions of Hunter heparitin sulfate have about the same characteristics of normal heparitin sulfate we have prepared an oligosaccharide from Hunter heparitin devoid of these regions. This was done by treating the heparitin sulfate with both heparitinases. The resulting oligosaccharide (MW 4000) contained only iduronic acid as the uronic acid moiety of its structure whereas intact Hunter heparitin contained both glucuronic and iduronic acids (Fig. 3).

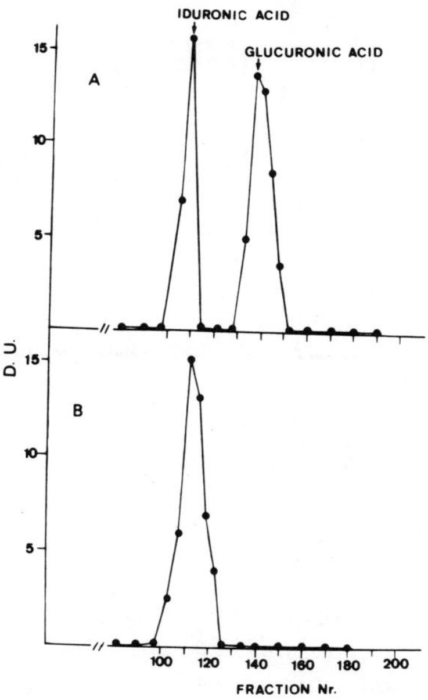

Fig. 3. Uronic acids of Hunter heparitin sulfate and Hunter oligosaccharide. A - Intact Hunter heparitin sulfate, B - Hunter oligosaccharide prepared as described in the text. The method used for the identification of uronic acids was that described by Fransson et al. (17).

This oligosaccharide was incubated with the heparinase and subjected to two-dimensional chromatography and electrophoresis (Fig. 4). Three main disaccharides were formed by action of the heparitinase, two with migrations similar to the disulfated disaccharide and one with the migration of monosulfated disaccharide. These compounds were prepared in large scale and analyzed. The results of the analyses confirmed these migrations. They contained one and two sulfates per hexosamine unit. The two disulfated disaccharides were then incubated with disaccharide sulfoesterase and glycuronidase. One of them was susceptible to the action of both enzymes forming glucosamine N-sulfate and keto acid and the other was susceptible only to the glycuronidase forming glucosamine 2,6-disulfate, and keto acid.

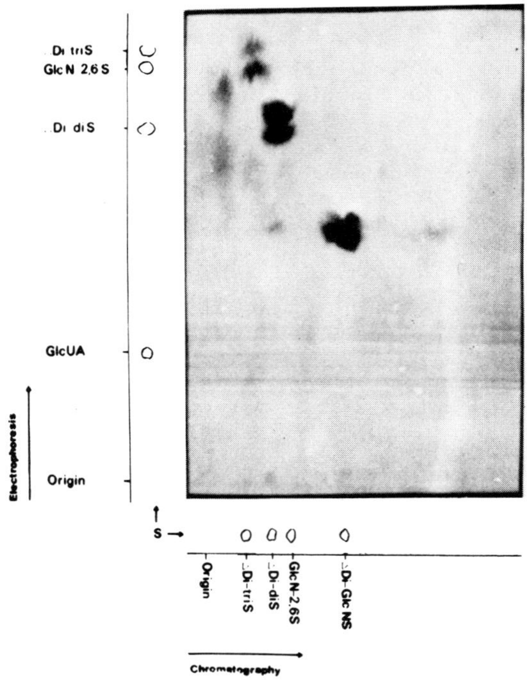

Fig. 4. Disaccharide products formed from Hunter oligosaccharide by action of heparinase. The Hunter oligosaccharide prepared as described in the text was incubated with heparinase as described in (9) and subjected to two-dimensional chromatography (isobutyric acid: 1 M NH_3) and electrophoresis (pyridine-acetate buffer, pH 3.7). The paper was stained with silver nitrate reagent. S = standards.

The relative amounts of the different disaccharide products formed by action of the enzymes upon heparitins and heparin are shown in Table I. These products were obtained from the three substrates in more than 90% yield. Fig. 5 shows the proposed structure of Hunter heparitin sulfate and the mode of action of the enzymes. The heparitinase II-susceptible region (10% of the total structure) and the trisulfated disaccharide from the heparinase-susceptible region (4% of the total structure) have been omitted from the drawing.

The results presented in this communication indicate that Hunter heparitin sulfate is a very complex structure containing at least nine different types of disaccharides. This would suggest that this heparitin is a mixture of sulfated mucopolysaccharides. Attempts to fractionate these compounds by methods similar to the ones used for beef lung heparitin

TABLE I

Disaccharide Products Formed From Heparitin Sulfates and Heparin by Action of Mucopolysaccharidases

Enzyme	Products	Substrates		
	%	Beef lung Heparitin	Hunter Heparitin	Heparin
Heparitinase I	ΔDi-GlcNAc	35	23	< 2
	ΔDi-GlcNAcS	16	5	< 2
	ΔDi-GlcNS	24	10	< 2
Heparitinase II	ΔDi-GlcNS	43	4	< 2
	ΔDi-GlcNS,6S	18	5	< 2
Heparinase	ΔDi-GlcNS	< 2	23	< 2
	ΔDi-US,GlcNS	< 2	10	< 2
	ΔDi-GlcNS,6S	< 2	11	3
	ΔDi-US,GlcNS,6S	< 2	6	52
	Tetra	< 2	< 2	40
	Yield (% of Total SMPS	96	97	95

sulfate were unsuccessful. This, however, does not rule out the possibility that the methods used were unsatisfactory, and the Hunter heparitin might indeed be a mixture of related compounds.

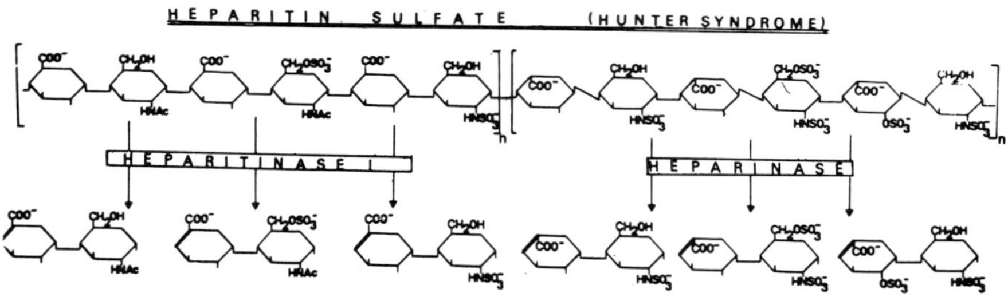

Fig. 5. Proposed structure of Hunter heparitin sulfate and the mode of action of the mucopolysaccharidases.

It has been proposed that a sulfoiduronate sulfatase is the enzyme defect of the patients with the Hunter syndrome. This conclusion was reached by analyses of Hunter fibroblasts in culture which did not degrade properly the sulfated mucopolysaccharides. This anomaly could be corrected by a purified extract that contained sulfoiduronate sulfatase activity (18).

The findings described in the present paper, that two-thirds of the iduronic acids of the Hunter heparitin sulfate are nonsulfated raises some questions regarding the proposed metabolic defect. If the proposal were correct we would expect that most of the iduronic acids would be sulfated in this heparitin (as in heparin) or that they would contain glucuronic acids (as in the heparitin from normal urine and beef lung). Our results showing that Hunter heparitin sulfate is a unique structure, not found in normal tissues, suggests on the the other hand that the metabolic error of this syndrome might be in the biosynthetic pathway.

III. STRUCTURE AND ENZYMATIC DEGRADATION OF CHONDROITIN SULFATE B FROM NORMAL TISSUES AND FROM PATIENTS WITH HURLER SYNDROME

Figure 6 shows the proposed structure of chondroitin sulfate B from pig skin and human skin and the mode of action of a chondroitinase B and a chondroitinase AC from *F. heparinum* upon this compound. The chondroitinase B releases from these chondroitins ΔDi-4S plus a dodecasaccharide (MW 3000) which is in turn degraded by the chondroitinase AC.

About one mole of dodecasaccharide was obtained per mole of chondroitin sulfate B either from human or pig skin. These results have been described in detail elsewhere (19-21). Hurler chondroitin sulfated B was also subjected to chondroitinase B degradation, and the products formed were analyzed by chromatography and polyacrylamide. The Hurler chondroitin sulfate B also produces ΔDi-4S as the main product of the reaction. Nevertheless no dodecasaccharide was obtained from this chondroitin (Fig. 7).

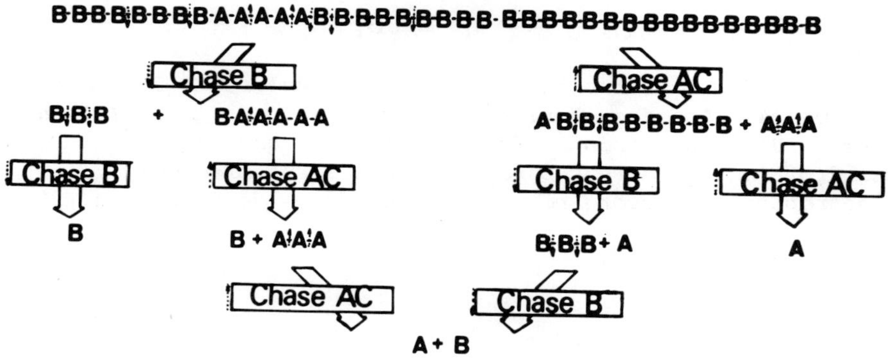

Fig. 6. Structure of chondroitin sulfate B and mode of action of chondroitinase B and chondroitinase AC. B, chondroitin sulfate B disaccharides; A, chondroitin sulfate A disaccharides.

These results show that Hurler chondroitin sulfate B is a different compound from the ones normally present in the tissues.

It has been suggested that the metabolic error of the Hurler syndrome is the lack of an iduronidase responsible for the normal catabolism of this compound (22). The results shown in this communication suggest on the other hand that the Hurler chondroitin sulfate B is an incomplete molecule lacking an oligosaccharide segment which is probably added in the biosynthetic process of the chondroitin sulfate B of normal individuals.

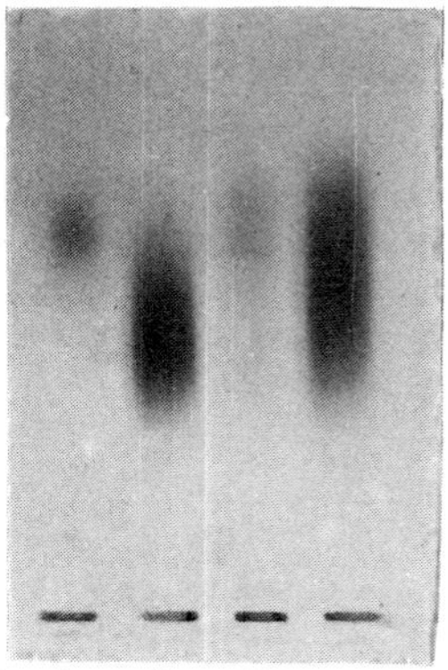

Fig. 7. Degradation of chondroitin sulfate B from normal tissues (A_1) and from Hurler syndrome (B_1). Pig skin (A) and Hurler (B) chondroitin sulfate B after incubation with chondroitinase B were subjected to polyacrylamide gel electrophoresis according to the procedures described in (20).

REFERENCES

1. Dietrich, C.P., Biochem. J. *108*, 647 (1968).
2. Dietrich, C.P., Biochem. J. *111*, 91 (1968).
3. Dietrich, C.P., Biochemistry *8*, 2089 (1969).
4. Perlin, A.S., Mackie, D.M., and Dietrich, C.P., Carbohyd. Res. *18*, 185 (1971).
5. Dietrich, C.P., Silva, M.E., and Michelacci, Y.M., J. Biol. Chem. *248*, 6408 (1973).
6. Dietrich, C.P., and Dietrich, S.M.C., Cienc. Cult. *26*, 55 (1974).
7. Silva, M.E., and Dietrich, C.P., Biochem. Biophys. Res. Commun. *56*, 965 (1974).
8. Dietrich, C.P., Nader, H.B., and Perlin, A.S., Carbohyd. Res. *41*, 334 (1975).
9. Silva, M.E., and Dietrich, C.P., J. Biol. Chem. *250*, 6841 (1975).
10. Silva, M.E., Dietrich, C.P., and Nader, H.B., Biochim. Biophys. Acta *437*, 129 (1976).
11. Dietrich, C.P., Nader, H.B., Britto, L.R.G., and Silva, M.E., Biochim. Biophys. Acta *237*, 430 (1971).
12. Dietrich, C.P., and Nader, H.B., Biochim. Biophys. Acta *343*, 34 (1974).
13. Linker, A., and Sampson, P., Biochim. Biophys. Acta *43*, 366 (1960).

14. Linker, A., and Hovingh, P., J. Biol. Chem. *240*, 3724 (1965).
15. Hovingh, P., and Linker, A., J. Biol. Chem. *245*, 6170 (1970).
16. Warnick, C.T., and Linker, A., Biochemistry *11*, 568 (1972).
17. Fransson, L., Rodén, L., and Spach, M.L., Analyt. Biochem. *21*, 317 (1968).
18. Bach, G., Eisenberg, F., Cantz, M., and Neufeld, E.F., Proc. Nat. Acad. Sci. *70*, 2134 (1973).
19. Michelacci, Y.M., and Dietrich, C.P., Biochem. Biophys. Res. Commun. *56*, 973 (1974).
20. Michelacci, Y.M., and Dietrich, C.P., Biochem. J. *151*, 121 (1975).
21. Michelacci, Y.M., and Dietrich, C.P., J. Biol. Chem. *251*, 1154 (1976).
22. Bach, G., Friedman, R., Weissmann, B., and Neufeld, E.F., Proc. Nat. Acad. Sci. *69*, 2048 (1972).

THE METABOLISM OF MACROMOLECULAR HEPARIN[a]

Alan A. Horner and Edward Young

Department of Physiology
University of Toronto

This paper presents evidence that macromolecular heparin is a unique protease-resistant proteoglycan. It is comprised of heparin chains, which are much larger than those of commercial heparin, linked through alkali-labile glycosidic linkages involving the hydroxyl groups of serine residues to a peptide core comprised entirely of equimolar proportions of serine and glycine.

The actions of four macromolecular heparin depolymerases on macromolecular heparin from rat skin are described. These are (a) a rat plasma enzyme with a pH optimum of 6.0, (b) depolymerase 1 from rat small intestine with a pH optimum of 7.4, (c) depolymerase 2 from rat small intestine with a pH optimum of 6.0, and (d) an enzyme from mouse mastocytoma with a pH optimum of 5.0. Activities (a) to (d) give products of successively smaller size.

The involvement of heparin in lipoprotein lipase metabolism is discussed. An experiment demonstrating the presence of two discrete heparin fractions in rat adipose tissue is described. These heparins are comparable in size to the products formed by the action of the rat plasma depolymerase on macromolecular heparin from rat skin.

Finally the possible role of lipoprotein lipase, and by association heparin, in atherogenesis is considered. An experiment in which feeding an atherogenic diet to squirrel monkeys caused the accumulation of high molecular weight heparin in their small intestines is described. It is suggested that this is an example of a situation in which impaired macromolecular heparin depolymerase activity may have pathological consequences.

I. INTRODUCTION

Macromolecular heparin is a term that was first used to describe a high molecular weight heparin product isolated from rat skin in our laboratory (1). The term has since been applied to high molecular weight heparin isolated from rat peritoneal mast cells (2), monkey tissues (2,3), and mouse

[a]*Supported by the Ontario Heart Foundation and the J.P. Bickell Foundation*

ISBN 0-12-484850-8

mastocytoma (4). Before discussing the metabolism of these high molecular weight forms of heparin it is necessary to update the present concept of their structure.

II. THE STRUCTURE OF MACROMOLECULAR HEPARIN

It was previously shown that macromolecular heparin from rat skin (RS heparin) with a molecular weight of the order of 1 million was resistant to digestion by pronase and papain. After one digestion with pronase the amino acid content was 0.7%. After a second digestion with pronase the only amino acids in the preparation were serine and glycine, each at a concentration of approximately 0.02 μmoles/mg (1). This corresponds to an amino acid concentration of only 0.35% by weight. By comparison with classical proteoglycans from cartilage with a protein content of approximately 10% (5), RS heparin did not seem to have an adequate protein content to support the concept of a protein core being responsible for the structural integrity of a multichain macromolecular heparin. On the basis of degradation studies with ascorbate-which released heparin chains of the same order of size as commercial heparin from a higher molecular weight ascorbate-resistant fraction that contained a high proportion of the total amino acids and neutral sugars, it was postulated that a polysaccharide core held together the entire multichain complex. Recent studies indicate that this concept was incorrect. In fact macromolecular RS heparin appears to be a proteoglycan with two unusual features: (a) the individual heparin chains have molecular weights in the range 40 to 100 x 10^3, much larger than commercial heparins; (b) structural integrity is maintained by a unique polypeptide comprised entirely of equimolar proportions of serine and glycine, which is resistant to the common broad spectrum proteases such as papain and pronase. The polysaccharide chains are attached to the serine residues in the same way as in other proteoglycans. This new model is based on a collaborative study involving the Toronto and Uppsala laboratories, in which macromolecular RS heparin has been degraded (a) with tritiated borohydride using the methodology originally developed by Robinson and Hopwood in their work with cartilage proteoglycans (6), (b) with nitrous acid by the method of Cifonelli and King (7), and (c) with a mastocytomal endoglycosidase prepared from mouse mastocytoma (4). This work will be described fully elsewhere (Robinson, Horner, Höök, Ögren, and Lindahl, manuscript in preparation). The salient features are as follows. Heparin chain weights were estimated by analyses of components of the linkage-to-protein region using a highly purified RS heparin preparation. The serine content of 0.021 μmoles/mg corresponded to a chain weight of 42 x 10^3 while the xylose content of 0.014 μmoles/mg corresponded to a chain weight of 63 x 10^3. Degradation with 0.5 *M* KOH in the presence of tritiated borohydride gave a product with a tritiated xylitol content corresponding to a chain weight of 93 x 10^3. Analytical ultracentrifugation (8) of this product gave a molecular weight value of 66 x 10^3. When the alkali-degraded product was chromatographed on DEAE-cellulose, analytical ultracentrifugation of the heparin that was recovered gave a molecular weight value of 81 x 10^3. Therefore it appears that the heparin chains released from the intact starting material by treatment with alkali have molecular weights of the order of 40 to 100 x 10^3. Approximately two-thirds of the serine in the starting material was destroyed by alkali. Glycine was not destroyed, but most of it was released from the macromolecular structure and separated from the heparin chains by chromatography on DEAE-cellulose. The glycine that was not released from the heparin was approximately equimolar to the serine that was not released from the heparin. Therefore between 2 out of 3 and 4 out of 5 of the serine residues in macromolecular heparin appear to be involved in glycosidic linkages to xylose in the same way as in other proteoglycans, that is, they are susceptible to β-elimination.

When macromolecular heparin was degraded with nitrous acid, gel filtration gave a nitrous acid-resistant core fraction containing only 2-4% of the uronic acid in the starting material, yet containing more than 90% of the neutral sugars and amino acids. The molecular weight of this product was approximately 20 x 10^3, and electrophoresis indicated a very low sulfate content. Furthermore, this nitrous acid-resistant core was susceptible to alkaline degradation, giving a polydisperse mixture of very low molecular weight products when fractionated on Sephadex G-50, a gel from which the core was excluded.

Treatment of macromolecular RS heparin with the mastocytomal endoglycosidase gave products in the same molecular size range as commercial pig mucosal heparin. Therefore this enzyme must act at several sites along each chain, the number of cleavages being dependent on the true molecular size of the alkali-degraded chains. Final evidence for a proteoglycan structure was obtained in experiments in which synthetic poly (glycyl-serine) accepted ^{14}C-xylose when incubated with UDP-^{14}C-xylose in the presence of a microsomal fraction prepared from mouse mastocytoma tissue. These data strongly support the concept of a unique proteoglycan structure. However, it is still necessary to actually isolate the polypeptide core.

The data also support and amplify the results of Yurt, *et al.* (9), who isolated a macromolecular heparin from rat peritoneal mast cells with a molecular weight of the order of 750 x 10^3, which was degraded by 0.5 *M* NaOH to products with a molecular size of the order of 40 x 10^3. The macromolecular heparin from this source was resistant to digestion with papain, pronase, pancreatin, trypsin, chymotrypsin, subtilisin, and elastase. If labeled with ^{3}H-serine, one-third of the label stayed with the heparin product isolated after degradation with alkali.

III. THE MACROMOLECULAR HEPARIN DEPOLYMERASES

These are enzymes that break down macromolecular heparin to smaller products, the smallest of which are still in the same general molecular size range as commercial heparin. These are therefore not catabolic enzymes in the general sense because the products are still biologically active. Rather they are enzymes that release physiologically active chains from a macromolecular multichain precursor form of heparin. Ögren and Lindahl have described a similar enzyme from mouse mastocytoma and presented evidence that it is an endoglucuronidase (4). They have called this *heparin-liberating enzyme* (10), which is a useful descriptive title. As this chapter will indicate, there are at least four mammalian enzymes which depolymerize macromolecular heparin. Three of these have been studied in our laboratory using ^{35}S-labeled macromolecular heparin prepared from rat skin as substrate. These studies amplify an earlier report of a heparin depolymerase activity in rat intestine that was assayed at pH 7.4 using unlabeled macromolecular RS heparin (11). It was shown in this earlier work that the products were on average of higher molecular weight than commercial pig mucosal heparin, and that repeated redigestion increased the proportion of lower molecular weight products but did not alter their overall size range. This is indicative of cleavage by an endoglycosidase at a limited number of specific sites rather than a random type of cleavage. It was also found at this time (Horner, unpublished observations) that depolymerase activity was much lower at pH 6.0 than at pH 7.4 using buffers containing phosphate or acetate ions. In more recent work using tris-maleate buffers, optimum depolymerase activity has been found at pH 6.0. In this case the heparin chains released from the ^{35}S-labeled macromolecular substrate are on average slightly smaller in size than commercial pig mucosal heparin. These points are illustrated in Fig. 1, which shows gel filtration patterns for products of digestion at pH 7.4 and pH 6.0 fractionated on the same column of Bio-Gel Al.5 m with pig mucosal heparin run through the same column for comparative purposes.

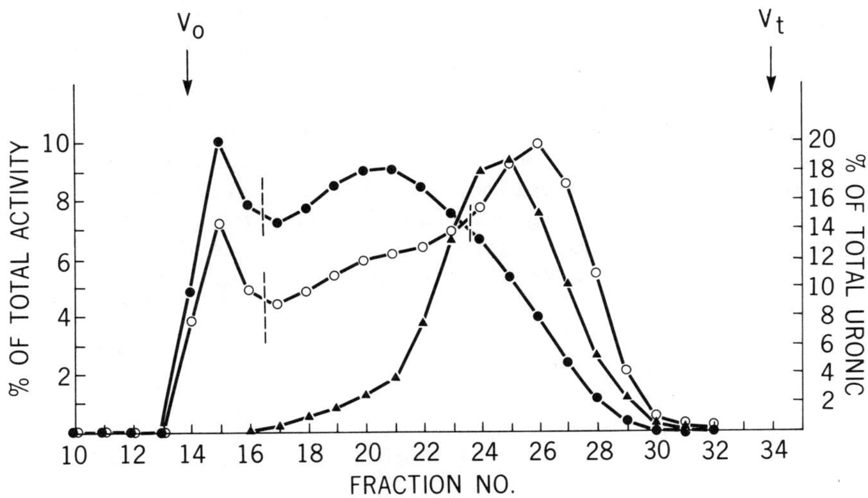

Fig. 1. Gel filtration of products of intestinal depolymerases 1 and 2 on a column of Bio-Gel A-1.5 m agarose gel granules equilibrated with 1.0 M NaCl. Samples of macromolecular ^{35}S-RS heparin were incubated with the 12,100 x g supernatant from homogenates of rat small intestine at pH 7.4 (●) and pH 6.0 (O). The radioactivity in each fraction is expressed as a percentage of the total radioactivity in each sample (left ordinate). Commercial pig mucosal heparin (▲) was run through the same column and quantified in terms of uronic acid content (12).

This type of experiment suggests that rat small intestine contains two depolymerases with different pH optima. The first enzyme, depolymerase 1, acts on the macromolecular substrate to give products that are mainly larger than PM heparin. This type of product is subsequently degraded further by a second enzyme, depolymerase 2, giving products that are slightly smaller than PM heparin. Both depolymerases appear to be active at pH 6.0. The activities of these two enzymes are dissociated by incubation at pH 7.4. At this pH there is very little depolymerase 2 activity. In previously published experiments (11), products of depolymerase 1 were fractionated by gel filtration. It was shown that the products ranged from inhibitors to activators of lipoprotein lipase (LPL) extracted from rat heart and assayed in an *in vitro* system. Similar results have been obtained with LPL extracted from rat adipose tissue (Horner, unpublished observations). High molecular weight heparins inhibited or failed to activate LPL in this system, and only products of the same order of molecular size as commercial pig mucosal heparin activated the enzyme. We have not tested the products of depolymerase 2 in this way but would expect them to be more active than the heparin chains released by depolymerase 1.

When macromolecular RS heparin was injected into rats it showed relatively poor LPL-releasing activity compared to pig mucosal heparin. Furthermore, LPL activity appeared in the plasma only after a lag period. Maximal activity was observed 7 minutes postinjection rather than 1 minute postinjection in the case of pig mucosal heparin. This suggested that a plasma depolymerase had to act on the macromolecular heparin

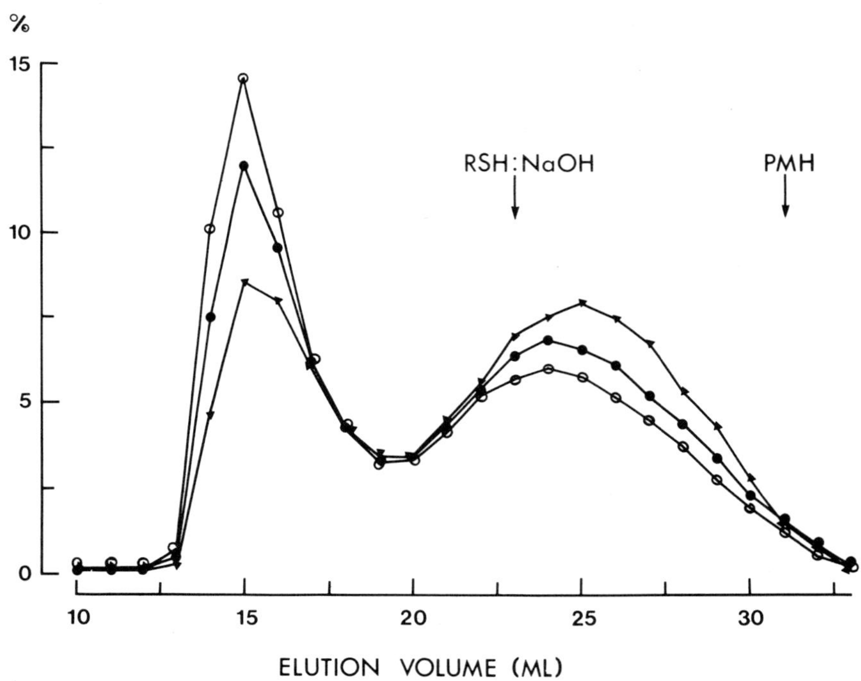

Fig. 2. O, ●, and ▼, samples of macromolecular ^{35}S-RS heparin fractionated on a column of Bio-Gel A-15m after 1, 2, and 3 incubations, for 18 hr at 37°C, with rat plasma at pH 6.0. The peak positions of other heparins run through the column are shown by arrows. RSH:NaOH, macromolecular ^{35}S-RS heparin depolymerized in 0.5 M NaOH; PMH, pig mucosal heparin.

before low molecular weight products were available to activate or release LPL. We have now demonstrated depolymerase activity in plasma using ^{35}S-labeled macromolecular RS heparin as substrate. To fractionate the products of depolymerase activity in plasma it was necessary to use Bio-Gel A-15m which has a higher molecular weight exclusion limit than the gel used to fractionate products of the intestinal depolymerases.

Figure 2 shows the fractionation by gel filtration of the products of three successive incubations of macromolecular ^{35}S-RS heparin with plasma that has been dialyzed against 0.05 *M* Tris-maleate-0.001 *M* EDTA, pH 6.0. These elution patterns clearly show that successive digestions increase the proportion of lower molecular weight products but do not cause a shift in their overall size distribution. The products of this depolymerase are appreciably larger than the products of the two intestinal depolymerases. This is best shown by recovering the heparin chains fractionated on Bio-Gel A-15m, rerunning them on Bio-Gel A-1.5m and running the products of the intestinal depolymerases through the same column for comparative purposes. This is illustrated by Fig. 3. Heparin

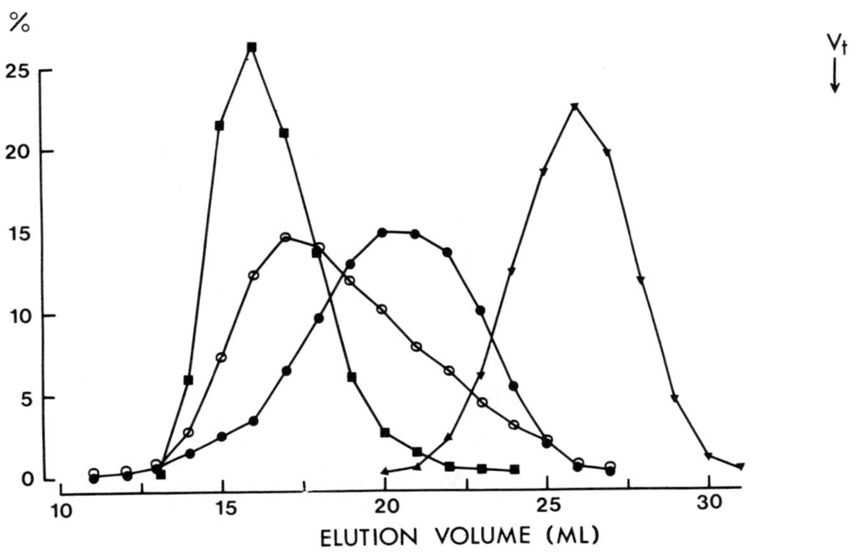

Fig. 3. Gel filtration on a column of Bio-Gel A-1.5 m of (a) macromolecular ^{35}S-RS heparin depolymerized in 0.5M NaOH (■) and (b) heparin chains released from macromolecular ^{35}S-RS heparin by the following rat enzyme activities: O, plasma depolymerase at pH 6.0; ●, intestinal depolymerase 1 at pH 7.4, and ▼, intestinal depolymerase 2 at pH 6.0.

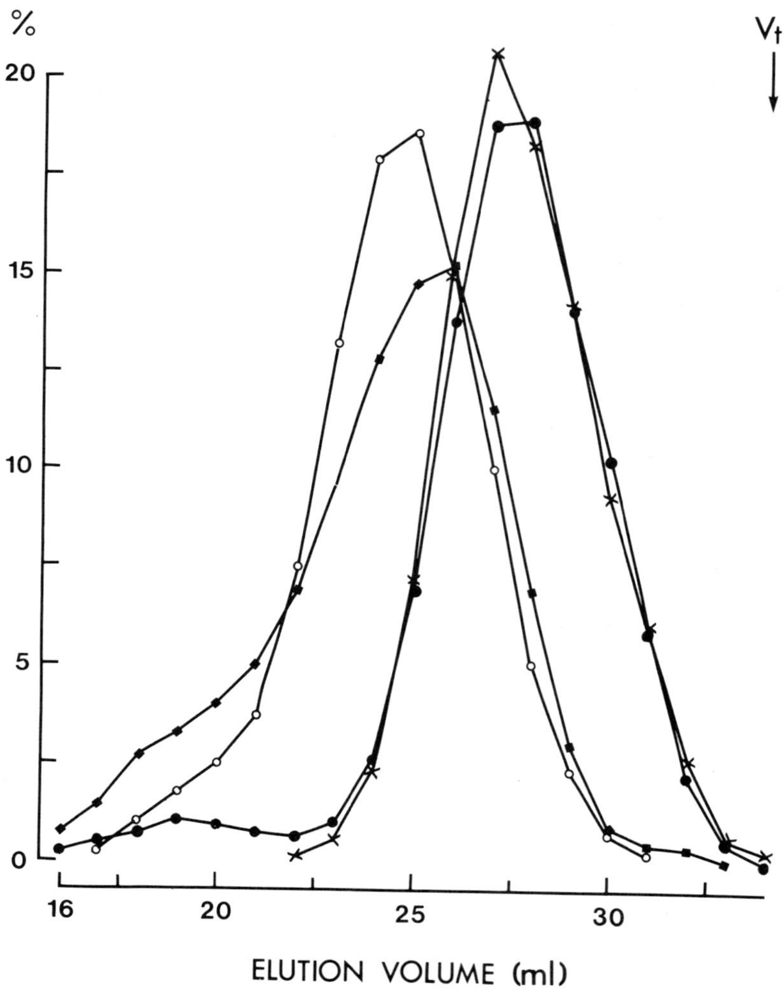

Fig. 4. Gel filtration on a column of Bio-Gel A-1.5 m of the following heparin products: (a) commercial pig mucosal heparin (0), (b) heparin chains released from macromolecular ^{35}S-RS heparin by rat intestinal depolymerase 2 activity at pH 6.0 (■), (c) product (b) after incubation with the mouse mastocytomal endoglycosidase at pH 5.0 (x), and (d) macromolecular ^{35}S-RS heparin after incubation with the mouse mastocytomal endoglycosidase at pH 5.0 (●).

chains released from macromolecular RS heparin by the action of 0.5 *M* NaOH were also run through this column. This clearly shows that the depolymerase that is active in plasma at pH 6.0 produces a much larger product than the enzyme, which is active in intestine at pH 6.0 and that the former products are of similar size to the individual heparin chains in the proposed model for a heparin proteoglycan.

We have also studied the action of the mouse mastocytomal endoglycosidase, which has a pH optimum of 5.0 (4), using a sample generously supplied by Dr. Lindahl. The results of our experiments are shown in Fig. 4, which illustrates gel filtration patterns for products fractionated on Bio-Gel A-1.5m. Using macromolecular ^{35}S-RS heparin as substrate, the rat intestinal depolymerase 2 produced heparin chains which were on average slightly smaller than pig mucosal heparin. These chains were degraded to an even smaller product by the mastocytomal enzyme. However, if macromolecular RS heparin was treated directly with the mastocytomal enzyme, the products were in exactly the same relatively low molecular weight range.

The concept of the mode of action of the 4 enzymes that have been described is summarized in Fig. 5, which illustrates a portion of the proposed proteoglycan structure for macromolecular heparin in which four out of every five serines are involved in glycosidic bonds to heparin chains. This figure is of course a deliberate oversimplification, intended purely to show how stepwise depolymerization to progressively smaller products is catalyzed by different enzymes. It is proposed that (a) the plasma enzyme active at pH 6.0 acts in or near the protein linkage region. Further studies are necessary to find the precise site of action and this hypothesis is presently based solely on the size of the products. (b) Intestinal depolymerase 1 acts approximately halfway along each heparin chain releasing products about half the size of the chains in the intact macromolecule. (c) Intestinal depolymerase 2 acts at two additional sites on each heparin chain to release smaller products. (d) The mouse mastocytomal endoglycosidase acts at possibly all the same sites as the rat enzymes already described, plus additional sites so that even smaller products are formed. This implies that the mastocytomal enzyme has less stringent specificity requirements than the enzymes from normal rat tissues.

IV. FUNCTIONS OF ENDOGENOUS HEPARINS

The physiological role of endogenous heparin is still unknown. The significance of the stepwise depolymerization of macromolecular heparin is therefore inevitably shrouded in mystery: a situation that allows us to speculate freely.

Early stages in the depolymerization process may be involved in the release of heparin from the mast cells into the circulation: the endogenous heparin associated with platelets and erythrocytes in the rat is in the same size range as the products of intestinal depolymerase 1 (13). Tissues may have specific cell-surface receptors for heparin chains of a particular size. The binding of heparin at a cell surface may initiate specific physiological reactions directly, or further depolymerization may first be required, involving other depolymerases. The *later* enzymes in the depolymerization sequence may curtail the action of an active weight form. The smaller products may be the natural substrates for catabolic enzymes which completely inactivate heparin by further depolymerization. Endoglycosidases which degrade heparin to

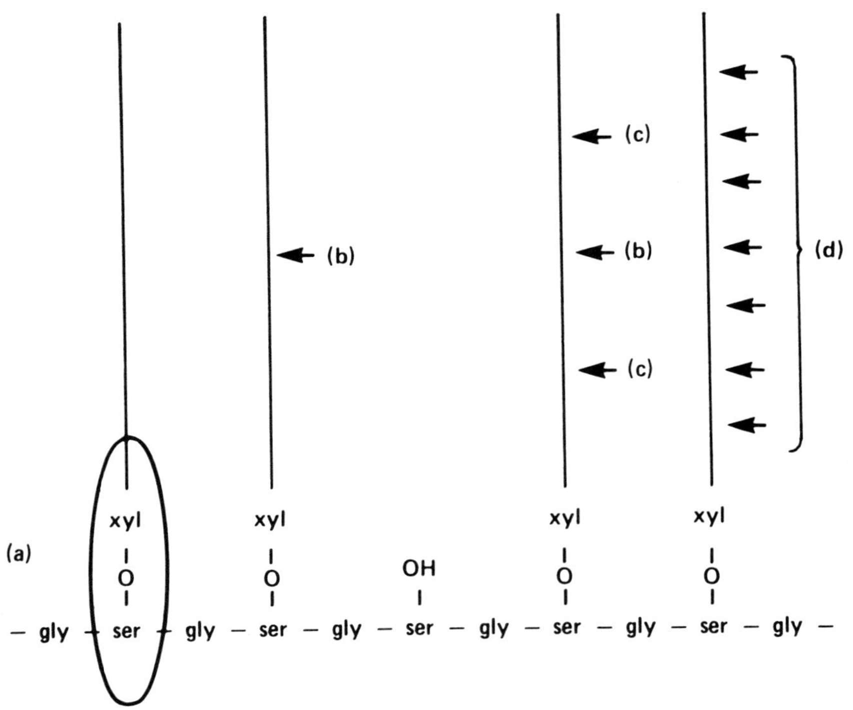

Fig. 5. Schematic representation of a segment of the proposed proteoglycan structure of macromolecular heparin. The vertical bars represent heparin chains in the molecular weight range 40 to 100 x 10^3*. This structure is depolymerized enzymically to successively smaller products by (a) a plasma depolymerase, (b) intestinal depolymerase 1, (c) intestinal depolymerase 2, and (d) the mastocytomal endoglycosidase of Ögren and Lindahl (4).*

oligosaccharides have recently been found in lysosomes isolated from rat liver (14) and rat spleen (15).

A. Heparin and Lipoprotein Lipase

It is not yet known if endogenous heparin is involved in LPL metabolism. There are even conflicting reports on the effect of heparin on purified LPL *in vitro*. Chung and Scanu (16) have recently shown that the activity of a highly purified LPL preparation from rat heart is increased three times by an optimal concentration of heparin, with rat serum added to provide excess apolipoprotein C-II as activator (17). Conversely, Olivecrona and co-workers (18) found that heparin had no effect in a test system containing highly purified bovine milk LPL and apolipoprotein C-II. These investigators have also presented evidence that LPL on endothelial surfaces is probably bound to a heparan sulfate proteoglycan. Olivecrona (19) has suggested that the role of endogenous heparin may be to displace proteins from heparan sulfate binding sites. This suggestion is compatible with a theory recently proposed by Felts, et al. (20). These workers suggest that after hydrolysis of triglycerides in chylomicrons and very low density lipoproteins by LPL on the vascular endothelium, the cholesterol-rich lipoprotein remnants are displaced into the blood stream still bound to LPL. The LPL-remnant complex is then recognized and sequestered by the liver. Endogenous heparin may cause the displacement from the endothelium and may also form part of the remnant complex carried to the liver.

Davies, et al. (21) have presented evidence based on *in vitro* experiments, that supports the view that heparin is required for the conversion of the lower molecular weight form of LPL synthesized within adipocytes to the high molecular weight physiologically active form which is transported to the endothelial surface.

We are continuing to study the possible role of endogenous heparin in LPL metabolism, stimulated by the demonstration that different molecular weight fractions from enzymically depolymerized rat skin heparin have dramatically different effects on LPL activity *in vitro*(11). In this context we have recently obtained evidence which indicates that active heparin metabolism is occurring in adipose tissue. After injecting inorganic ^{35}S-sulfate into male rats, ^{35}S-heparin was recovered from the combined epididymal and perirenal adipose tissues. The experimental procedure was similar to that used previously to demonstrate ^{35}S-heparin in rat blood (13). This endogenous heparin was separated into two well-resolved fractions by gel filtration on Bio-Gel A-15m. These two fractions had the same specific radioactivity. The elution pattern was very similar to that of macromolecular RS heparin depolymerized in plasma at pH 6.0 (see Fig. 2). We believe that this is the first reported isolation of heparin from adipose tissue, although it has been known for some time that this tissue contains mast cells. Hellman, *et al.* (22) used standard histological techniques to show the presence of mast cells (3 mast cells per 1000 adipocytes) in epididymal fat from normal mice and Jennings, *et al.* (23) detected ^{35}S-labeled mast cells in rat epididymal fat by autoradiography.

The only practical source from which to isolate intact mast cells is the peritoneal cavity. In the two cases in which the molecular size of rat peritoneal mast cell heparin has been estimated by gel filtration (2,10), a single peak of macromolecular heparin was found. It is therefore interesting to speculate that the lower molecular weight heparin fraction isolated from rat adipose tissue may be heparin that has been released from the mast cells.

B. Heparin, Lipoprotein Lipase, and Atherogenesis

In 1973 Zilversmit proposed that the formation of atherosclerotic plaques involved the accumulation of cholesterol-rich lipoprotein remnants, formed by the action of LPL on chylomicrons and very low density lipoproteins, within the arterial endothelium (24). This theory requires that LPL be present within the walls of large arteries, and this was subsequently demonstrated (25). Zilversmit has recently shown that the hypercholesterolemia in cholesterol-fed rabbits is due, at least in part, to a rise in the concentration of chylomicron remnants (26).

If endogenous heparin is required for the release of LPL-remnant particles from the endothelium, as discussed in section IV. A, then a deficiency of heparin would exacerbate the deposition of remnants within the arterial wall. This situation could arise if the activity of the macromolecular heparin depolymerase system was impaired.

The following recent study demonstrated, in an indirect manner, the impairment of the macromolecular heparin depolymerase system in an experimental situation which may be relevant to the process of atherogenesis. Previous work with cynomolgus monkeys (2) and squirrel monkeys (3) in our laboratory has shown that different tissues have different proportions of high and low molecular weight heparins. We assume that these differences correlate with different depolymerase activity levels in the tissues. In both species of monkey, the highest proportion of low molecular weight heparin was found in the small intestine, which we therefore assume has the highest depolymerase activity. The accumulation of high molecular weight heparin in this tissue would provide a dramatic demonstration of impaired depolymerase activity. A feeding experiment was therefore planned to examine the effect of an atherogenic diet on heparins in the small intestines of squirrel monkeys.

Six young feral female Bolivian squirrel monkeys were obtained commercially. Three received a synthetic atherogenic diet containing butter (25.5% w/w) and cholesterol (0.5%). Three received a control diet containing corn oil (8%). These diets were developed by Portman and co-workers (27,28). After a one year feeding period each animal received an intraperitoneal injection of sodium ^{35}S-sulfate and was sacrificed 24 hr later. ^{35}S-heparins were recovered from the small intestines by digestion with pronase and precipitation with cetyl pyridinium chloride (1) and purifed by digestion with chondroitinase ABC (29) followed by gradient elution from DEAE-cellulose at pH 2.5 (1). Purity was confirmed by gel electrophoresis (30) and autoradiography of the dried gels, and by a specific nitrous acid degradation procedure for N-sulfated glycosaminoglycans (31).

The purified ^{35}S-heparins were fractionated on a column of Sephadex G-200. The elution patterns are shown in Fig. 6. Fig. 6 (b) clearly shows the presence of a high molecular weight heparin fraction in the monkeys fed the atherogenic diet. This type of heparin is only present in traces in control animals (Fig. 6 (b)).

One cholesterol-fed monkey (J) had severe atherosclerosis (fibrous plaques throughout the thoracic and abdominal aorta). A second animal (K) showed numerous fatty streaks. There was no visible atherosclerosis in the third animal in this group (L). This variability is not surprising, for there is known to be a genetic factor involved in susceptibility to atherosclerosis in squirrel monkeys. The plasma cholesterol concentration values indicate that the experimental group contained only one *hyperresponder* (monkey J) and two *hyporesponders* to cholesterol feeding (32). Also with monkeys not bred in captivity we could not control the age variable, which is undoubtedly important.

However, in spite of the small number of monkeys used, some novel findings were made. The greatest accumulation of macromolecular heparin was observed in the monkey with advanced atherosclerosis. The absence of visible atherosclerosis in monkey L suggests that failure to depolymerize macromolecular heparin may be a metabolic defect which precedes the development of atherosclerosis.

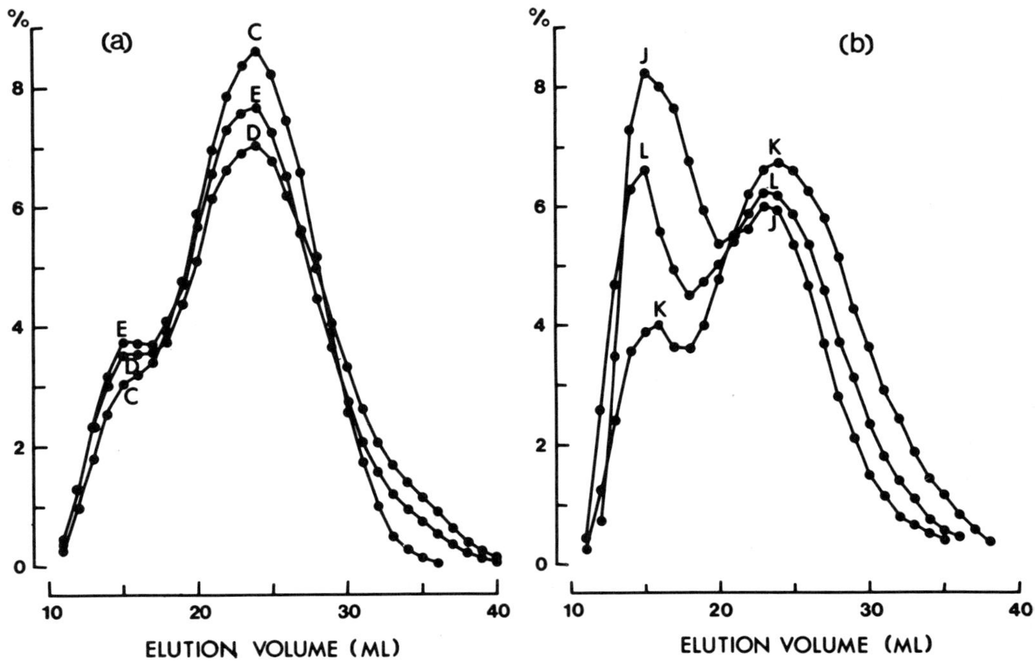

Fig. 6. Gel filtration on a column of Sephadex G-200 (bed volume 35 ml), equilibrated with 1.0 M NaCl, of ^{35}S-heparins recovered from the small intestines of squirrel monkeys. The radioactivity in each fraction is expressed as a percentage of the total radioactivity applied to the column. (a) The elution patterns of ^{35}S-heparins from three monkeys fed a control diet containing corn oil. The plasma cholesterol concentrations of monkeys C, D, and E were 155, 166, and 144 mg/dl, respectively. (b) The elution patterns of ^{35}S-heparins from three monkeys fed an atherogenic diet containing butter and cholesterol. The plasma cholesterol concentrations of monkeys J, K, and L were 585, 341, and 356 mg/dl, respectively.

This type of feeding experiment cannot establish whether changes in heparin molecular weight distribution patterns are a cause or an effect of atherosclerosis. However, it does indicate that the heparin depolymerization process can be altered, directly or indirectly, by diet. If endogenous heparin plays a role in LPL metabolism, and LPL is involved in atherogenesis, any impairment of the heparin depolymerization mechanism has profound pathological implications.

We do not intend to imply that impaired heparin depolymerization is a sine qua non for the development of atheroslerotic lesions. It may however be one causative factor which has not previously been considered; for the existence of macromolecular precursor forms of heparin, and of enzymes involved in their breakdown, are quite recent findings. The pathological implications of this study must remain conjectural until the physiological role of heparin has been elucidated.

REFERENCES

1. Horner, A.A., J. Biol. Chem. *246*, 231 (1971).
2. Horner, A.A., Fed. Proc. *36*, 35 (1977).
3. Horner, A.A., in "Heparin: Chemistry and Clinical Usage" (V.V. Kakkar and D.P. Thomas, eds.), p. 34. Academic Press, London, 1976.
4. Ögren, S. and Lindahl, U., J. Biol. Chem. *250*, 2690 (1975).
5. Davidson, E.A., in "Metabolic Conjugation and Metabolic Hydrolysis" (W.H. Fishman, ed.), Vol. 1, p. 337. Academic Press, New York, 1970.
6. Robinson, H.C., and Hopwood, J.J., Biochem. J. *133*, 457 (1973).
7. Cifonelli, J.A., and King, J., Carbohydr. Res. *21*, 173 (1972).
8. Chervenka, C.H., Anal. Biochem. *34*, 24 (1970).
9. Yurt, R.W., Leid, R.W., Austen, K.F., and Silbert, J.E., J. Biol. Chem. *252*, 518 (1977).
10. Ögren, S., and Lindahl, U., Biochem. J. *154*, 605 (1976).
11. Horner, A.A., Proc. Natl. Acad. Sci. U.S.A. *69*, 3469 (1972).
12. Bitter, T., and Muir, H.M., Anal. Biochem. *4*, 330 (1962).
13. Horner, A.A., FEBS Lett. *46*, 166 (1974).
14. Arbogast, B., Hopwood, J.J., and Dorfman, A., Biochem. Biophys. Res. Commun. *75*, 610 (1977).
15. Höök, M., Pettersson, I., and Ögren, S., Thromb. Res. *10*, 857 (1977).
16. Chung, J., and Scanu, A.M., J. Biol. Chem. *252*, 4202 (1977).
17. Brown, W.V., Levy, R.I. and Fredrickson, D.S., Biochim. Biophys. Acta *200*, 573 (1970).
18. Olivecrona, T., Bengtsson, G., Marklund, S.-E., Lindahl, U., and Höök, M., Fed. Proc. *36*, 60 (1977).
19. Olivecrona, T., Fed. Proc. *36*, 113 (1977).
20. Felts, J.M., Itakura, H., and Crane, R.T., Biochem. Biophys. Res. Commun. *66*, 1467 (1975).
21. Davies, P., Cryer, A., and Robinson, D.S., FEBS Lett. *45*, 271 (1974).

22. Hellman, B., Larsson, S., and Westman, S., Acta Physiol. Scand. *58*, 255 (1963).
23. Jennings, M.A., Florey, H.W., Robinson, D.S., and Salaman, M.R., Ann. N.Y. Acad. Sci. *103*, 313 (1963).
24. Zilversmit, D.B., Circ. Res. *33*, 633 (1973).
25. Dicorleto, P.E., and Zilversmit, D.B., Proc. Soc. Exp. Biol. Med. *148*, 1101 (1975).
26. Zilversmit, D.B., Ann. N.Y. Acad. Sci. *275*, 138 (1976).
27. Portman, O.W., and Andrus, S.B., J. Nutr. *87*, 429 (1969).
28. Portman, O.W., Alexander, M., and Maruffo, C.A., J. Nutr. *91*, 35 (1967).
29. Yamagata, T., Saito, H., Osami, H. and Suzuki, S., J. Biol. Chem. *243*, 1523 (1968).
30. Horner, A.A., *in* "Heparin Structure, Function and Clinical Implications" (R.A. Bradshaw and S. Wessler, eds.), p. 85. Plenum Press, New York, 1975.
31. Lindahl, U., Bäckström, G., Jansson, L., and Hallén, A. J. Biol. Chem. *248*, 7234 (1973).
32. Clarkson, T.B., Lofland, H.B. Jr., Bullock, B.C. and Goodman, H.O., Arch. Path. *92*, 37 (1971).

HEPARIN FROM RAT PERITONEAL MAST CELLS

Jeremiah E. Silbert

Veterans Administration Outpatient Clinic and Tufts University School of Medicine

Roger W. Yurt, and K. Frank Austen

Harvard Medical School and Robert B. Brigham Hospital

The native structure of heparin in tissues is poorly understood, but differs from a conventional proteoglycan structure, such as that of chondroitin sulfate (1), which consists of multiple glycosaminoglycan chains attached by xylosyl-serine linkages to a large protein core. For example, mouse mastocytoma heparin occurs primarily as single glycosaminoglycan chains apparently attached to peptide fragments (2). Pig intestinal mucosa heparin has also been found in this form and at least some of the single chains are attached to peptide fragments by xylosyl-serine bonds (3). In contrast, heparin from rat skin is found as a higher molecular weight molecule and the term "macromolecular" heparin has been used (4). It has been suggested, but not demonstrated, that rat skin heparin consists of glycosaminoglycan chains connected to a polysaccharide core rather than to a protein core. In addition it appears that this molecule is attached to peptides in some fashion. The single chain mouse mast cell tumor heparin may be the product of endoglycuronidase action on the macromolecular species (5).

A problem that has been encountered in pursuing studies on heparin is in obtaining the molecule from tissues without using harsh procedures that might degrade a native structure. One source from which heparin can be obtained under mild conditions is rat peritoneal mast cells. These cells release heparin-containing granules as well as histamine and biologically active peptides upon immunologic challenge (6). We have previously described the extraction and partial characterization of heparin from concentrated normal rat peritoneal mast cells (7). The heparin is of high molecular weight, and in this respect similar to the "macromolecular" heparin isolated from rat skin. The rat peritoneal mast cell heparin

ISBN 0-12-484850-8

is readily degraded by alkali to a lower molecular weight species, but is resistant to a variety of proteases (7). Synthesis of this heparin *in vitro* indicates a time-related growth in size over a period of 4 hours or more to a final product similar in apparent molecular weight to the heparin formed during *in vivo* synthesis. These data will be reviewed and the mechanism of growth during *in vitro* synthesis will be analyzed further.

I. EXPERIMENTAL PROCEDURES

Materials and methods used for further experiments were the same as those described previously (7). Cells from 40 to 50 male or female Sprague-Dawley rats, each weighing 200 to 300 g, were collected by lavage of the peritoneal cavity of each rat with 20 ml of Tyrode's buffer containing 0.1% gelatin and 50 mg/l of commercial heparin. Mast cells were concentrated by centrifugation on Metrizamide gradients. For double labeling experiments, 0.2 mC of $[^{35}S]$ sulfate and 1.0 mC of L-$[^{3}H]$ serine were used *in vitro* with 4 x 10^7 to 5 x 10^7 cells in an otherwise standard procedure (7).

Heparin was extracted by freezing and thawing the cells six times followed by the addition of NaCl to bring the solution to a final molarity of 1.0.

II. RESULTS

The mast cell extract was applied directly to a column of Dowex 1 equilibrated in 1 *M* NaCl, and eluted with 1.0, 3.0, and 4.0 *M* NaCl (8) as shown in Fig. 1. Portions of each fraction were assessed for ^{35}S, protein (by absorbance at 280 nm), uronic acid (9), and metachromasia (10).

The 1.0 *M* NaCl effluent contained a major portion of the total protein and approximately two thirds of the ^{35}S but was essentially without uronic acid or metachromasia. The material eluting with 3.0 *M* NaCl contained a small amount of protein, and one third of the ^{35}S. The ^{35}S chromatographed exactly with the material showing metachromasia and the presence of uronic acid indicating $[^{35}S]$ sulfate incorporation into the heparin-like material present. The heparin-like material was characterized as heparin by virtue of its susceptibility to specific heparinase (7) and was then used as starting material for further characterization. It had a low anticoagulant activity when compared to commerical heparin based on the uronic acid content. Chromatography on Sepharose

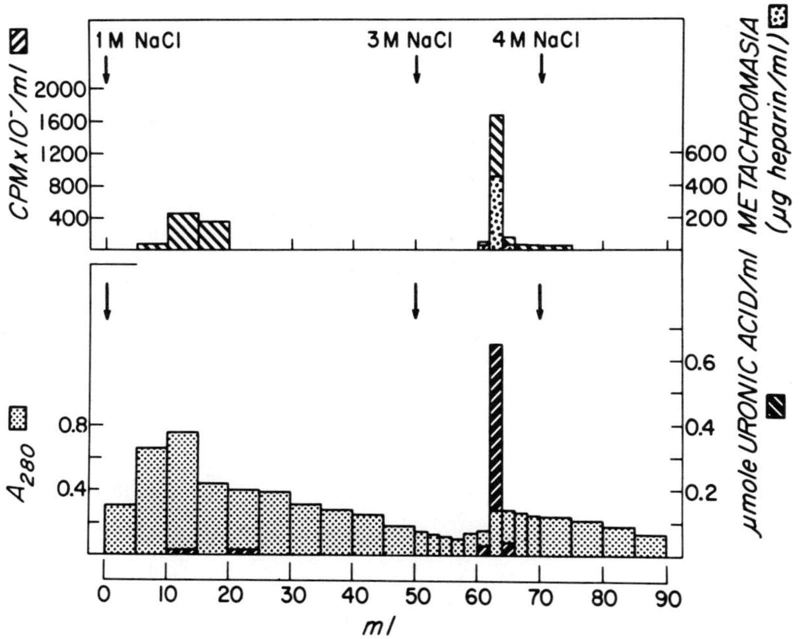

Fig. 1. Dowex 1 chromatography of ^{35}S-labeled material from concentrated rat mast cells. A 2 ml sample was applied to a 1 x 30 cm column of Dowex 1 and eluted by stepwise addition of 1 M, 3M, and 4 M NaCl. Ten 5 ml, ten 2 ml, and four 5 ml fractions were collected at a flow rate of 10 to 15 ml per hour. Fractions were assayed for ^{35}S and metachromasia (upper panel) and for protein and uronic acid (lower panel). The width of each bar equals the fraction volume.

4B indicated an average molecular size of approximately 250,000 to 750,000 after 4 hours of *in vitro* synthesis. This molecule was not measurably decreased in size by treatment with proteolytic enzymes but was decreased to an average molecular size of approximately 40,000 by treatment with 0.5 *M* NaOH at room temperature overnight.

Samples of the [^{35}S] heparin and alkali-treated [^{35}S] heparin were chromatographed on a column of DEAE-cellulose. Native [^{35}S] heparin began to elute with the ascending limb of the commercial heparin but was also found in later fractions (Fig. 2A). The alkali-treated [^{35}S] heparin eluted at a lower ionic strength closer to the profile of commercial heparin (Fig. 2B).

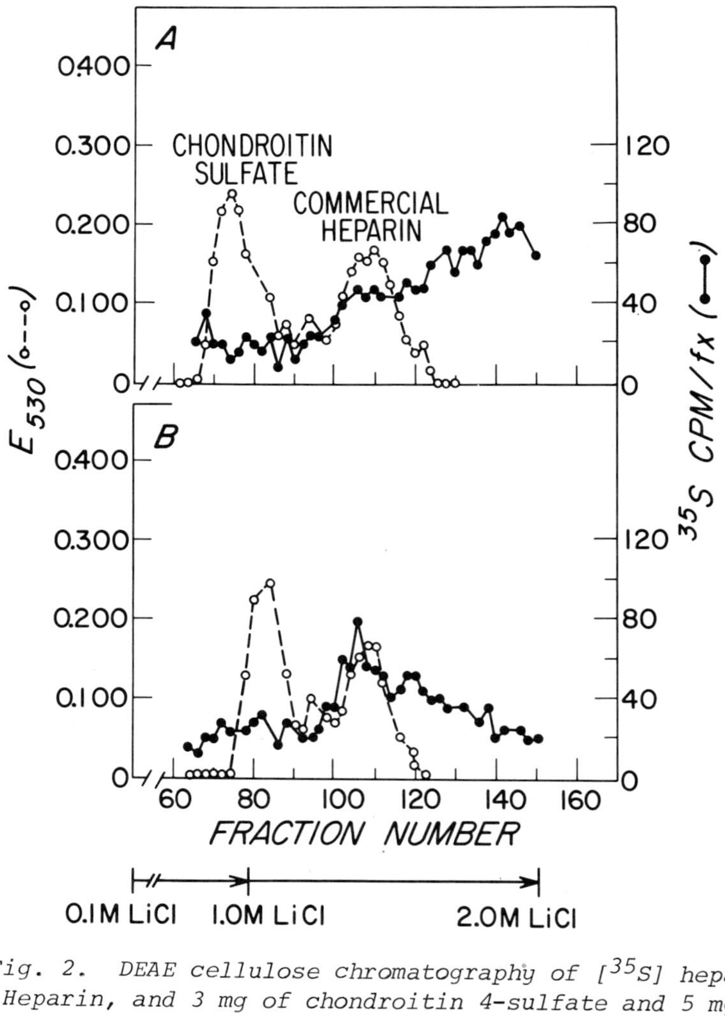

Fig. 2. DEAE cellulose chromatography of [^{35}S] heparin. [^{35}S] Heparin, and 3 mg of chondroitin 4-sulfate and 5 mg of commercial heparin as standards were eluted from a 1 x 5 cm column of DEAE cellulose by a 0.1 M to 1.0 M LiCl logarithmic gradient, followed by a similar gradient of 1.0 M to 2.0 M LiCl. For this gradient the mixing flask contained 125 ml of 0.1 M LiCl and the reservoir contained 1 M LiCl, which was changed to 2 M LiCl at fraction 61. Two ml fractions were collected at 10 to 15 ml per hour and assayed for radioactivity (●——●) and uronic acid content (O--O). A) [^{35}S] Heparin, B) [^{35}S] Heparin after treatment with 0.5 M NaOH. Figure modified from Fig. 1 of (7).

The marked reduction in size caused by alkali treatment suggested that the native heparin might be a proteoglycan with alkali-labile linkages of glycosaminoglycan to protein. In order to investigate this point further, mast cells were doubly labeled by incubation with L- [^{3}H] serine and [^{35}S] sulfate. When chromatographed on Dowex 1, as previously described, there was a peak of ^{3}H in the 3.0 *M* NaCl eluate coincident with ^{35}S and metachromasia. Tritiated material was also found to have a wide distribution similar to the protein shown in Fig. 1. The fractions in the 3.0 *M* eluate were dialyzed, lyophilized, and rechromatographed under the same conditions. After rechromatography, the 3.0 *M* NaCl eluate showed a distinct peak of ^{3}H-labeled material. After dialysis and lyophilization, an aliquot was filtered on Sepharose 4B

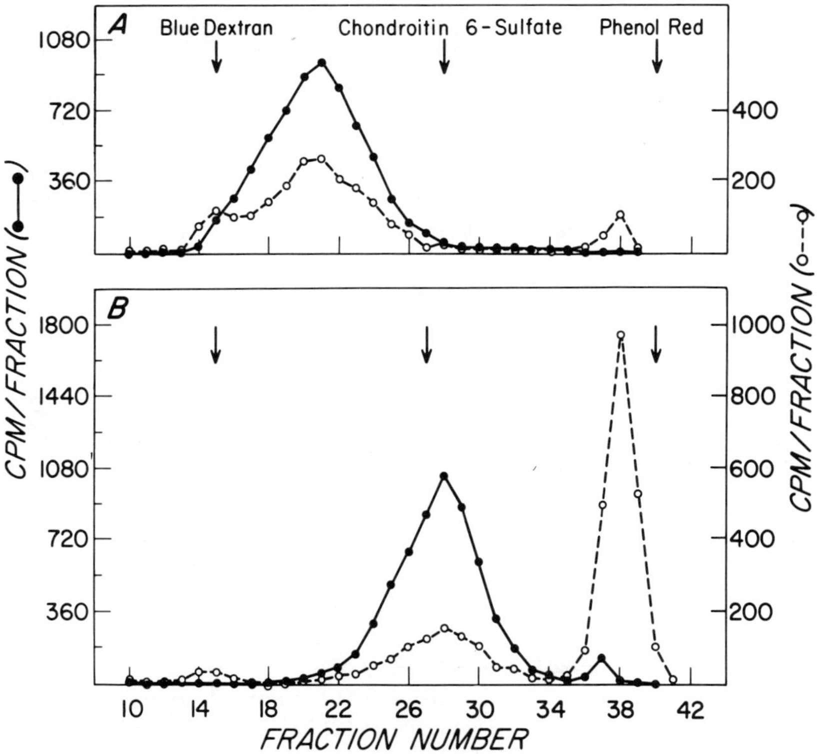

Fig. 3. Filtration on Sepharose 4B of [^{3}H, ^{35}S] heparin. Samples of mast cell heparin and internal standards of phenol red, blue dextran, and chondroitin 6-sulfate (approximately 60,000 M_r) were filtered on a 1 x 60 cm column of Sepharose 4B with 2.0 M NaCl eluant at a flow rate of 4 to 5 ml per hour. One ml fractions were collected and assayed for ^{35}S (●——●), and ^{3}H (O--O). A) [^{3}H, ^{35}S] Heparin, B) [^{3}H, ^{35}S] Heparin after treatment with 0.5 M NaOH. Figure from Fig. 4 of (7).

(Fig. 3A), and both ^3H and ^{35}S were in similar fractions. After alkali treatment, the [^{35}S] heparin was reduced in size to an approximate molecular weight of 40,000 based on the chondroitin 6-sulfate standard of average 60,000 M_r. Approximately one third of the ^3H-labeled material cochromatographed with the ^{35}S peak, while the other two thirds of the ^3H presented in a completely separate further retarded peak

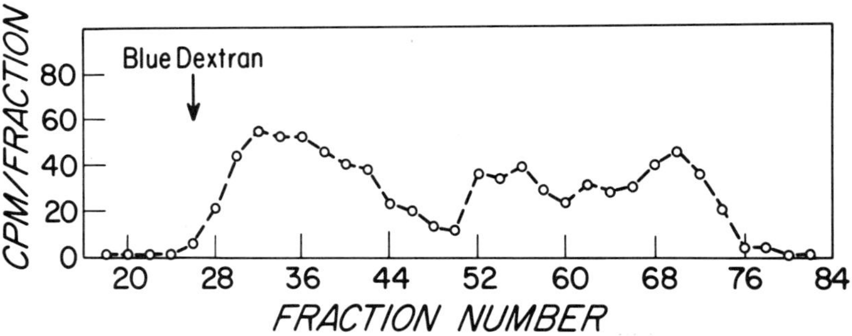

Fig 4. Sephadex G-25 gel filtration of fractions 37 to 40 from Fig. 3B. The concentrated sample together with blue dextran marker was applied to a 1 x 30 cm column of Sephadex G-25 equilibrated in 0.1 M ammonium acetate. The flow rate was 2 to 3 ml per hour and 0.5 ml fractions were collected and assayed for ^3H.

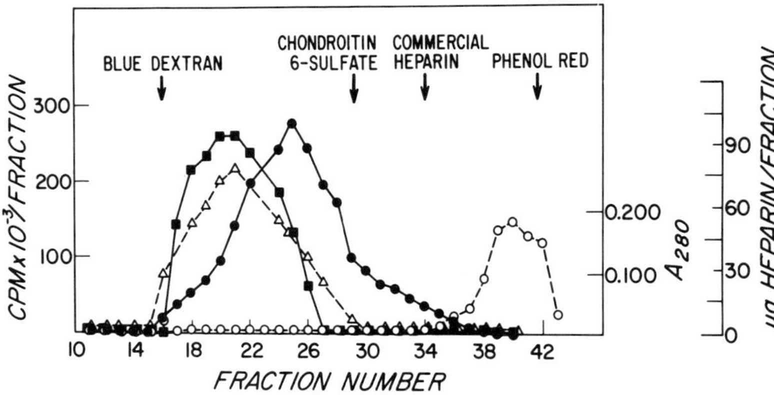

Fig. 5. Gel filtration of rat peritoneal mast cell heparin on Sepharose 4B. The mast cell heparin and a standard of phenol red were filtered on a 1 x 60 cm column of Sepharose 4B with 2.0 M NaCl eluant at a flow rate of 4 to 5 ml per hour. One ml fractions were collected and assayed for ^{35}S (●—●), metachromasia (■—■), uronic acid (Δ--Δ), and protein (O--O). The positions of blue dextran, chondroitin 6-sulfate (approximately 60,000 M_r), and commercial heparin (approximately 12,000 M_r), which were filtered separately on the same column, are shown. Figure from Fig. 2 of (7).

with essentially no ^{35}S (Fig. 3B).

Fractions containing the separated ^3H-labeled product were pooled, lyophilized, resuspended in 0.1 M ammonium acetate buffer, pH 8.0, and applied to a column of Sephadex G-25, Peaks of ^3H were found at 40%, 65%, and 89% column bed volume (Fig. 4) where polypeptides of less than 4000 M_r would filter.

Heparin synthesized during two hours of *in vitro* labeling of mast cells was compared to stored mast cell heparin measured chemically. Newly synthesized *[*^{35}*S]* heparin was distinctly

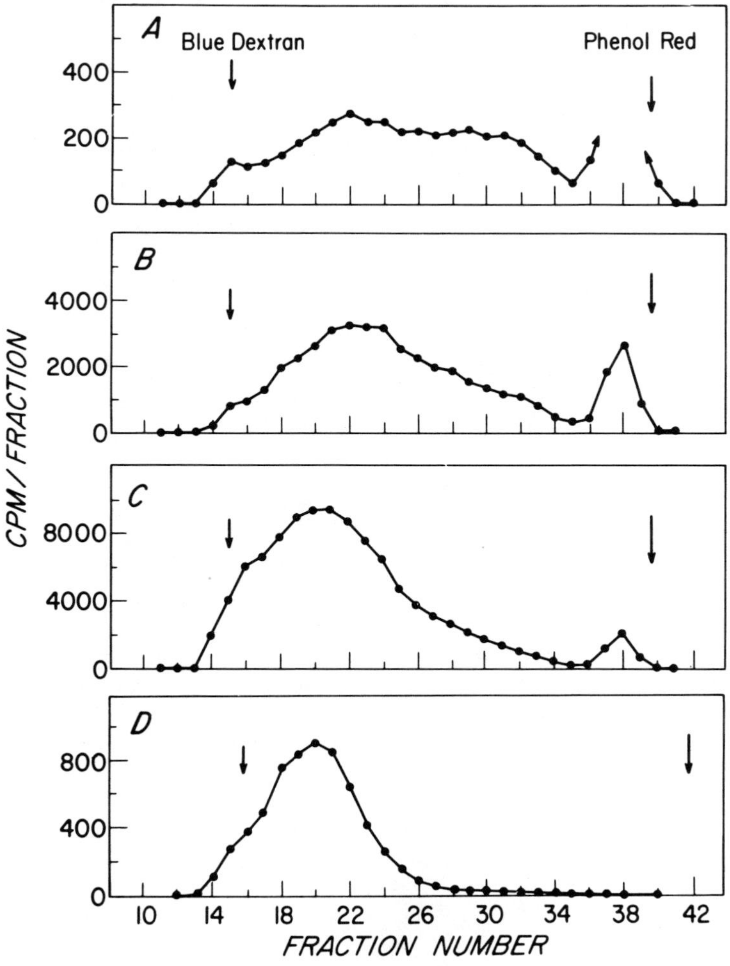

Fig. 6. Gel filtration on Sepharose 4B of [^{35}*S] heparin formed during timed incubations. [*^{35}*S] Heparin was isolated and filtered as in Fig. 4 with internal standards of blue dextran and phenol red.* In vitro *incubations were for (A) 1 hour, (B) 2 hours, (C) and 4 hours, while* in vivo *labeling (D) was carried out for 14 days. Figure from Fig. 3 of (7).*

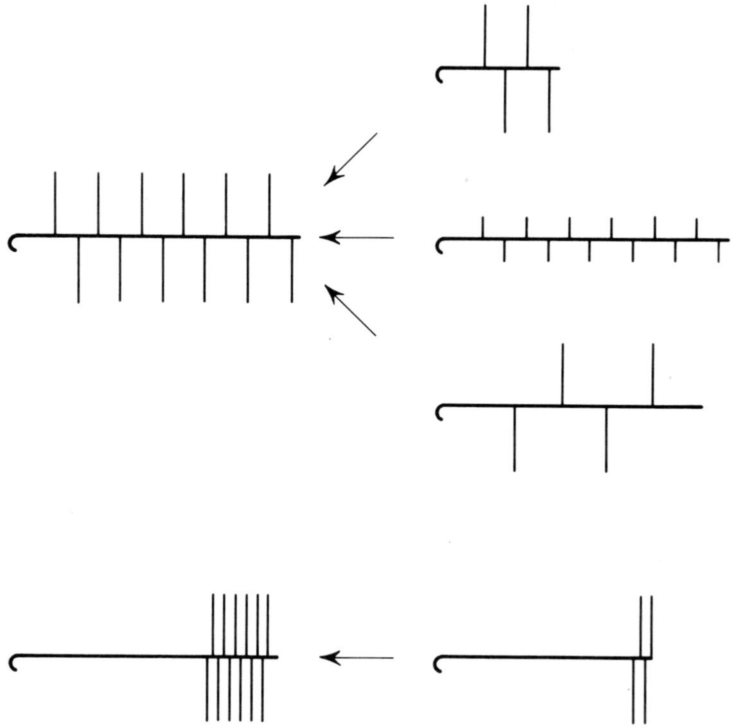

Fig. 7. Diagramatic representation of proteoglycan growth with time. (A) The heparin proteoglycan grows in size with time by assembly from essentially identical small proteoglycan subunits; the ratio of glycosaminoglycan to protein would remain the same for all sizes. (B) The large protein core does not change in size while the glycosaminoglycan chains elongate; the ratio of glycosaminoglycan to protein would increase with size. (c) The large protein core does not change in size while more glycosaminoglycan chains are added with time; the ratio of glycosaminoglycan to protein would increase with size. (d) Small glycosaminoglycan-peptide subunits are added to an original proteoglycan subunit containing a large protein core; the ratio of glycosaminoglycan to protein would increase with size.

smaller (Fig. 5). Longer incubations of mast cells with ^{35}S sulfate were, therefore, conducted to see if larger heparin would be formed. ^{35}S Heparin formed in the one, two, and four hour incubations grew in size relative to the time of incubation (Fig. 6). At the end of a fourteen hour *in vitro* incubation (not shown) the pattern was identical to that of ^{35}S heparin formed two weeks after injection of ^{35}S sulfate *in vivo*. Thus it appeared that the heparin was a proteoglycan of considerable size heterogeneity and grew considerably up to several hours during synthesis. Four possibilities to account for this growth in size are illustrated in Fig. 7.

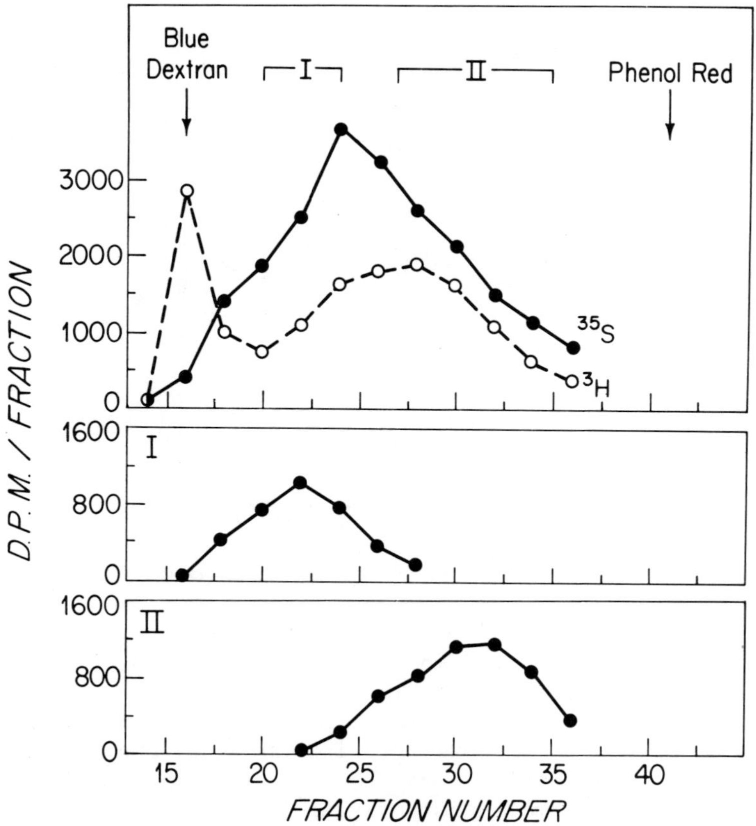

Fig. 8. Gel filtration of [^{3}H, ^{35}S] heparin on Sepharose 4B. The chromatography was conducted as in Fig. 3. Rechromatography of selected fractions is shown in the lower graphs. ^{35}S (●—●), ^{3}H (O--O).

The ratio of ^{35}S to ^{3}H was determined in fractions from a Sepharose 4B chromatogram of [^{3}H] serine [^{35}S] sulfate-labeled proteoglycan (Fig. 8, upper panel). Exclusive of the area of contaminating protein at the V_o and V_1, there was a linear variation of the ratio of [^{35}S] sulfate to [^{3}H] serine (Fig. 9). Thus the amount of glycosaminoglycan relative to protein was shown to increase with increasing size of the proteoglycan. This effectively eliminates possibility A, Fig. 7, that the proteoglycan is assembled from equal small proteoglycan subunits.

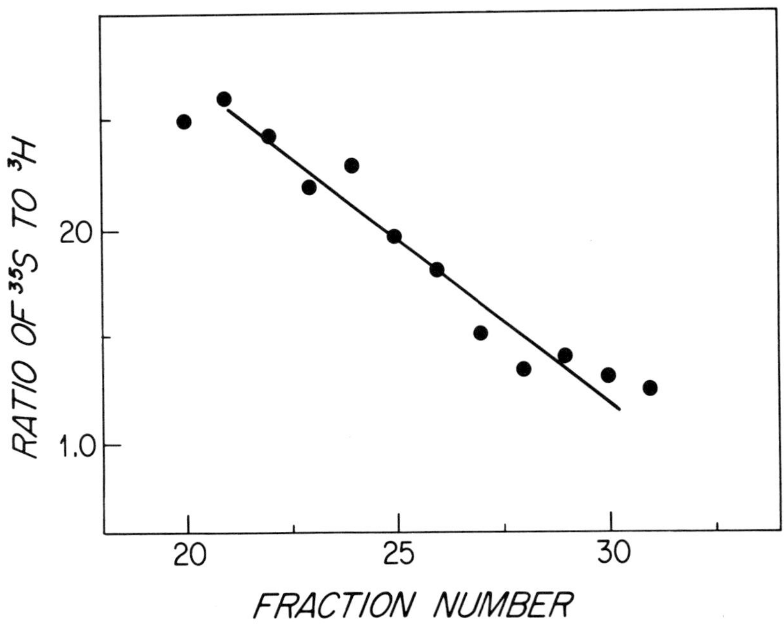

Fig. 9. Ratios of ^{3}H to ^{35}S for fractions from Fig. 8.

Both large and small proteoglycans were obtained from the Sepharose 4B chromatogram, and rechromatography of these pooled fractions is shown in Fig. 8, lower panels. The proteoglycans were then treated with 0.5 *M* NaOH overnight and chromatographed on Sepharose 6B (Fig. 10). It can be seen that the free glycosaminoglycan chains thus produced, from both the large and small proteoglycans, are approximately the same size. This effectively eliminates possibility B, that the glycosaminoglycan chains grow in size with time. This leaves possibility C, that more chains are added with time, or possibility D, that with time small proteoglycan subunits are added to a starting proteoglycan subunit that contains a large extra protein core.

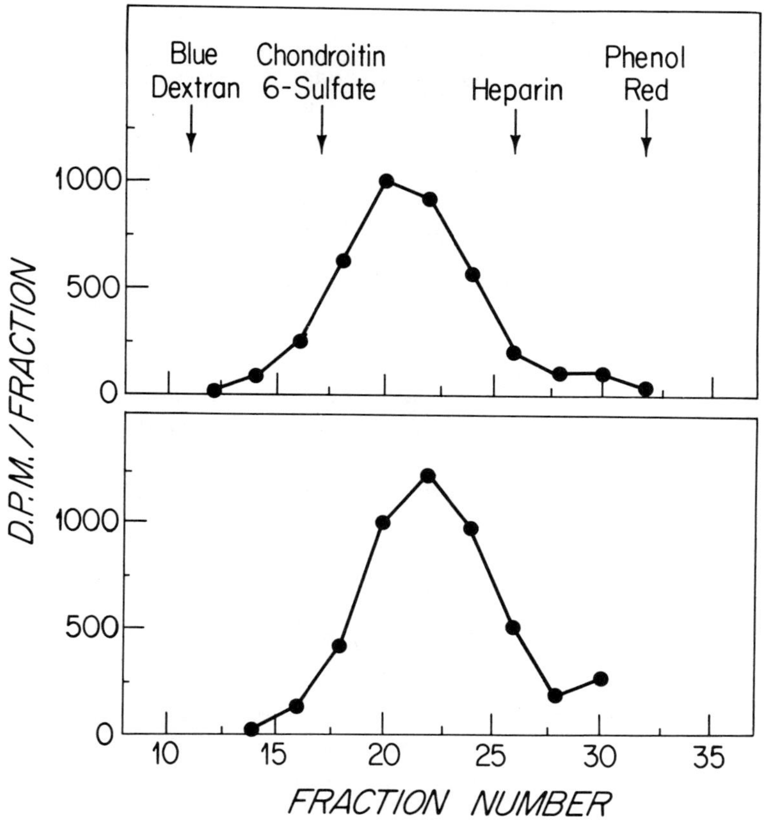

Fig. 10. Gel filtration on Sephadex 6B of NaOH-treated I) large [^{35}S] heparin and II) small [^{35}S] heparin.

III. DISCUSSION

A simple technique avoiding proteolytic enzymes or prolonged alkali treatment has been used to obtain heparin in a native form from rat peritoneal mast cells. The molecule was much larger (approximately 750,000 M_r) than the heparin found in commercial preparations or that found in preparations from mouse mast cell tumors (2) and bovine liver capsule (11,12). In this respect rat peritoneal mast cell heparin was similar to the "macromolecular" heparin previously found in rat skin (4).

Alkali is known to cleave the xylosyl-serine linkages that occur in proteoglycans such as chondroitin sulfate. Furthermore, in heparin preparations a xylosyl-serine component has been found in single glycosaminoglycan chains attached to peptides (3). It is likely that the alkali-labile linkages in rat peritoneal mast cell heparin are also xylosylserine and that the heparin is a proteoglycan. The resistance to degradation by proteolytic enzymes is unusual for proteoglycans as is the apparent assembly of the molecule over a several hour period. Moreover the growth of heparin by addition of glycosaminoglycan chains is related to its availability for release from the cells, since the larger molecules are preferentially released by immunologic challenge (6).

The rat peritoneal mast cell material fulfills criteria for heparin such as metachromasia, high charge, and susceptibility (or resistance) to degradation by specific polysaccharidases. Nevertheless, as previously reported by other investigators (13), it has a low anticoagulant activity. In this respect it may be comparable to the heparin of low anticoagulant activity recently shown to be present as a large proportion of commercial heparin preparations (14).

REFERENCES

1. Lindahl, U., and Rodén, L., *in* "Glycoproteins" (A. Gottschalk, ed.), Vol. A, pp. 491-517. Elsevier, Amsterdam, 1972.
2. Ogren, S., and Lindahl, U., Biochem. J. *125*, 1119-1129 (1971).
3. Lindahl, U., Cifonelli, J., Lindahl, B., and Rodén, L., J. Biol. Chem. *240*, 2817-2820 (1965).
4. Horner, A., J. Biol. Chem. *246*, 231-239 (1971).
5. Ogren, S., and Lindahl, U., J. Biol. Chem. *250*, 2690-2697 (1975).
6. Yurt, R.W., Leid, R.W., Jr., Spragg, J., and Austen, K.F., J. Immunol. *118*, 1201-1267 (1977).
7. Yurt, R.W., Leid, R.W., Jr., Austen, K.F., and Silbert, J.E., J. Biol. Chem. *252*, 518-521 (1977).
8. Slorach, S.A., Acta Physiol. Scand. *82*, 91-97 (1971).
9. Bitter, T., and Muir, H.M., Anal. Biochem. *4*, 330-334 (1962).
10. Jaques, L.B., Monkhouse, F.C., and Stewart, M., J. Physiol. *109*, 41-48 (1949).
11. Lindahl, U., Biochem. J. *116*, 27-34 (1970).
12. Serafini-Fracassini, A., Branford-White, C.J., and Hunter, J.C., FEBS Letters *32*, 116-118 (1973).
13. Schiller, S., and Dorfman, A., Biochim. Biophys. Acta. *31*, 278-280 (1959).
14. Lam, L.H., Silbert, J.E., and Rosenberg, R.D., Biochem. Biophys. Res. Commun. *69*, 570-577 (1976).

STRUCTURAL CHARACTERISTICS OF HEPARINS REVEALED BY ELECTROFOCUSING

N.M. McDuffie and N.W. Cowie

Department of Physiology
University of Saskatchewan

The application of electrofocusing to heparin and related mucopolysaccharides provides some insights that influence our understanding of the structure and biological action of these compounds. The process can be used analytically or preparatively. Fractions obtained have been partially characterized structurally, chemically, and assessed for biological activity.

I. INTRODUCTION

There is now general agreement that heparin, the naturally occurring mucopolysaccharide, is polydisperse. Most recent publications state or imply that *heparin is not a single chemical compound, but rather a family of compounds of diverse chain length (and molecular weight) possessing similar saccharide repeating units and functional groups* (1). The literature is replete with demonstrations of this polydispersity, ironically this is perhaps one of the most consistent findings among heparin investigators. As has been exemplified by my predecessors in this symposium, and as no doubt will be further emphasized by my successors, resolution and characterization of the structural heterogeneity of heparin preparations must be considered of paramount importance, if we are to clarify its possible physiological roles or if we expect to achieve more precise standardization and presumably more efficient utilization of the drug.

I must hasten to point out that the current standards and preparations, though less than perfect, have served well; however the methodology is perhaps now available to permit marked improvements in these materials.

II. ELECTROFOCUSING OF HEPARINS

Heparins, due to their substituent groups, are anionic polyelectrolytes and consequently bind tenaciously to cations. This characteristic has been used to prepare various derivatives and to explain many of its biological activities. Serendipitously Dr. Helena B. Nader observed that heparin preparations would interact with low molecular weight carrier

ISBN 0-12-484850-8

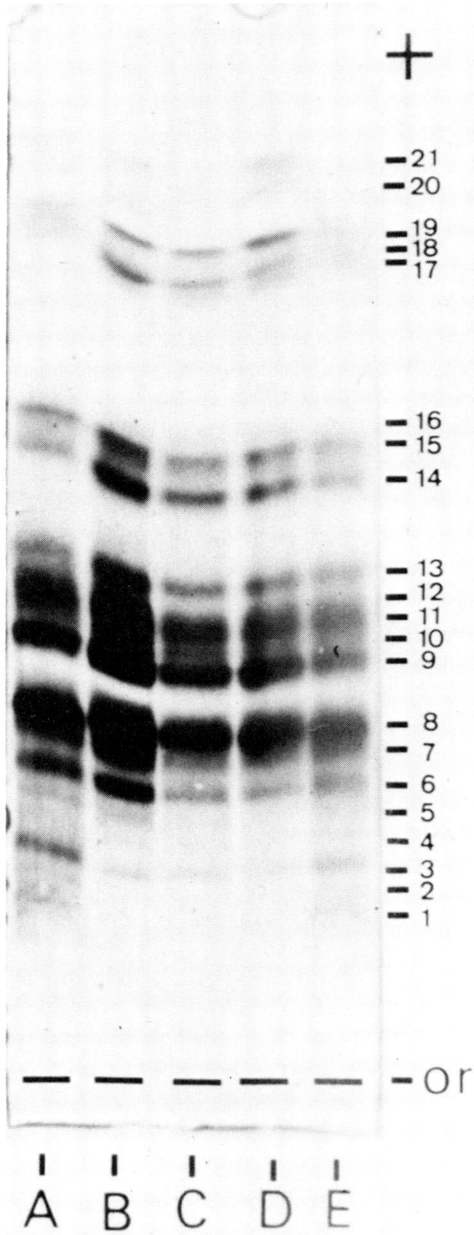

Fig. 1. Analytical electrofocusing patterns for five commercially available clinically effective heparins. A) Upjohn lot 76-RTS-12, B) Wilson lot 145493, C) BDH lot 4040, D) Riker lot N-3043, E) Upjohn lot ZX-320. Or = origin.

ampholytes (2). When heparin is subjected to electrophoresis in a natural pH gradient provided by amphoteric substances a large number of bands are observed (Fig. 1). In the example different preparations of clinically effective heparins have been subjected to electrofocusing in acrylamide gel (6%) containing LKB ampholyte, pH 3-5.5 (final concentration 2% W/V) (3). After 16 hr at a potential of 15 V/cm at 5°C, multiple bands are observed. The bands may be visualized as white zones or may be stained with Toluidine Blue reagent (3). Ten to two hundred μg of heparin preparation are routinely applied. An average of 22 bands may be observed between point of application and the anode.

The bands produced by electrofocusing may be cut from the gel and eluted by elevating the pH with NH_4OH. The eluates may be freed of ampholyte by use of gel filtration and ion-exchange resins, e.g., Dowex, Sephadex and DEAE-Sephadex, differential salt elution, and finally, dialysis. Through this process *purified* heparin fractions may be obtained for chemical, physical and biological studies. Early studies (3) indicated that fractions prepared in a similar fashion from lung heparin were of variable molecular weight (range 3-37,000 daltons) and demonstrated marked differences in anticoagulant potency in the USP assay (the % of each fraction was determined by scanning densitometry (Table I). The variation in molecular weight between fractions was approximately 1500-2000, which would be equivalent to the heparin hexasaccharide observed upon enzymatic degradation of heparin.

III. FACTORS AFFECTING THE PROCESS OF ELECTROFOCUSING OF HEPARIN

The parameters of the technique have been defined (3). Table II lists some important factors which affect the process.

A. Ampholyte

After testing different batches of ampholytes from different suppliers we have observed that the nature of the substituent groups on the amphoteres is quite important. Ampholytes with sulfo- and phospho- groups do not produce sharp bands but rather produce smears. Variable concentrations of ampholyte may be used in the gel, however 4% produces distortions in the bands and dissolution of bands upon destaining. Even with the same supplier, variation in number and type of amphotere occurs from batch to batch. We consistently use the same batch for analytical, comparative and preparative electrofocusing.

TABLE I Molecular Weight, Sulfate/Hexosamine Ratios, and Anticoagulant Potency of Heparin Fractions Obtained by Electrofocusing

Fraction	% Total Heparin	Molecular Weight	M_r Intervals Between Fractions	Anti-coagulant Potency	Sulfate/Hexosamine Molar Ratios[a]
1	5.2	37,500	7,500	--	3.28
2	6.9	30,000	500	--	2.56
3	2.2	29,500	4,500	--	2.81
4	1.3	25,000	1,500	1.9	2.26
5	3.0	23,500	2,500	1.1	2.94
6	4.3	21,000	1,500	2.2	2.89
7	2.2	19,500	1,500	1.8	3.01
8	3.5	18,000	2,000	0.6	2.59
9	4.4	16,000	2,000	1.3	2.45
10	10.9	14,000	2,500	1.9	2.75
11	4.4	11,500	1,000	1.6	--
12	10.9	10,500	1,000	1.6	2.94
13	5.2	9,500	2,200	--	--
14	1.7	7,300	1,300	1.3	--
15	11.3	6,000	1,200	0.4	--
16	8.7	4,800	200	--	--
17	2.2	4,600	250	<0.1	--
18	4.4	4,350	950	<0.1	--
19	5.2	3,400	200	<0.1	--
20	0.8	3,200	200	<0.1	--
21	1.3	3,000	--	<0.1	--
Heparin	--	--	--	1.0	2.75
Heparitin sulfate D	--	--	--	0.05	2.72

The relative potency of the fractions was measured in relation to unfractionated heparin, which was taken as 1.0 in the U.S.P. assay.

[a]Fractions 13-21 were still contaminated with ampholytes, which interfered with the hexosamine determinations.

TABLE II Factors which Affect the Electrofocusing Pattern of Heparins

Variable	*Remarks*
Ampholyte	*Amine and carboxyl groups essential; ampholytes with sulfo- and phospho-groups unsatisfactory*
	0.5,1,2 & 4% final concentrations in gel are workable, however, 4% produces distortions and instability of bands
	Amphoteres present may vary between batches
pH	*Banding patterns observed throughout the range of 3-5*
Molecular weight	*Higher molecular weight fractions precipitate at high pH, low molecular weight fractions at low pH*
Support	*Independent - can occur in batch, polyacrylamide, agarose or density gradient columns*
Time	*Running time for analytical gels = 12-16 hr, preparative gels = 72-120 hr*
Nature of heparin	*Variation may occur due to heparin source or mode of preparation*

B. pH

The actual pH of the gel produced by the amphoteres is determined by cutting 0.5 mm segments of gel, elution with distilled water and pH measurement. Under these conditions a smooth pH gradient is obtained over the length of gel (3). Complexation and band formation occurs in the pH zone of 2.8-4.5 (3).

C. Molecular Weight

Molecular weights of eluted fractions may be determined in polyacrylamide gel (4). An inverse correlation exists between distance migrated and molecular weight, hence high molecular weight species precipitate at high pH during electrofocusing, and low molecular weight species precipitate at low pH.

Banding patterns are observed throughout a broad range of pH. The bands require combination of heparin species with an amphotere of appropriate charge and size. Therefore, dependent on the chain lengths present in a heparin, differences in pattern may be observed. Conversely, variation in ampholyte species will produce alteration in patterns.

D. Support

The process is independent of the supporting medium. Indeed, the process may be successfully carried out in solution, gels, or in density gradient columns.

E. Time

Time of development of bands is dependent upon gel size and sample load. Nine ml analytical gels may require 12-16 hr for complete band development, using sample loads of 10-200 μg. Preparative gels of 350 ml volume and sample loads of up to 100 mg require 72-120 hr.

Loads in excess of those quoted lead to rupture of the gel when a potential is applied.

F. Nature of Heparin

As indicated above, variation in electrofocusing pattern may be expected with variations in chain length. This may be due to innate characteristics of the heparin or mode of preparation. Figure 2 shows electrofocusing patterns of canine mastocytomal preparations (5). Note the dissimilarities between the control (heparin and crude heparitin) and mastocytomal preparations. These preparations appear rich in high molecular weight materials.

Figure 3 shows patterns of porpoise and whale heparins kindly provided by Dr. Kimura and Yosizawa of Japan and Grant Barlow of Abbott Laboratories. Again note dissimilarities in the patterns produced. It would appear that the porpoise heparin contains primarily low molecular weight heparins, whereas the whale heparins are more variable in their distribution of chain lengths.

Hence the process of electrofocusing involves an interaction of variable molecular weight heparin components with carrier ampholyte to form complexes which precipitate at the pH appropriate of the pI of the complex. This procedure of analytical electrofocusing has now been applied to 50 different batches of commercial heparins of diverse origins, with similar results.

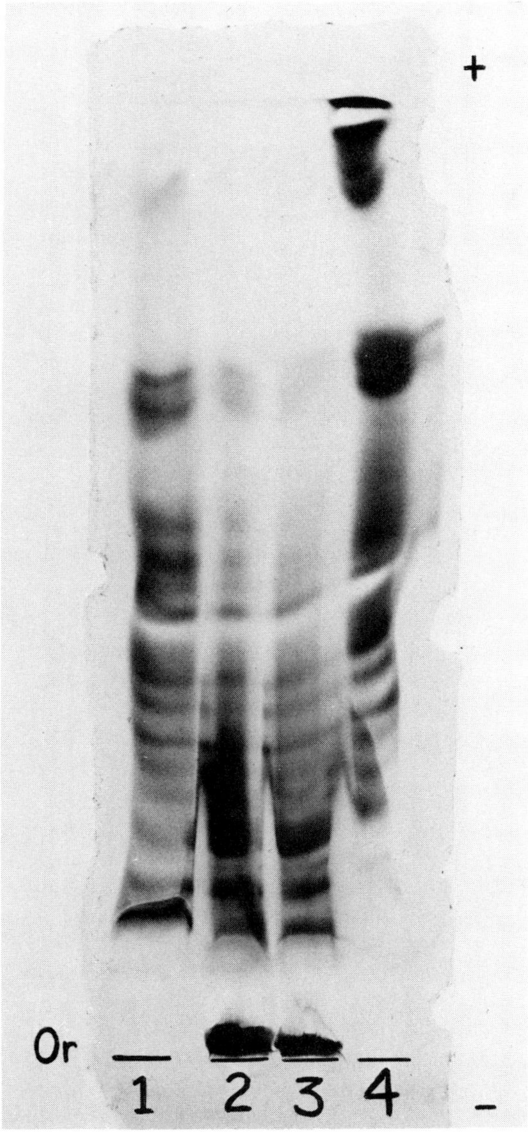

Fig. 2. Analytical electrofocusing patterns for canine mastocytomal extracts (5). 1) Reference heparin - Upjohn lot ZX-320, 2) Mastocytomal extract prepared by proteolysis, 3) Mastocytomal extract prepared with 2 M potassium acetate, 4) Crude heparitin sulfate reference. Or = origin.

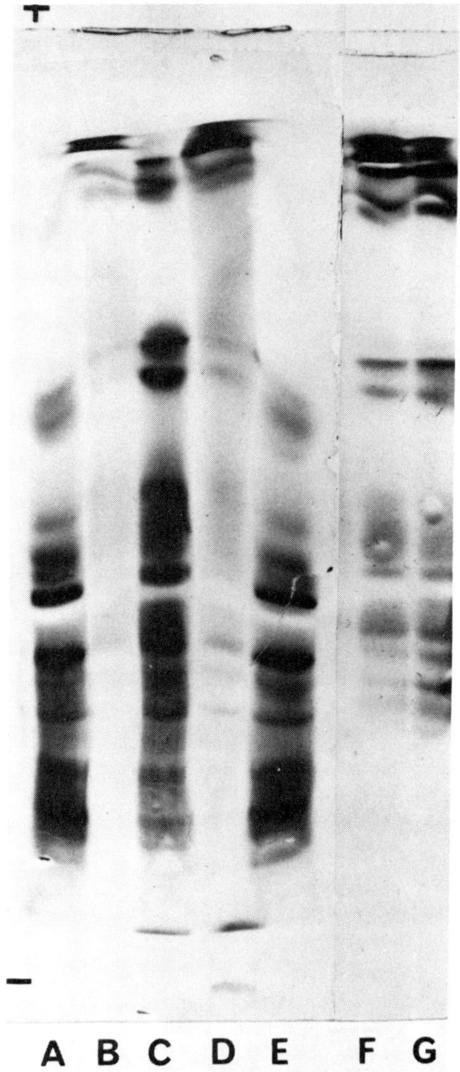

Fig. 3. Comparative analytical electrofocusing patterns for whale and porpoise heparins. A) Beef lung heparin (Upjohn lot ZX-320), B) Porpoise heparin (Barlow #1102-5), C) Whale heparin B (Kimura #1102-3), D) Whale heparin (Barlow #1102-4), E) Na Heparin (Abbott 1958), F) Whale heparin (Kimura #1102-1), G) Whale heparin (Yosizawa #1102-2).

G. Other Mucopolysaccharides

The results of electrofocusing of chemically related chondroitins and heparitins generally differ from heparins. Chondroitins show patterns atypical of heparin with only faint smears visible throughout the length of the gel and major banding at the anode. Heparitins, with the exception of fraction D, do not show banding, and D only yields bands comparable to the lower molecular weight fractions of heparin (3). Consequently this procedure may be used to qualitatively distinguish between these types of mucopolysaccharides.

As an example of the usefulness of the technique, Table III shows a range of mucopolysaccharides that have been subjected to analytical electrofocusing in our laboratory. Macromolecular heparin fails to penetrate the polyacrylamide gel and hence no pattern is obtainable.

TABLE III Various Mucopolysaccharides subjected to Analytical Electrofocusing

Commercial heparins
Whale heparins[a]
Macromolecular heparin - rat skin[b]
Ox lung heparin[a]
Sheep mucosal heparin[a]
Canine mastocytoma[a]
Canine liver heparin[a]
Porpoise heparin[a]
Commercial chondroitin sulfates - A,B,C
Heparitin sulfates - A,B,C,D[a]
Hyaluronic acid
Kerato sulfate
Standard mucopolysaccharides[c]

[a]*Indicates similarity to commercial heparin in electrofocusing*

[b]*Provided by A.A. Horner, U. of Toronto*

[c]*Provided by M. Matthews, U. of Chicago*

H. Chemical Modification of Heparins

We have previously reported (3) the results of N-desulfation, N,O-desulfation and O-desulfation of a lung origin heparin (Upjohn, lot #SH-042). The heparin hexasaccharide obtained by enzymatic degradation was also electrofocused. N, and N,O-desulfation drastically reduced the band numbers. O-desulfation is less deleterious, however the alkaline hydrolysis apparently did reduce the linkages and molecular weight of the heparin. It would appear that the N-sulfate is required for band formation.

I. Comparison of Heparin of Mucosal and Lung Origin

When electrofocused fractions are eluted from the gel and subsequently exposed to polyacrylamide electrophoresis a range of molecular weights are obtained. This is true of heparin of mucosal or lung origin. An important difference exists, however, between lung and mucosal heparins. This is summarized in Figure 4. Unfractionated lung heparin yields a *single* component in agarose, a diffuse band in polyacrylamide and 22 components upon electrofocusing. Unfractionated mucosal heparin yields *two* components in agarose, a diffuse band in polyacrylamide and 22 components upon electrofocusing. Lung heparin fractions derived from the electrofocusing procedure yield a single band in agarose, polyacrylamide and electrofocusing. Mucosal heparin fractions derived from the

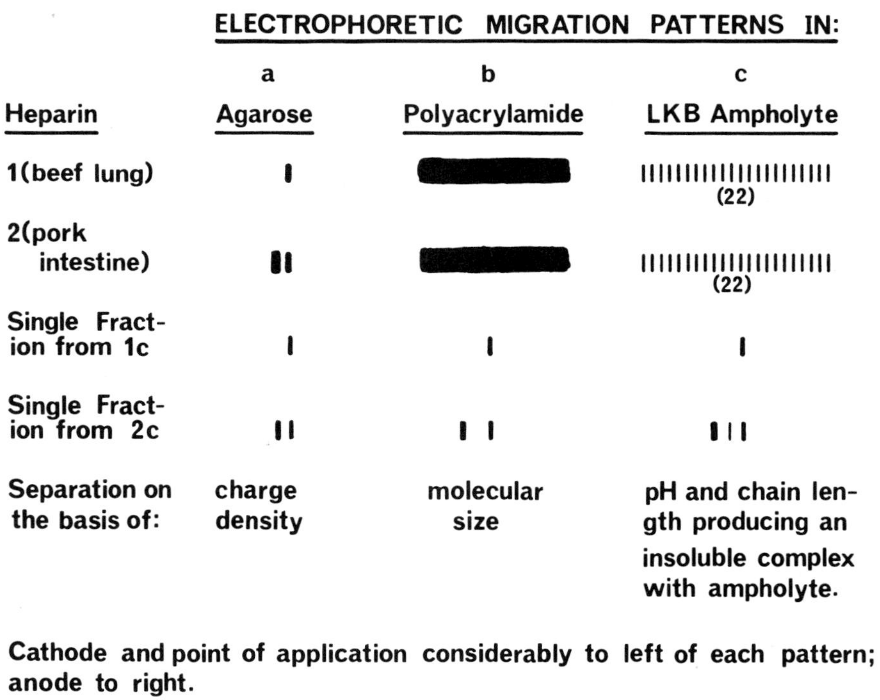

Fig. 4. Summary diagram of electrophoretic patterns obtained for different heparins prior to and following electrofocusing.

electrofocusing procedure yield *two* bands in agarose, *two* bands in polyacrylamide and a variable number of bands upon electrofocusing.

When molecular weights of the lung heparin fractions are determined in polyacrylamide gels, a family of different chain lengths are observed (Fig. 5). Molecular weight determinations of mucosal heparin fractions, containing 2 components, yield 2 families of differing chain legnths with a high degree of parallelism (Fig. 6). We earlier demonstrated that in mucosal heparin fractions the 2 components represented a monomer and dimer (6), since the higher molecular weight band was approximately twice the value of the lower (Table IV). This supposition was supported by conversion of the higher molecular weight form into the lower form by ascorbate.

Other molecular associations may be possible since upon re-electrofocusing the mucosal fractions may yield more than one component. This may be a technical artefact due to the vagaries of cutting the bands in preparative gels, however it only occurs with mucosal heparins. The nature of these associations remains unclear.

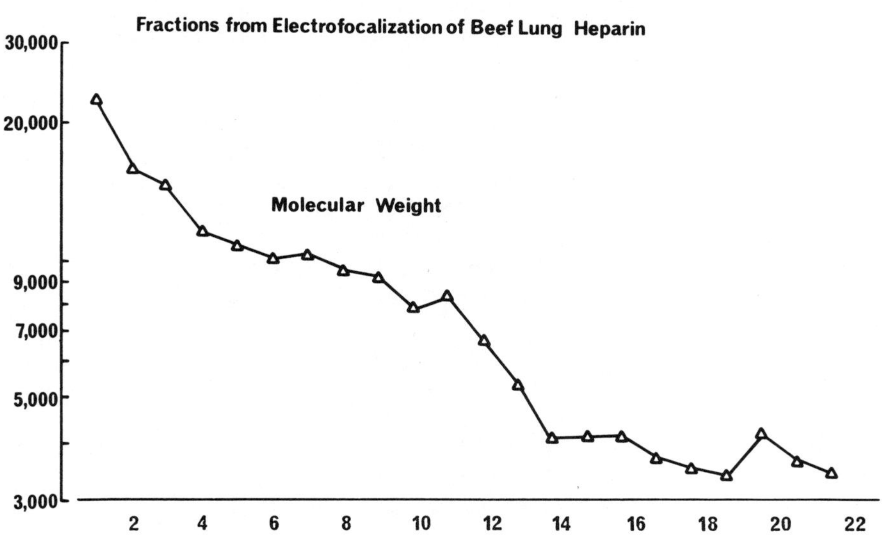

Fig. 5. Molecular weight analysis of fractions derived from beef lung heparin by preparative electrofocusing.

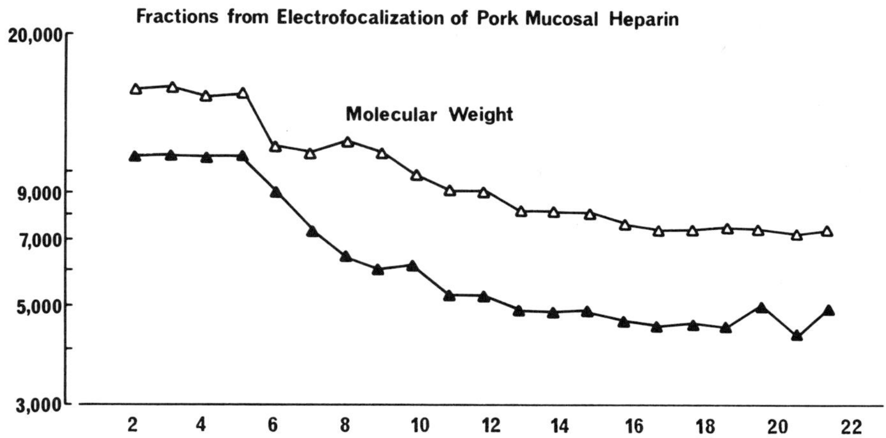

Fig. 6. Molecular weight analysis of fractions derived from pork mucosal heparin by preparative electrofocusing.

IV. HEPARIN FRACTIONS PRODUCED BY PREPARATIVE ELECTROFOCUSING

Heparins of lung origin (Upjohn, lot SH-042) and of mucosal origin (Lederle, lot 1804-B4740) were subjected to preparative electrofocusing. The recovery after purification was 75%. The fractions obtained have been subjected to molecular weight analysis, degradation by heparinase and heparitinase II from *Flavobacterium Heparinum,* microelectrophoretic analysis in agarose, scanning densitometry of the procedure (7), and more specifically, the Yin and Wessler technique of activated factor X inhibition (8). Preliminary data are also available on the effects of the fractions on induced release of labeled serotonin from dog platelets by a collagen derivative.

Figure 7 shows the results of degradation of the heparin fractions of mucosal origin with bacterial enzymes. All fractions are susceptible to the enzymes, although differences in quantity of products occur. Similar results were obtained with fractions of lung origin, as has been reported previously (3).

The percentage distribution of the various fractions (relative to the total material) obtained by preparative electrofocusing was determined in several ways.

A. Scanning Densitometry

Gels were scanned prior to elution and the proportions of each peak determined by computing integrator.

TABLE IV Molecular Weight of Heparin Fractions Obtained after Electrofocusing

Heparin Fraction (Electrofocusing)	Molecular Weight					
	Heparin (Pork Mucosal)					Heparin (Beef Lung)
	Source A[a]		Source B[b]		M.W. Ratio	
	Band I[c]	Band II[d]	Band I	Band II	II/I	
2	19,000	28,000	----	----	1.47	18,000
4	----	----	17,500	25,500	1.45	----
6	15,000	23,000	----	----	1.53	16,000
8	9,500	15,000	----	----	1.57	12,000
10	7,500	13,000	7,900	12,500	1.65	9,000
12	6,000	10,500	6,200	11,000	1.76	7,200
14	5,600	10,000	----	----	1.80	6,400
16	5,000	8,800	5,000	9,600	1.84	5,400
18	4,000	7,600	4,600	8,200	1.90	4,000
20	----	----	3,500	7,500	2.14	----
Average M.W. Ratio					1.71	

[a] Heparin preparation, Lederle, lot 1804-B4740
[b] Heparin preparation, Fisher, lot (H-19)732852
[c] I - fast-migrating heparin component
[d] II - slow-migrating heparin component

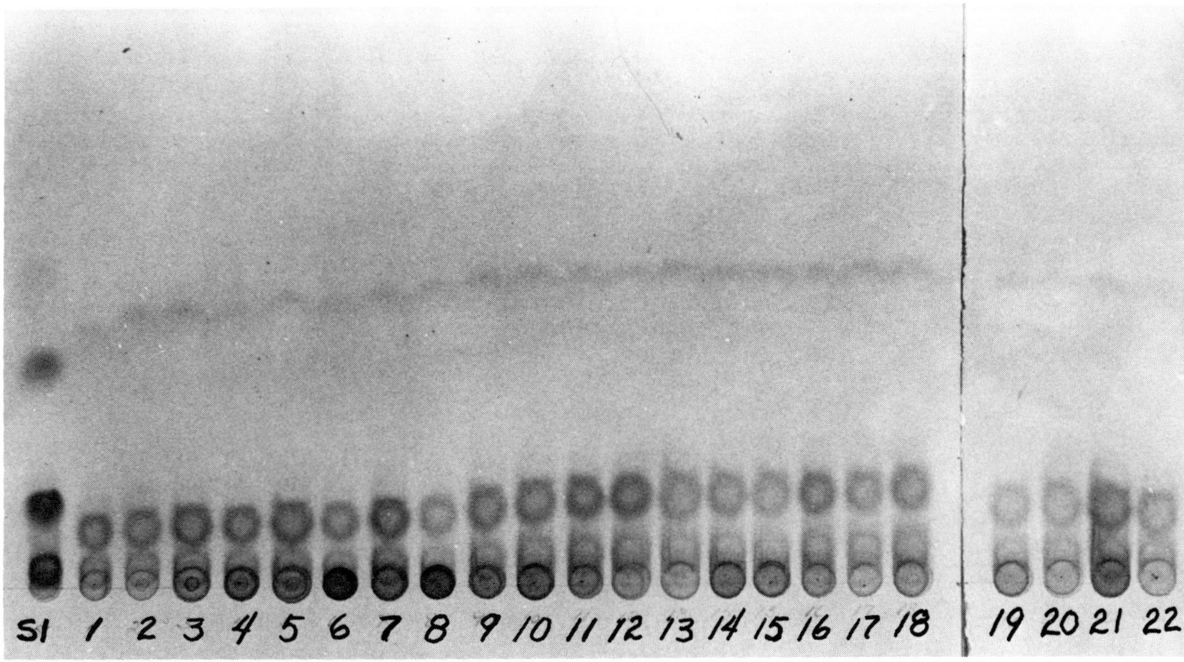

Fig. 7. Thin layer chromatogram of degradation products of mucosal heparin after incubation with enzymes of Flavobacterium Heparinum (Heparinase and Heparitinase II). S1 = unfractionated heparin and enzymes, #1 - 22 = heparin fractions and enzymes, incubation conditions as per Dietrich et al. (9), stained with Toluidine Blue reagent.

B. Electrophoresis in Agarose

The number of units of each fraction was determined by measuring the metachromatic activity of the fraction and metachromatic activity of a known amount of International Standard Heparin. The individual values per fraction were divided by the total units measured.

C. Anticoagulant Assays

The proportion of each fraction was calculated by measuring the total units available per fraction per assay system and dividing these individual totals by the grand total of units measured.

D. Gravimetric Determination

The *purified* fractions were lyophilized and the actual weights determined. Individual fraction weights were divided by the total weight of all fractions.

Although reasonable agreement was obtained for percentage distribution values between the densitometric measurement and the gravimetric determination, wide variations were present when units were determined by anticoagulant assays and metachromatically. This finding is not unexpected, since these methods either measured unrelated expressions of heparin activity or different stages of related phenomena, e.g., heparin effects on the general coagulation cascade with the USP assay and the selective Factor X inhibition of the Yin and Wessler assay.

Three examples of the calculated percentage distribution are presented in the lower panel (c) of Figure 8 for lung origin heparin. Also on this summary diagram are presented molecular weight analyses and relative anticoagulant potencies.

Since large variations were observed in percentage distribution by different methods, units obtained by anti-coagulant assays were expressed as *specific activities*, through dividing the units obtained per fraction by the number of milligrams determined gravimetrically. *Specific activities* were similarly determined for the parent unfractionated heparin.

Relative anticoagulant potencies were then calculated by dividing the individual *specific activities* of the fractions by those of the parent heparins.

In the case of lung heparins, relative potencies 2 to 3-fold greater than the unfractionated heparin were observed with the Yin and Wessler assay. With the USP assay the highest value was 1.23. Potencies equivalent to parent

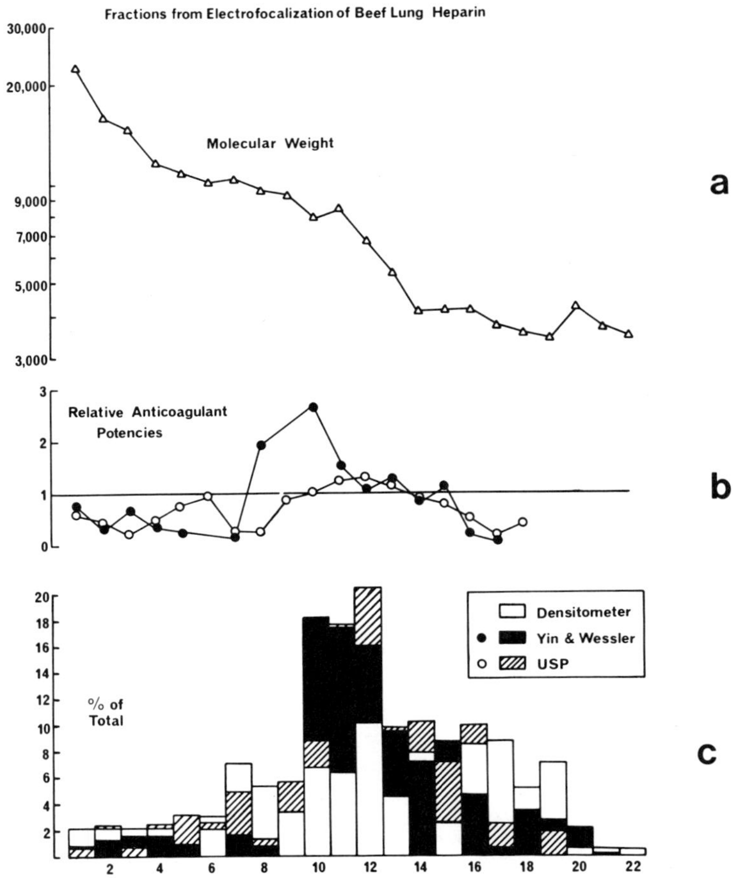

Fig. 8. Summary diagram for fractions derived from beef lung heparin. See text for details.

heparin were found in fractions 10 through 14 in the USP assay (M.W. 8000-4000). In the Yin and Wessler assay, equivalent or greater potencies were found in 8, 10 through 13, and 15 (M.W. 10,000-4000). These fractions account for 45% of the total material obtained, by weight.

Figure 9 shows a similar summary diagram for heparin fractions of mucosal origin. The data were calculated in the same fashion. For the USP assay, high potency fractions are: 5, 7, 10, 11 and 14, the highest value being 1.42. For the Yin and Wessler assay fractions 5, 7, 10, 11 and 14 (i.e., the same fractions) have high potency. The high value is 1.3. There is no readily discernible correlation with molecular weight. These fractions comprise 20% of the total material obtained, by weight.

Please note that in both examples several fractions have *no* activity and although there is good agreement between the anticoagulant assays for mucosal heparin, this is not quite true for lung heparin.

A comment about the calculation of *specific activity* is required. If the actual measured weight of the fractions is not used, but rather the defined relationship of weight to International Units is used, more fractions show very high potencies. We have used this calculation because it gives a conservative estimate of the high potency fractions and correlates actual weight with observed activity.

V. CONCLUSIONS

Heparin is a family of components of varying chain lengths. The results of analytical and preparative electrofocusing suggest multiple components of similar charge and variable weight.

The variation between chain lengths may be equivalent to the heparin hexasaccharide. Fractions produced by electrofocusing show consistent intervals between chain lengths. Our earlier data suggested an interval of molecular weight equivalent to the heparin hexasaccharide. The values obtained with our more recent preparative electrofocusing suggest a smaller interval, for a different beef lung preparation, as well as a narrower range of molecular species present. With mucosal preparations *two species* of heparin are present at each chain length. Monomeric and dimeric associations (at *least) are present in commercial preparations and others may be present naturally or pathologically.* The parallelism between the fast and slow migrating components is remarkable, with preparative and analytical electrofocusing using multiple mucosal preparations. The differences in intervals between chain lengths for our previous reports and the current data may

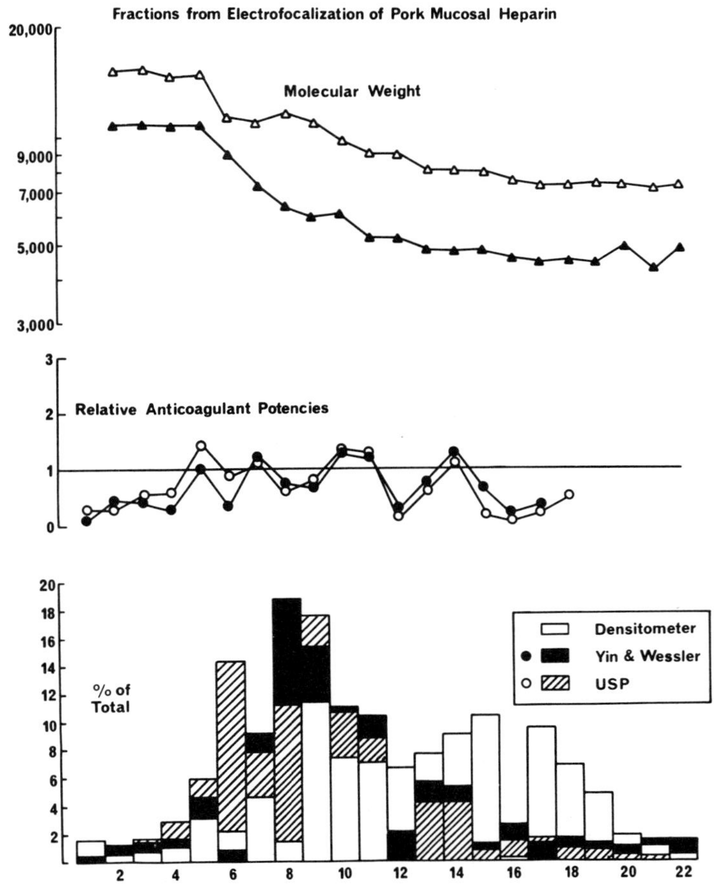

Fig. 9. Summary diagram for fractions derived from pork mucosal heparin. See text for details.

be indicative of side to side molecular associations that are not precisely monomeric and dimeric. Hence multiple chain associations may be feasible. This is further substantiated by the multiple band patterns observed upon re-electrofocusing of individual mucosal fractions.

Biological specificity may vary within the individual species of the heparin chain lengths. Our results clearly demonstrate that all components of a heparin preparation are *not* equally effective in a given biological test. This data is consistent with the findings of Lam *et al.* (10), and Höök (11). Our gravimetric analysis and determination of specific activity of the fractions suggests the total anticoagulant activity may be resident in 25-30% of the preparations (12).

Anticoagulant activity alone cannot be used to define heparins Since multiple pharmacological activities (13) have been reported for heparin and since only a small portion of the clinically effective material is active in anticoagulant tests, it is no longer feasible to define heparin solely in terms of anticoagulant activity.

Due to the complexity of the *molecule* we now know as heparin, *the concept of a known weight of heparin yielding a unit of activity must be re-evaluated in light of the possibility of varying amounts of antagonists or agonists being present in any preparation.*

VI. ACKNOWLEDGEMENTS

These studies were supported by the MRC grant MA5641, and were carried out with the capable assistance of Miss W. Joan Madland and Mr. Kevin McDuffie.

VII. REFERENCES

1. Kiss, J., *in* "Heparin Chemistry and Clinical Usage" (V. Kakkar, and D.P. Thomas, eds.), p. 3. Academic Press, London, 1976.
2. Nader, H.B., McDuffie, N.M., and Dietrich, C.P., Biochem. Biophys. Res. Comm. *57*, 488 (1974).
3. McDuffie, N.M., Dietrich, C.P., and Nader, H.B., Biopolymers *14*, 1473 (1975).
4. Hilborn, J.W., and Anastassiadis, P.A., Anal. Biochem. *39*, 88 (1971).
5. Jaques, L.B., Sue, T.K., McDuffie, N.M., and Presnell, K.R., J. Amer. An. Hosp. Ass. *13*, 359 (1977).
6. Dietrich, C.P., Nader, H.B., and McDuffie, N.M., Anais. Acad. Bras. de Ci. *47*, 2 (1975).

7. Pharmacopeia of United States of America. Heparin Sodium, p. 609, 1965.
8. Yin, E.T., Wessler, S., and Butler, J.V., J. Lab. Clin. Med. *81*, 298 (1973).
9. Dietrich, C.P., Silva, M.E., and Michelacci, Y.M., J. Biol. Chem. *248*, 6408 (1973).
10. Lam, L.H., Silbert, J.E., and Rosenberg, R.D., Biochem. Biophys. Res. Comm. *69*, 570 (1976).
11. Höök, M., Björk, I., Hopwood, J., and Lindahl, U., FEBS Letter *66*, 90 (1976).
12. Cowie, N.W., "Isolation and Characterization of Heparin Fractions Prepared by Electrofocusing". M.Sc. Thesis. Univ. of Saskatchewan, Saskatoon. Sept. 15, 1976.
13. Ehrlich, J., and Stivala, S.S., J. Pharmac. Sci. *62*, 517 (1973).

A CONTRIBUTION TO THE PROBLEM OF HEPARIN

P. Bianchini

Opocrin Research Laboratories

In a recent paper (1), we showed by electrofocusing that heparins extracted from various organs can be resolved into several components, thus confirming the results of Nader *et al.* (2) and McDuffie *et al.* (3).

We also observed that the heterogeneity of heparins is associated with modifications of biological activities both *in vitro* on the anticoagulant activity (IU), on the activated

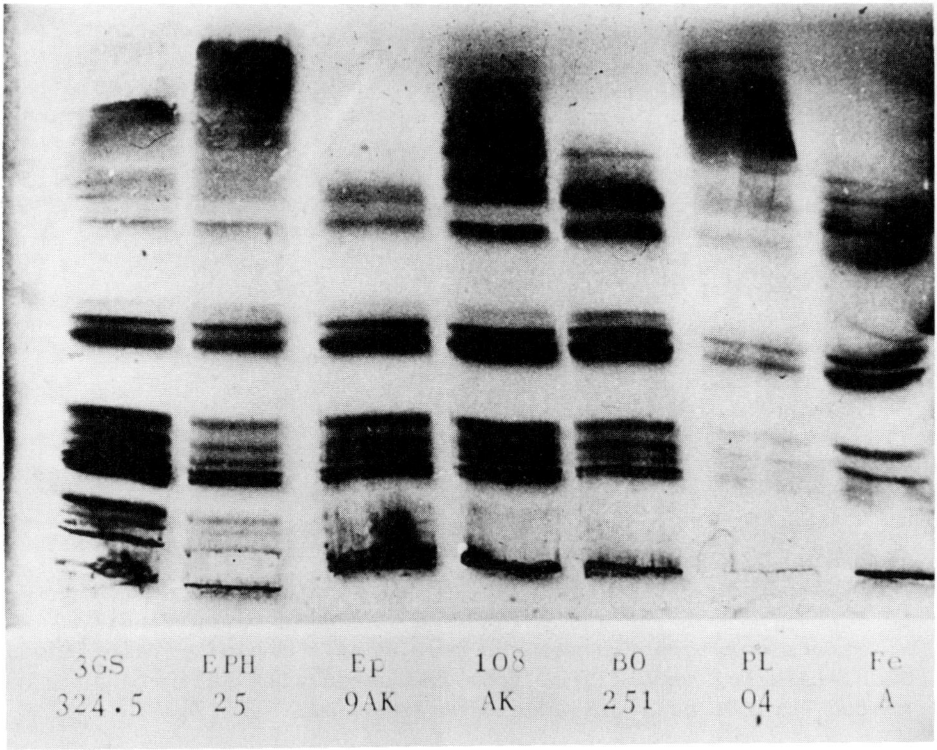

Fig. 1. Electrofocusing of heparins from different organs. Fractionation on polyacrylamide gel slabs containing 1.5% ampholyte from LKB - Sweden - (pH 2.5-6). Staining with Toluidine Blue.

ISBN 0-12-484850-8

partial thromboplastin time (APTT), thrombin time (TT), inhibition of platelet factor 4 (PF4) and complement hemolytic system (CH 50), and *in vivo* on the activation of lipoprotein lipase (LPL) and the prolongation of APTT.

In particular electrofocusing indicates that the different heparins contain several fractions that focalize in the same position as a result of specific binding with ampholines, but are present in different amounts and can be clustered into 4-5 groups (Fig. 1). Some heparins seem to contain low molecular weight fractions.

Paper chromatography (4) has confirmed the existence of these groups of fractions that we have shown to be active on LPL release (Fig. 2).

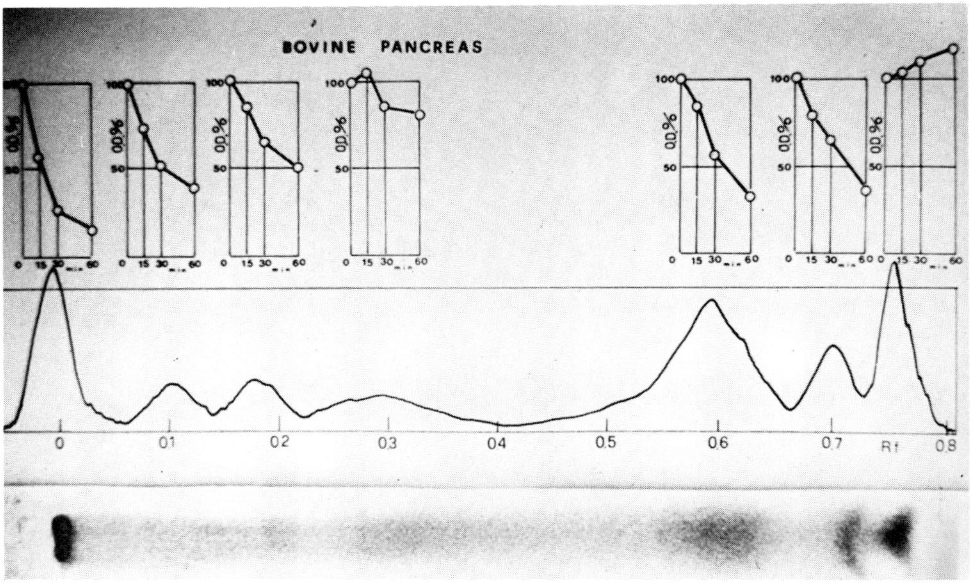

Fig. 2. Paper chromatography (Whatman 3MM) of heparin from pancreas. I° solvent system Isopropanol/Water/Ammonia 50:50:1, II° solvent system Ethanol/Water/Ammonia 50:50:1. Fractions corresponding to the metachromatic bands (Toluidine Blue staining) were eluted from the paper with saline and tested for LPL activity according to Ediol Test (7,8).

Heparins with different activity ratios also have been fractionated on Sephadex G50 gel chromatography columns, employing distilled water as eluent in order to maximize the interactions between the polysaccharide components and the cross-linked dextran. The results obtained from the fractionation of a heparin from pancreas are summarized in Figs. 3, 4, and 5.

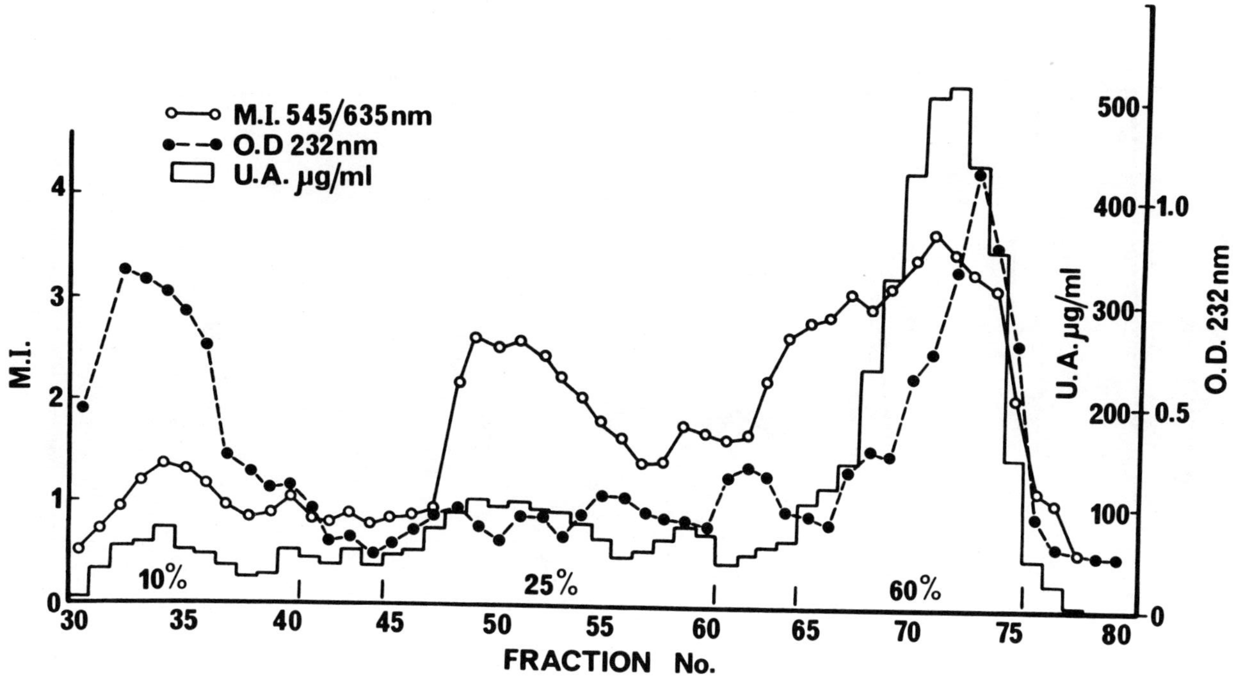

Fig. 3. Gel chromatography of heparin from pancreas (100 mg) on G50 Sephadex column (2.5 x 100 cm) which was eluted with water. Effluent fractions (5 ml) were analyzed for metachromatic index (M.I. 545/635 nm), optical density (O.D. 232 nm), and uronic acids (U.A. μg/ml).

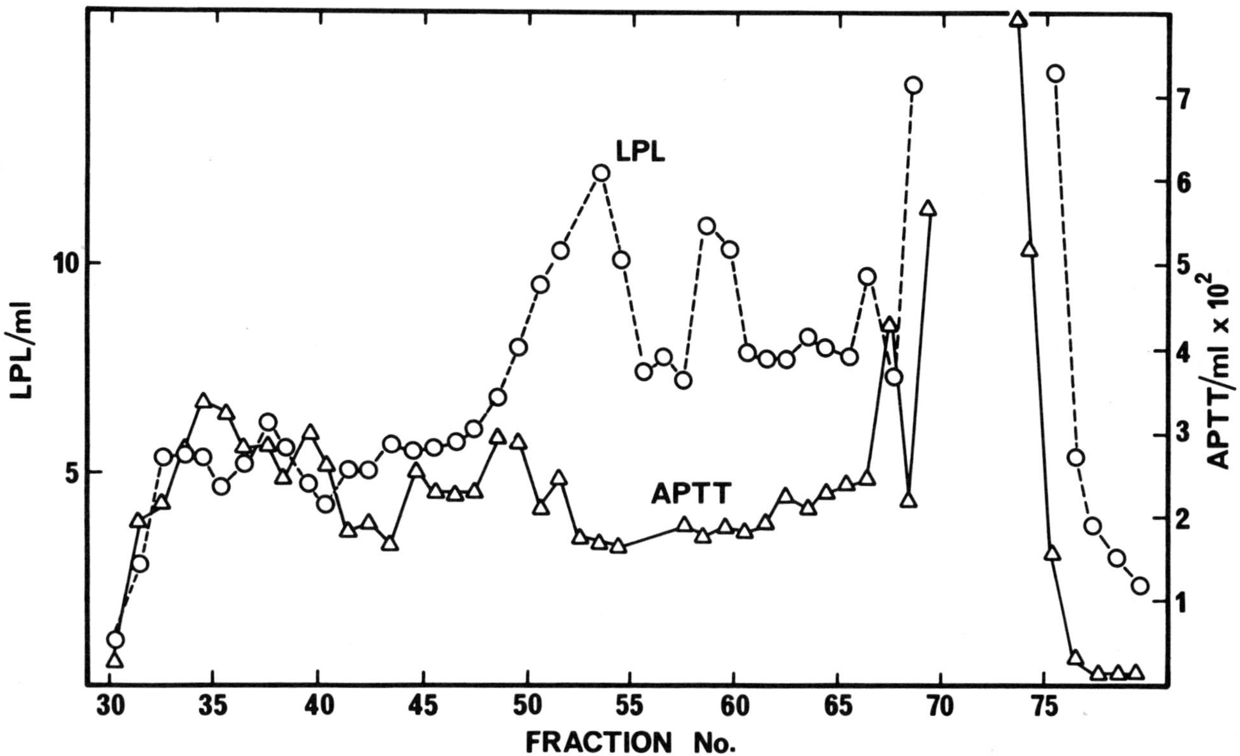

Fig. 4. The same effluent fractions as in Fig. 3 analyzed for LPL (7)(8) and APTT (9) activities.

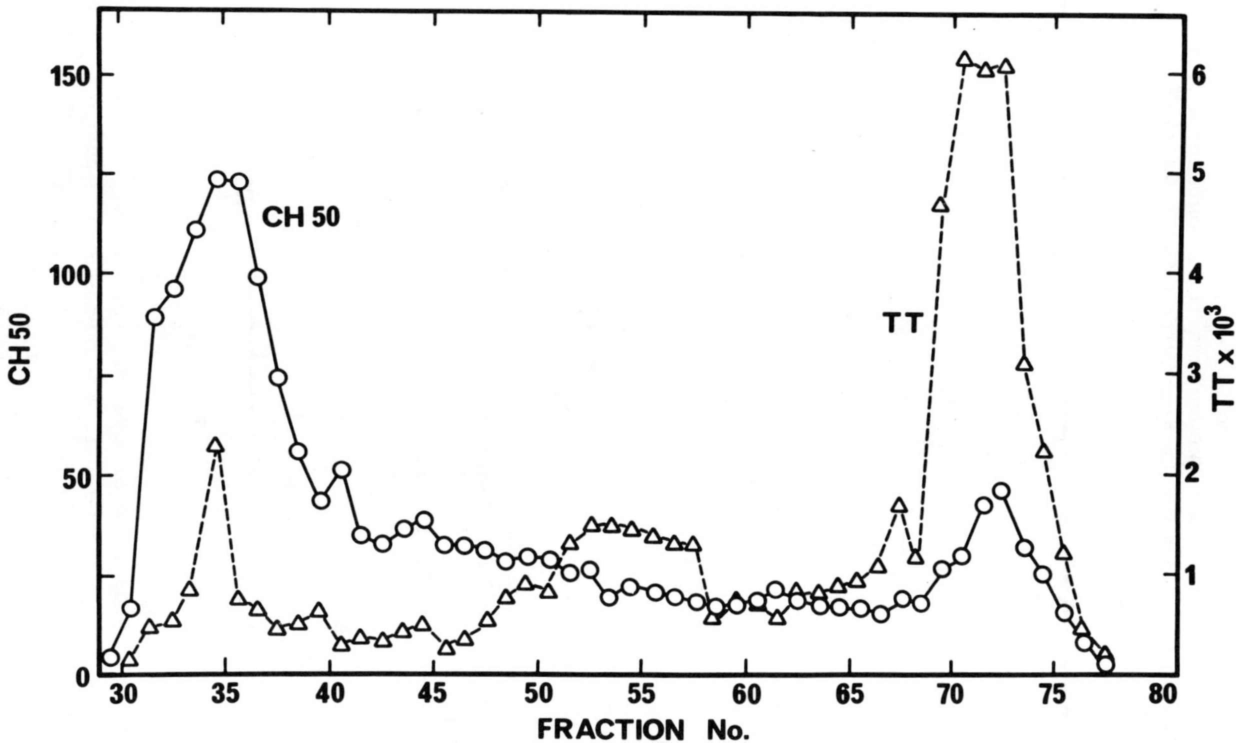

Fig. 5. The same effluent fractions as in Fig. 3 analyzed for thrombin time (TT) (10) and anti-complement activity as inhibition of immune hemolysis (CH 50) (11).

It is quite clear that uronic acid, metachromasia and O.D. 232 nm are located in three zones. The zone close to the void volume contains about 10% of the total uronic acid, a slight activity in LPL, APTT, and TT, but a high immune hemolysis inhibiting activity (CH50).

The central zone of the column that contains about 25% of the total uronic acid is subdivided into 3-4 fractions

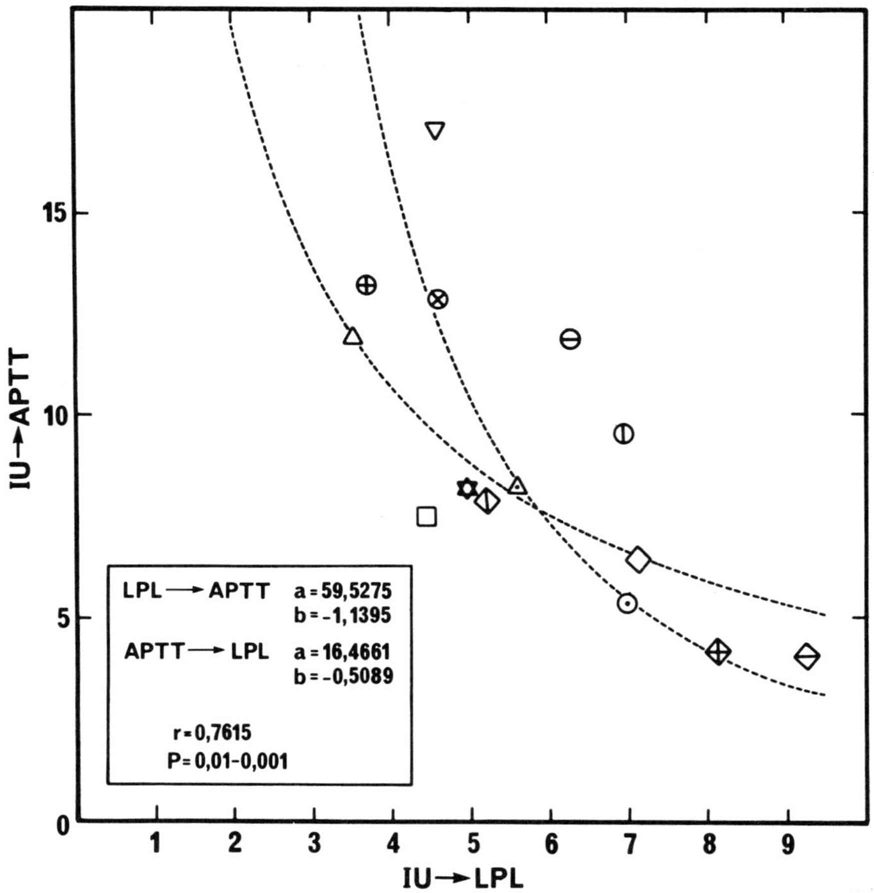

Fig. 6. Heparins extracted from different organs. Correlation curves between LPL and APTT in vivo - Sprague Dawley rats are given heparin intravenously. (Heparins from: ▽ Liver; ⊕ Lung; ⊖ Beef intestinal mucosa; ⊙ - ⦶ - ⊗ - Pig intestinal mucosa; □ Pig duodenum; △ - △ Beef pancreas; ◇ - ◇ Beef placenta; ⬖ - ⬖ Human placenta; ✡ Int. Standard WHO - pig intestinal mucosa).

and is mainly active on the LPL releasing system and less on TT. Finally, the zone with the highest retention volume contains about 60% of the uronic acid, high APTT, TT, and LPL activities but low anti-complement activity.

From *in vivo* experiments one observation is relevant: the different heparin doses (expressed in IU) required to have the ED50 for LPL and to prolong the APTT to 50 sec are described by an inverse correlation curve, as Fig. 6 shows. This figure also suggests that some heparins (e.g., those extracted from bovine liver and bovine pancreas) are more active on LPL release than on APTT at the same doses expressed in IU, while other preparations (e.g., heparins extracted from bovine and human placenta) show an inverse relationship.

Such behaviour supports the hypothesis that two types of heparin exist, with different active sites and different affinity for antithrombin III and LPL, and thus, presumably, with different physiological roles.

In vitro, i.e., in absence of the LPL releasing system, heparin is completely available for antithrombin III, whereas *in vivo* there will be a competition between the two systems.

Such a competition is in good agreement with the existence of a *high affinity heparin* and a *low affinity heparin* for antithrombin III (5,6).

The facts mentioned above clearly call attention to the meaning of the term *heparin*. This term should be understood to be the name of a family of compounds differing not only in their molecular weights, but also in their structures and thus in their biological activities. In particular, it seems justified to think that this family includes substances with a prevailing activity on either hemocoagulation, or on LPL release, or on the cytolytic system of complement. It may therefore be possible to employ different heparin *fractions* in the treatment of thromboembolic diseases, of dislipidemia, and of some immunocomplex diseases.

REFERENCES

1. Bianchini, P., Osima, B., Rimini, V., and Macchi, M., Eur. Symp. on Advances in Coagulation, Fibrinolysis, Platelet Aggregation and Atherosclerosis. Palermo (Italy) Oct. 1976 in press.
2. Nader, H.B., McDuffie, N.M., and Dietrich, C.P., Biochem. Biophys. Res. Comm. *57*, 488 (1974).
3. McDuffie, N.M., Dietrich, C.P., and Nader, H.B., Biopolymers *14*, 1473 (1975).

4. Bianchini, P., Osima, B., and Rimini, V., Seminario Naz. Studi sull' Eparina - Fano (Italy) September 1975.
5. Höök, M., Björk, I., Hopwood, J., and Lindahl, U., FEBS Lett. *66*, 90 (1976).
6. Riesenfield, J., Höök, M., Björk, I., Lindahl, U., and Ajaxon, B., Fed. Proc. *36*, 39 (1977).
7. Bianchini, P., Casetta, R., Osima, B., and Casarini, A., Biochem. Exp. Biol. *10*, 159 (1972).
8. Bianchini, P., Guidi, G., and Osima, B., Biochem. Exp. Biol. *10*, 243 (1972).
9. Proctor, R.R., and Rapaport, S.I., Am. J. Clin. Path. *36*, 212 (1961).
10. Biggs, R., and McFarlane, R.G., *in* "Human Blood Coagulation and its Disorders" (R. Biggs and R.G. McFarlane, eds.), Blackwell Scientific Publications, Oxford, 1962.
11. Basevi, A., and Furlan, S., Giorn. Mal. Inf. Parass., *8*, 480 (1956).

DISCUSSION

Wednesday, July 6th, 1977, 2:30 p.m.

SILBERT, Boston I have a question for Dr. Dietrich concerning the nonreducing terminals of the chain. Did you say you had isolated single hexosamines also in the course of degradation?

DIETRICH, São Paulo I isolated disaccharides.

SILBERT, Boston Only disaccharides, there were no single hexosamines?

DIETRICH, São Paulo Yes, we had glucosamine N-sulfate, glucosamine 2,6, disulfate, etc., but these were due to degradation by the heparinase and glycuronidase.

SILBERT, Boston Have you ever looked at the degradation in the absence of the glycuronidase to see if you do have a single hexosamine cleaved off from the nonreducing end by means of your enzymes? Do you know what would happen if you had a trisaccharide for example, would the heparinase enzyme cleave off free hexosamine, or does it have to have uronic acid on it?

DIETRICH, São Paulo No, we have not done that exact experiment. We have not looked for glucosamine N-sulfate without the use of the glycuronidase, we expected the amounts would be very small.

SILBERT, Boston The reason I ask is very specific, to determine which is the nonreducing terminal sugar. In the case of chondroitin sulfate it's a mixture of uronic acid and acetyl hexosamine and I wonder if it's a mixture in the case of heparin. This then leads one on to another step as to the specificity of synthesis. Is synthesis more or less random in terms of when the chain is finished or is there a specific ending to the chain?

DIETRICH, São Paulo I understand, I think that the borohydride reduction experiment might say something about that... 80% of the nonreducing terminal is uronic acid, and perhaps 50% glucosamine, I don't know!

SILBERT, Boston So you're suggesting that perhaps it's a mixture but you're not sure.

ISBN 0-12-484850-8

DIETRICH, São Paulo Perhaps it's a mixture, I'm not sure. If we consider the yields, one would expect a much higher yield.

SILBERT, Boston It's very difficult.

DIETRICH, São Paulo If you have 10% yield, which is twice as much as would be expected, perhaps instead of the suggestion that I made about dimerization of heparin we have a heparin tetrameter. Then, it would appear to be a ball rather than a chain.

LINDAHL, Uppsala Could I just make one short addition to that - probably it would be difficult to get an idea of the chain termination mechanism during biosynthesis by looking at the nonreducing terminals of heparin chains as you find them since these degradation products evidently have been cleaved by endoglycosidases and I'm a bit surprised to hear as much as 80% of the chains would end with a uronic acid since the only endoglycidase investigated so far turned out to be an endo-glucuronidase and would give the nonreducing terminal of glucosamine.

DIETRICH, São Paulo We were also surprised!

LINKER, Salt Lake City I think I have a partial answer to Dr. Silbert's question. I seem to remember that the trisaccharide that was hexosamine at the nonreducing end is not degraded by the heparinase. However, we should get the trisaccharide - we haven't found any trisaccharide but we do also find a saturated disaccharide at least in heparan sulfate which we assumed was from the nonreducing end. The yields of this we didn't pay much attention to, we just assumed that it came from the nonreducing end.

LINDAHL, Uppsala If I understood you correctly, you found non-sulfated iduronic acid in samples and deduced from this finding that these iduronic acids have been introduced as such on the nucleotide sugar level rather than being formed by epimerization. This is evidently not the case since the true substrate for the epimerase is a polymer consisting of alternating units of glucuronic acid and N-sulfated glucosamine - if this is incubated with the epimerase a portiòn of the uronic acids, about 10 to 15%, are converted to iduronic acid with no need for sulfation, however, if there is opportunity for sulfation by including PAPS in this mixture, the yield of iduronic acid increases and this iduronic acid will then be sulfated. So I don't think that there is any contradiction in that finding.

DIETRICH, São Paulo Yes, I was referring to a previous paper, by your group, in which you thought at one time that there would be a link between the sulfation and the epimerization.

LINDAHL, Uppsala There still is such a link.

DIETRICH, São Paulo I don't understand.

LINDAHL, Uppsala Sulfation is not the prerequisite for epimerization but it promotes epimerization - this I think would provide the basis for saying that there is a link between sulfation and epimerization.

DIETRICH, São Paulo An indirect one - yes, because you could then have a polymer with iduronic acid and no need for sulfation of it. It could be the case of chondroitin sulfate B.

LINDAHL, Uppsala It seems to be exactly the same thing in chondroitin sulfate B. Without sulfation there is some iduronic acid formed, in the presence of sulfation the yield of iduronic acid decreases presumably due to sulfation of the iduronic acid as it's formed but the main point is there is no need for UDP - iduronic acid in either of these two cases.

DIETRICH, São Paulo But in the case of chondroitin sulfate B you might have 2% sulfation of the total iduronic acid residue in the structure. You can have probably a pure polymer with no sulfation but containing iduronic acid.

LASKER, New York Both Dr. Dietrich and Dr. Linker prepare heparinase from a variety of different heparins, probably both use mucosal heparin. Then use the heparinase to degrade a variety of different heparins, pig heparin, bovine heparin, whale heparin, etc.; I wonder to what extent the differences in the heparinase introduce both qualitative and quantitative differences in your results.

DIETRICH, São Paulo I don't know if Dr. Linker has a different opinion, we have only one single heparinase that degrades either the beef lung type of heparin or the mucosal type of heparin, etc., and in our hands, the heparin that we have shown in the slide is much simpler than the heparin that was shown by Dr. Linker. We do not find three types of tetrasaccharides, we were able to find only one type of tetrasaccharide. In Dr. Linker's hands the tetrasaccharide containing iduronic acid without sulfate is not degraded by heparinase, in our hands a similar compound, not the same compound, but a similar compound like Hunter's heparitin sulfate is degradable by the heparinase. This compound contains iduronic acid nonsulfated in the structure, I don't know how I can explain this type of difference.

LASKER, New York Is there a spectrum of heparinases that you produce from the Flavobacterium growing on heparin? Does it vary from one batch to another?

DIETRICH, São Paulo No, it doesn't. As a matter of fact bacteria may be grown in heparitin sulfate. They may be grown in disaccharide, the N-acetylated disaccharide shown to be one of the products formed from heparitin sulfate by the action of heparitinase. This disaccharide is enough to induce the three enzymes. The heparinase and the two heparitinases. I think we published that five or six years ago.

UVNÄS, Stockholm Mast cell granules show different solubility from different animals and as far as I can understand it the mast cell granule in the rat is composed of a water insoluble complex between heparin and a strongly basic polypeptide. In other animals, like the dog, mast cell granules are readily soluble in water. The mast cell granule dissolves in sodium chloride. One molar sodium chloride yields a break between the heparin and the basic polypeptide. The different solubilities of the granules from various species could be explained by assuming heparin of different sulfation in different species with more or less stable complexes between heparin and basic polypeptide formed. My question is, are there any differences in sulfation between heparin from different animal species? Perhaps some mast cells do not contain heparin at all, but other mucopolysaccharides?

LINKER, Salt Lake City The last slide I showed indicated different degrees of sulfation. Lung heparin is more highly sulfated than mucosal heparin. That's actually within the same species of beef or pork. In the rabbit, lung, intestine or liver, (which are excellent tissue sources in beef), we could not isolate any significant amounts of heparin. Dr. Jaques, I think, has pointed out that the rabbit does have mast cells and has also pointed out that in the rabbit mast cells there probably is not heparin but a different glycosaminoglycan. This prompts the extremely basic question, what is the function of heparin in mast cells, and can this function be taken over by another type of sulfated polymer? That's a very difficult thing to answer at the moment, I think that certainly there are large variations in sulfation that are found in different heparins and certainly in different types of mast cells.

Now to get back to the point about the heparinase and getting somewhat different results. I have very carefully called this a purified heparinase and not a pure heparinase. In terms of activity, we find that it acts on heparins, it does not act on heparan sulfate, however, so we have a fair amount of specificity, but if you are bold enough to run it on acrylamide gel you get three to four bands from the purified material and if you are even bolder and run isoelectrofocusing, I shudder to think how many bands you would get - so these are not highly purified enzymes that either I, or Dr. Dietrich probably work with. They are purified in the sense of the activities, but they are certainly not pure enzyme preparations. The crude enzyme preparations contain glycuronidases, various kinds of sulfatases, heparinase - we find only one heparitinase though I am quite certain that Dr. Dietrich is quite correct that there is a different type of heparitinase that we have missed because we use a different isolation procedure.

SILBERT, Boston I would like to address myself to Dr. Uvnäs' question. We don't have a direct measurement of the sulfate content of the rat peritoneal mast cell heparin. However, if we look at its size, which we do have a measure of, and compare it with other heparins and observe its behavior on ion exchange columns, it appears to be very highly sulfated. On a DEAE Cellulose column it elutes after commercial heparin; its size is larger but it is not as large as mouse mast cell heparin which appears at nearly the same point. We know that the latter is highly sulfated, having actually measured the sulfate content. We can confirm that the granules are insoluble unless salt is used. They are insoluble in water but with one molar salt the heparin is solublized, but I don't know that we can say that it's because of binding to anionic protein. It could just as easily be the sort of binding that one sees in proteoglycan aggregation; e.g., chondroitin sulfate proteoglycan may be disaggregated with high salt. Although it probably is binding to protein we really don't know the nature of this binding, and it may be unrelated to the sulfate content of the heparin.

PADAWER, New York I'm interested in the possible other functions of these enzymes, particularly the ones that are native to mammalian tissues rather than the ones that are derived from bacteria. Is there any evidence that instead of just acting as either depolymerases or endoglycosidases, some of these enzymes might work in the opposite direction? Could they in some way pull the reaction, or might they act as transferases, allowing large pieces of the chains to be transferred from one part to another? I would also like to ask Dr.

Horner, whether he has perchance looked in mast cells themselves for the presence of the depolymerase since this would connect with some statements he has in the literature that he believes that the macromolecular heparin has to be degraded to a small molecular weight before it becomes active, and that those species that lack this ability are the ones that come down with atherosclerosis?

HORNER, Toronto These ideas have occurred to me and we do intend to pursue them, but like the heparin field the mast cell field is also full of problems of definition. No, we have not looked at enzymes in the mast cells. We have degranulated mast cells but by compound 48/80, and the produce which is released from the mast cells under those conditions is not degraded at all, it is still the same one million molecular weight size. It is possible that it is released in the macromolecular form and then degraded. I mention again the preliminary data I gave this morning that in adipose tissue one finds both macromolecular heparin and low molecular weight heparin of the type released by the plasma enzyme at pH 6, again suggestive of depolymerization outside the mast cells, but this is very preliminary.

LINDAHL, Uppsala Could I add a comment to Dr. Padawer's question. We have actually found the enzyme intracellularly in neoplastic mast cells from mouse. Now these are neoplastic, we don't know really what this represents, but we followed the intracellular metabolism of the newly synthesized heparin. It is formed in a particulate fraction sedimenting at 20,000 G and is then transferred into another fraction, presumably the mast cell granules, which sediments at 1000 G and in this 20,000 G fraction one finds the endoglycosidases or endoglucuronidase that degrades the macromolecular heparin. It has actually been isolated in particles which behaved on silica density gradients centrifugation like lysosomes and the storage form in the mast cells granules is clearly degraded. The whole degradation process seems to be completed within five to six hours after the biosynthesis.

DIETRICH, São Paulo Still on the question of Dr. Padawer. We did isolate a sulfaminidase from mammalian tissues, which removed one single sulfate from normal heparin, not macromolecular heparin. This was done with radioactively labeled N-sulfated heparin and this enzyme is a sulfaminidase. Later on it was shown to be deficient in San Filipo's Syndrome. If you inject heparin intraperitoneally into rats, 50% appears as inorganic sulfate in the urine of the animal after 24 hours. This suggests that perhaps the sequential degradation of heparin in mammalian tissues is completely different from the sequential degradation in bacterial systems. Since the latter occurs only at the monosaccharide level, and mammalian sulfaminidase desulfation seems to occur at the polysaccharide level. A question for Drs. Horner and Linker. Does macromolecular heparin appear in all tissues or, is its distribution limited to only *certain tissues?*

HORNER, Toronto Obviously a survey needs to be done of many tissues, there is no reason to postulate the macromolecular complexes are of the same molecular size in all species, but they may follow the same general scheme. I would point out for instance that the commonest commercial heparin, pig mucosal heparin, upon analysis and calculation of the molecular weight by end-group analysis, obviously was a much bigger molecule. There is always a twofold difference between the molecular size that would be expected (from end-group analysis) and the molecular size actually found by physical measurements. That then would suggest that the chains in pig mucosal heparin were at some stage at least twice as long as they are in the final product available commercially.

DIETRICH, São Paulo The reason for the question is that I did do some work on the extraction of heparin and I'm trying to do a comparative study on the distribution of heparin. With rat tissues, skin and liver, we were able to find the macromolecular type of heparin. (We used the standard method of Scott with potassium acetate.) We did find the macromolecular heparin in rat skin specifically, but in all of the other tissues, human tissues, beef lung, and dog tissue we did not find any type of macromolecular heparin.

A curious thing happened with the macromolecular heparin of rat tissues, perhaps you can comment upon. After extraction of macromolecular heparin, we did ascorbic acid degradation and we found the depolymerization that you have observed, but subsequently we found a spontaneous reassociation of the same heparin. After ascorbic acid depolymerization we ran it on an agarose electrophoresis system similar to yours. Then we extracted the band containing the depolymerized heparin and reran it again - in agarose. We again found a polymerization type that is a slow migrating compound. Do you have any comment about this?

HORNER, Toronto I have definitely never found that. I would like to get back to some of the other things you said about the existence of macromolecular heparins in other tissues. I did at one time look at human tissue, although sampling problems exist, I did find traces of macromolecular heparin in liver and lung. We then went to monkey tissues, which are available in great numbers at Connaught Laboratories because they kill vast numbers of monkeys to get the kidneys for polio vaccine manufacture - in this case it is possible to get tissues which are frozen in liquid nitrogen within 30 seconds of sacrifice of the animals, and under those conditions you can find large proportions of macromolecular heparin, as I showed on one of my slides, in many tissues. So I think that macromolecular heparin in tissues breaks down rapidly post-mortem.

LINDAHL, Uppsala Could I add one comment here which I think could be of interest - as you say - you look in certain tissues and you find no trace of macromolecular heparin. We recently did a gel chromatographic separation of commercial pig mucosal heparin which had been treated under mild conditions - if you just analyze it as such it has fairly low molecular weight. Perhaps one serine on every three chains, and this would certainly not indicate macromolecular heparin. If you take the high molecular weight fractions, around 35,000, and analyze these, they account for a small proportion of the total material but contain serine and glycine amounting to seven to eight residues per polymer chain. This could then very well represent the remainder of the macromolecular heparin with part of the protein core and most of the chains cleaved off by endoglycosidase.

BENTLEY, Portland I have a comment directed to Dr. Horner's observations that there may be several different depolymerases and it's possible that this observation is due to perhaps limiting quantities of enzyme. If, for example, you treat chondroitin sulfate proteoglycan with commercial cathepsin D or with liver lysosomal preparation containing a lot of cathepsin D, you can degrade this substance to a product of about the same size as papain produced, about 20,000 molecular weight. If you make the same sort of enzyme preparation from tumors or a tumor preparation that we use, the degradation product barely penetrates sepharose 6B, so that it looks like a very large product, and this occurs regardless of the length of time that you incubate with the enzyme. We thought perhaps it was incomplete degradation because the enzymes hadn't been there long enough. That wasn't the case. If you concentrate this tumor lysosomal preparation by freeze drying and then dissolving in a smaller amount of material, you get the same product, 20,000 molecular weight. Now if you do the converse, if you make the concentration of papain limiting so that you go to vanishingly small concentrations of papain, you don't get a very small amount of 20,000 molecular weight product and a large amount of sepharose 6B excluded substrate. You get an intermediate product. So I wonder whether if you used a depolymerase from one source, it apparently gives you a large molecular weight product and then concentrated that material somehow, or just used more enzyme, would you get the same product as that from a depolymerase from another source?

HORNER, Toronto Yes, Peter, I feel very strongly that you do, and I guess that I didn't explain it very well for you to have asked that question. In some of the graphs that I showed incubated once, twice, and three times, the products were purified each time and started anew with fresh enzyme. It wasn't just the case of incubating for longer times with the same preparation, and in those cases starting off with the fresh enzyme at the same substrate to enzyme ratio there was no sign at all of the tendency to go to lower molecular weight products.

LINDAHL, Uppsala Dr. Horner, since you are up there, could you comment a little on substrate specificity of different endoglycosidases.

HORNER, Toronto Pure speculation, of course. Your mastocytomal enzyme seems to be able to do alone that which a rat seems to require three different enzymes to produce, and which isn't quite as degraded. I suggest that it is to do with constituents in the neighborhood of the linkages which are actually cleaved, which vary and cause specificity differences with the mammalian enzymes, but not with the mastocytomal for some reasons for which we have no explanation. I don't think that your enzyme is going for different linkages from ours because we have taken the product of your mastocytomal enzymes and incubated it with our enzymes and if they were going for different linkages we should then get smaller molecular weight products still, but we do not see that.

LINKER, Salt Lake City While the subject is still being discussed, I would like to say something about this endoglucuronidase which has a very curious specificity which is almost as unusual as the anticoagulant specificity because as several of us have pointed out there is quite a bit of glucuronic left in the 10,000 - 15,000 molecular weight heparin and yet this does not seem to be degraded further. Therefore, it must depend upon the surrounding groups not only on the presence of glucuronic acid itself. I was going to make one other point, that everyone here has probably forgotten, that Dr. Meyer and I many years ago isolated an endoglucuronidase from leeches that acts on hyaluronic acid. This enzyme does not act on heparin, heparan sulfate, or even completely desulfated heparan sulfate, which may have to do with the linkage position which is 1,3 in one case and 1,4 in the other.

I am still bothered by the question that Dr. Lindahl asked me this morning about the tritium, and I really didn't give a very good answer, perhaps because I don't have one. Actually, if all the heparin chains had glucuronic at the end which would be labeled by treating with sodium borotritiide and then treating with periodate, we should get almost entirely very low molecular weight fragments from the reducing end which we don't seem to get. However, we have not been terribly careful at this point yet to see what we really have at the ends, in other words, we might have some chains that certainly have xylosylgalactose at the end, and I was mostly interested in the internal type of uronic rather than the end one.

BECK, Bern I have a question for Dr. McDuffie and perhaps Dr. Horner would like to comment on this too. I am a complete outsider, but since we are trying to talk to each other, I would also like to understand some of the basics. I believe that each of the speakers was referring to molecular size with respect to some of these products and I noticed that Dr. Horner obtained very large differences concerning molecular size based on constituent measurement. On one of your figures, you showed elution patterns from preparative isoelectrofocusing and actually, I believe, with decreasing molecular size you got a secondary peak. Could this be accounted for by secondary interactions between the eluted products which by themselves are not complete homogeneous or do you think that there are other reasons for that?

McDUFFIE, Saskatoon The elution products vary in homogeneity with the mucosal or the lung preparations. For this reason, I don't believe the peak differences seen with the lung heparins. With the preparative electrofocusing system, using lung heparin, we find in these large gels we have sharp bands with diffuse trails that follow. We do not always obtain straight patterns across the entire gel width. Hence, we have variation in our cutting and variation of the molecular weight analysis. Also, with the mucosal heparins, we have the phenomenon that occurs upon reelectrofocusing, that of multiple association, under our conditions we are uncertain if this is a reassociation that occurs after the processing or as a result of the processing. Hence, the nature of the association is unclear. We have reported monomeric and dimeric associations but other associations are conceivable. After analytical electrofocusing of different batch preparations of mucosal heparin, large variations in molecular weight 3000 to 40,000 or 4000 to 20,000 may be observed, although not nearly as much variation in biological activity is recorded.

LINDAHL, Uppsala Dr. McDuffie, your suggestion of dimers is hard to fit into a biosynthetic scheme as it exists now. I wonder if I understood you correctly, you find the dimers preferentially in mucosal preparations. I think that it is true that in mucosal preparations you find much higher proportions of linkage region components in general than you do in lung preparations. Is there a possibility that the two bands could be very similar to each other but differ by the presence of a linkage in a polypeptide fragment, one which is not present in the other. The question is, have you separated these two and done analysis for amino acids and neutral sugars?

McDUFFIE, Saskatoon No, we have not done analysis for amino acids or neutral sugars. In the original studies we simply separated the components and measured uronic, hexosamine, and sulfate ratios, but we propose to do large scale preparative agarose electrophoresis prior to large scale preparative electrofocusing and will subsequently be able to produce the components of each monomer or dimer in individual fractions for analysis. We are now accumulating the monomers and the dimers before and after electrofocusing to determine differences. We haven't enough material yet to make those analyses.

MEYER, New York Dr. Dietrich mentioned dimers in one of his oligosaccharide fractions. What did he mean by a dimer? Is there any chance for covalent linkage, namely for branching in the molecule? Is there any evidence for branching in this molecule? With regard to the 0.05 *M* sodium hydroxide effect which Dr. Silbert showed, are there ester linkages in heparin? Did he try hydroxylamine, for example?

DIETRICH, São Paulo There are two types of dimers - one of them was mentioned by Professor McDuffie in regard to mucosal heparin. This dimer is defined by the molecular weight difference in polyacrylamide gel electrophoresis between the two types of materials that appear at the same point during electrofocusing. We thought also that it was a dimer in a very special type of linkage, because of the change in electrophoretic migration in agarose gel electrophoresis. We have two components, one fast migrating and one slower migrating one. If you do hexosamine-sulfate ratios of these two components, after separating them you'll find that the hexosamine-sulfate ratio is the same. So, somehow the sulfate group should be involved in this type of aggregation or dimer formation, and in this sense I think that this answers the questions of Professor Lindahl about the presence of peptides on this type of material. This should not be the case, because if we have the peptide or piece of peptide and 80 negative charges, that will not effect the migration of these compounds in electrophoresis. What I think now is that you have some kind of association between two heparin molecules, in the case of beef lung heparin, which is through some sort of sulfate bridge.

SILBERT, Boston Just an answer about 0.05 *M* NaOH. I think I probably wasn't clear enough in my presentation. The alkali that was used for cleaving the proteoglycan was 0.5 *M*, the usual amount. The 0.05 *M* had no effect at all. That was not used routinely, it was the 0.5 *M* that was. No other method was tried, no hydroxylamine.

PERLIN, Montreal I want to go back to the question of the enzyme specificity. It's universal to talk about the cleavage of certain linkages and in my opinion with endoglycosidases, and that's a very weak opinion, it may be a little misleading to think of linkages. Unless one is talking about, for example, eliminases where the linkage between the carbon and oxygen bond, it's a question of which side of the linkage the break takes place and glycosidases generally speaking (from what one knows using heavy water ^{18}O experiments) the bond broken usually is the C1O1 bond. If the bond breaks there, what one is really looking at is a product which does not tell you what the linkage was *because you are breaking the linkage*. You can't really examine that linkage once it has been broken. So to talk about specificity in terms of the linkage broken can be a little misleading. One can only talk about the product that is isolated, and therefore one looks at the residue at the reducing end which has resulted from the C1O1 bond having been broken. One can say that a particular type of sugar, is specific, for the enzyme, although we know that enzymes usually required rather large surfaces sometimes and may in fact be associated with several units. I say this because some years ago, we examined polysaccharides which have mixed linkages but using well defined enzymes, for example, a cellulase or laminarinase. We all thought of laminarinase as breaking 1,3 linkages because they hydrolyse polysaccharides which consist of glucose having β 1,3 linkages. If you put that enzyme on a polysaccharide which in fact has both 1,3 and 1,4 linkages, it does not break a 1,3 linkage, it breaks a 1,4 linkage. What it releases is the residue that is three substituted. That is, the reducing end of the oligosaccharide has a three substituted glucose. So that when you talk about specificity, really one can think in terms of the three substituted glucose or cellulase attaching a four substituted β glucose residue, it may in fact require also 1,4 linkages elsewhere, but it's a little bit misleading to simply talk about splitting linkages and specificity. I think that the enzymes that Dr. Linker referred to, the difference between glucuronidases, which may or may not attack two different polymers even though it's an endoglycosidase, of course, could very well be related to the fact that in one case the glucuronic acid residue has a linkage to it from a residue in the sequence which is in fact attached to a different position. I think one might give that some thought in thinking of specificity.

LINDAHL, Uppsala I think that's a very important point, and actually now in a large number of laboratories there are a large number of endoheparitinases, as we call them, from various tissues being isolated and characterized. In the cases where these have been studied they seem to be endoglycuronidases. They haven't been defined as to glucuronitic or iduronitic linkages, but in most of these cases, the size of the end product seems to differ just as described by Dr. Horner. It must be that the substitution pattern of the sugar residues in the vicinity of the linkage determines the distance. In this context, it's really surprising what a very large number of different specificities - can be - or specific information has been implanted in this polysaccharide molecule which is supposedly composed by at least a partly random mechanism. This goes not only for the interaction with antithrombin or lipoprotein lipase or other proteins but also with enzymes of this kind.

PADAWER, New York I would like to ask Dr. McDuffie to perhaps enlighten me a little more about these ampholytes in his system, particularly in analogy to that we might have *in vivo*. I gather that what was necessary was carboxyl and amino groups, although I don't know what the molecule is that we are talking about, but it strikes me that in the mast cell granules, or for that matter as Dr. Uvnäs will probably discuss, the binding of histamine which gives us these amino groups in addition to carboxyl groups in the protein and I wonder whether what you are using as a method for looking at the purified heparins might have a role within the cell similar to what you have been talking about here, but something that might tell us something about what the function of heparin might be within the cell. Do we have an electrofocusing kind of system within the mast cell granule which helps the mast cell do whatever it is that it is supposed to be doing?

McDUFFIE, Saskatoon It is an interesting thought and we have had it before. Ampholytes are oligoethylene oligoamines that are polymerized with acrylic acid yielding derivatives of acrylic acid with amine and carboxyl groups, available. Some manufacturers suggest sharper resolution is attainable by substituting sulfate groups and phosphate groups and depending upon the isoelectric point of the protein used, sharper distinctions in certain pH ranges are possible. Unfortunately, there is no sharp synthetic process for producing these. The process is very simply to mix the oligoamines with the acrylic acid, percolate them for 20-24 hours at 70°C and polymerization occurs. The manufacturer selects those amphoteres which give a smooth pH gradient, bottles them, gives them a batch number, and that's the material. Molecular weights are described only in so far as the individual ampholytes are reported not to exceed a molecular weight of 1000, the number of ampholytes in the system is not determined. Thus the variability between batches may be large. We examined diamines from ethylene diamine up to decane diamine (Dr. Dietrich has published this work) in terms of using these materials as selective retardants of some mucopolysaccharides in an agarose system. We have also looked at acids of varying carbon lengths to determine if they could influence the process alone. I am convinced that the whole process of electrofocusing involves critical spacings of the amine groups on the ampholytes permitting binding of the sulfate groups on heparin. Hence N-desulfation of heparin abolishes the phenomenon. If sulfate in the ampholyte is increased, this impedes the binding of the sulfate of the heparin to the amine, blocking proper fractionation. A number of proteins have been demonstrated to bind the heparin, and in some instances this has been correlated with the amount of N-sulfate present. So I think in answer to your question, yes, the N-sulfate is very important for binding of heparin to a variety of agents - I feel that this definitely can happen in the body, if indeed you have the proper configuration present. The mast cell may be a prime candidate. One problem, and I think some of this will come out tomorrow, is that it is very difficult to correlate numbers of mast cell with heparin distribution throughout the body - so it may not purely be a mast cell phenomenon, it may be the critical spacing on any molecule that has the proper charge to permit heparin to bind.

LINDAHL, Uppsala Dr. Perlin, the bacterial eliminases are used for structural work, they would be even more useful, I think, if we knew the exact substrate specificity of these linkages. Now, for instance, with the heparinase, when you don't get disaccharide but get higher oligosaccharides, it is generally believed that this is due to under sulfation, lack of sulfates. My question would be is there any possibility that it could be a matter of confirmation of the sugar residues? For instance, if there would be occasional iduronic acid residues in *Cl* instead of *lC* chair confirmation, first how would that effect enzyme specificity, - or enzyme action, that might be difficult to answer? My second question is, could there be a small number of such residues?

PERLIN, Montreal Well, the information one has from NMR spectroscopy, of course is a time-average picture. If there were few residues, and it's awfully hard to visualize why that should be, I wouldn't say that that could not be possible. I think one would certainly not pick it up in the splitting pattern one sees. Due to the time-averaged situation, one would simply have either a very slight decrease in the coupling constant or a very slight increase in the coupling constant, and since one can't really relate coupling constants to dihedral angles that closely, a percentage, 10 or 15 percent either way would just simply not be picked up. One would have to speculate, I think rather rashly, to say that you could pick it up. I can't see why of course, some residues should have different confirmation than others if the chain is reasonably homogeneous. Although there has been recent evidence in looking at something like cyclohexamylose that one of the sugar residues is a slightly different shape than the other five in the solid state. It is rather surprising that this doesn't show up in the NMR spectrum in solution. Again there you would have a time-averaged situation, but there must be a tendency for that odd confirmation to be achieved in solution as well. It would be lost however, I think in the time-averaged picture.

LINDAHL, Uppsala One would assume, would one, that the glucuronic acids initially introduced into the heparin have *Cl* confirmation?

PERLIN, Montreal The *Cl* D confirmation would be the one certainly adopted by glucuronic acid residues unless there is some very severe restraint.

LINDAHL, Uppsala Right, and then the question is the chain confirmation. Would that occur as the *C5* carbon is epimerized or as the iduronic acid is 2-sulfated? In the latter case it might be conceivable that some iduronic acid residue remain in the *Cl*.

PERLIN, Montreal Well, electrostatic interactions, of course, really are very important, they have quite high energies and if through space attractions were such as to somehow hold some interaction between a carboxyl group in one residue and some other functionality, a free amino group, certainly not hydroxyl or sulfate groups. You would have to visualize some sort of interaction which would constrain the residue and keep it in that confirmation. I would expect that as the uronic acid moiety is being generated, the iduronic acid would simply flop over into the other confirmation. Certainly, in looking at sulfated iduronic acids or free iduronic acids the evidence is that these prefer the *1C* confirmation by a long shot.

DISCUSSION

SUE, Saskatoon I have a few words from Dr. Jaques regarding Dr. Linker's comments in the previous discussion. I think Dr. Linker indicated that we found mast cells in rabbits. Actually we found few mast cells in rabbits; instead we found quite a lot of blood basophils. These blood basophils don't contain heparin but chondroitin sulfate. We have found chondroitin sulfate and heparitin sulfate containing mast cells in chickens. We haven't found heparin yet. After extracting the mucopolysaccharides from dog skin mast cell tumor, 50% of the mucopolysaccharides found are not heparins.

BECK, Bern Is there any compelling evidence that these funny amino acids glycine and serine, if I understood correctly, are bound by true covalent peptides in your macromolecular heparin? And if so, how do you account for the genetic coding of the underlying either oligopeptide or protein? Do you think there is, for instance, a protease in tissue responsible for cleaving off this particular part of a larger protein which might be a repeating sequence? Is there any evidence that such a thing exists in tissues?

HORNER, Toronto Many of your questions are not answerable, but let's point out that macromolecular heparin is isolated after proteolytic digestion, and if we are going to get some meaningful information about the protein core, we must isolate the native proteoglycan. It contains those amino acids which bind the heparin chains, but I'm sure that there is another protein component as well, possibly something like in the diagram for the cartilage proteoglycan which Dr. Silbert showed, but if there was such a thing containing other amino acids it would be lost in the way in which we prepare the molecule.

LINDAHL, Uppsala I could add regarding your question as to the demonstration of regular peptide bonds, this has not yet been done. The polypeptide as such has not been isolated, but we have obtained a synthetic peptide with alternating ser-gly residues and have studied the properties of this peptide as acceptor for the mastocytomal xylosyltranserasse and it seems to work quite well as an acceptor provided that you go up to a molecular weight of 2 decapeptides. Small oligopeptides do not seem to work.

ROSENBERG, Boston Does the glycine seem to be important in such a primer, or could you substitute other residues?

ISBN 0-12-484850-8

LINDAHL, Uppsala I don't know.

BIANCHINI, Modena I have a question for Dr. Horner. We isolated a high molecular weight heparin from pancreas that is without anticoagulant and lipoprotein lipase releasing activity but is active on the complement system (evaluated as immune hemolysys). Have you similar data or not?

HORNER, Toronto No, I have no information on that whatsoever. I am aware that there are a lot of papers coming out recently on the action of heparin in the complement system, but nobody has even written to me yet for a sample of macromolecular heparin to see what it does in that system.

PADAWER, New York I find myself a little bit like a fish out of water here because my innate thinking is more along morphological lines than along the obviously chemical ones which have so far been emphasized. Tomorrow in my talk I will be foolhardy enough to suggest that the mast cell does not secrete its granules and that, therefore, the heparin that is inside the granules stays inside the mast cell, so that I find myself a little bit in trouble with all of these suggestions of how and what is happening to it once it is outside of the cell which I don't believe normally happens. Now, one interesting piece of datum that was given to us by Dr. Silbert before struck me, namely that within two hours he found roughly one-tenth of one percent of the total heparin in the mast cell becoming sulfated and this would mean that 100% of the mast cell heparin would be changed over in approximately 2.54 years, which is also roughly the life span of the rat, and this falls very neatly within the kind of arguments that I have used, which have been primarily morphological arguments, that indeed mast cell granules can be accounted for if properly tagged for at least 10 months - I presume I could continue - but I did not go beyond that, still it looks as if they stay within the mast cell. The second problem which I have is that I'm impressed, and you have succeeded in convincing me that we don't really know what heparin is except that we know what it isn't and it isn't one compound. That being the case, how can we, or can you tell me how I can link the mast cell heparin, for instance, with the heparin that is found either in association with lipoprotein lipase or that in the blood or that in platelets? My difficulty is that I suddenly feel that the rug has been pulled from under me and I can no longer try to think of the organism as a whole when I use the word heparin since there may be many sources. We are now faced with the real question, where is heparin made other than the mast cell and I would gather from what has been said here, that the vast majority of heparin, certainly that which you extract from various places, certainly from blood, probably does not come from mast cells, so where are we?

SILBERT, Boston This is opinion. I believe the heparin *is* made by mast cells and I think this is how I would define heparin. Heparin is a molecule which has these certain characteristic chemical compositions of high sulfate content, glucosamine, uronic acid, and perhaps a bizarre sort of proteoglycan structure, *is* made in mast cells, *is* stored in granules. Other proteoglycans that are similar I would classify as heparan sulfate; that material which appears to have smaller amounts of sulfate, usually, and seems to have a more characteristic proteoglycan structure. There is some work coming out in the literature now which seems to indicate that the heparan sulfate proteoglycan probably is similar to the chondroitin sulfate proteoglycan. I think that there is a difference, I think that mast cells do make a specific compound heparin. I don't think that this simplifies things at all.

LINDAHL, Uppsala Well, in a way, if we define heparin as something being made by mast cells it certainly couldn't be produced by any other cells.

SILBERT, Boston It could be, but I don't think it is. We've looked at some basophils also, I should add, the guinea pig basophils do not make heparin. Whether basophils in other animals do I don't know.

McDUFFIE, Saskatoon A question to Drs. Silbert and Padawer. If we are going to assume that the mast cell is the normal site of heparin, then are we to assume that the tissues used for regular commercial production are loaded with mast cells and indeed are they always demonstrably loaded with mast cells?

LINDAHL, Uppsala That's a good question. How about the mast cell content of pig intestinal mucosa for instance?

PADAWER, New York The richest source of mast cells is the lining of many organs.

MAHADOO, Saskatoon I understand Dr. McDuffie has been saying that heparin consists of some 20, 22 molecular species, and Dr. Horner suggested that heparin exists as a macromolecule and can be degraded into smaller functional units. I'm tempted to think that maybe heparin in the body starts as small sub units, possibly the lower molecular species. Dr. McDuffie found with electrofocusing that these sub units can be complex and perhaps they end up as the macromolecule of

Dr. Horner. I wonder if I can have some comments on that?

HORNER, Toronto I'm sure I didn't wish to imply that any of the products of my enzymes were single molecular weight species. I'm sure that if you took any of those and gave them to Dr. McDuffie to do electrofocusing he would get different patterns and if his electrofocusing presumably works on the basis of molecular weight, they would overlap. The point is that the polydispersity is a natural function of the molecule and the polysaccharide parts of these molecules are not made on a template. The switching off of the biosynthetic process is not precise at any distinct molecular weight, therefore, if you assume the action of the depolymerases I have discussed, you would get different proportions or products depending on the molecular size of the substrates. Hence, there is no reason why macromolecular heparin should not contain chains varying considerably in molecular size and therefore giving different products with degradative enzymes. I know for a fact that macromolecular heparin is polydisperse over a different magnitude range in just the same way as commercial heparin is polydisperse. In commercial heparin one is dealing with the individual chains after they have been split off from the protein backbone. I think we tried to show that in Dr. Lindahl's slide of enzymes acting at different places on different chains. No, they're not precise in terms of molecular weight at all. The molecular size range of commercial heparins can go from as low as 3000 or 4000 up to 30,000 and those could all exist bound to the same protein backbone. Their relative proportions could depend on some physiological stimulus. I refer you to Dr. Silbert's work showing how slowly the label in normal mast cells seems to go in until it's evenly distributed throughout the macromolecule. If there was some stimulus for the release of heparin that process might speed up and you'd get different proportions of molecular species.

McDUFFIE, Saskatoon I would tend to concur with Dr. Horner. I wouldn't be at all surprised if there is a great variation. I must admit to our own limitations because when we used Dr. Horner's sample, which he graciously provided, as I indicated it didn't penetrate the gel and due to pure laziness we didn't go to the batch process and I think that should be the next step. On the basis of what is being said today here I think we need to look at some of these *natural forms of the proteoglycan* - and put them into the electrofocusing system but I'll hasten to add that we cannot use the system as I presented it to you today. We now must go on to an entirely different system because that system is afunctional because of the penetration limitation of the gel. The possibility of low molecular weight components complexing to form a macromolecular material requires study.

LINDAHL, Uppsala If you take one of the bands, isolate on a preparative scale, and rerun it single - does it focus on just the same place in the gradiant?

McDUFFIE, Saskatoon It does if it's the lung heparin. If it's the mucosal heparin, it essentially focuses in the same place as well, but other components appear with the mucosal heparin bands that focus along the gradient, which doesn't appear to occur with the lung heparin.

ROSENBERG, Boston It's very important that if you are going to test the homogeneity of the band on rerunning it that you use precisely the same concentration of component on the rerun as you had initially in the total sample or else it's really not a valid test of the band running true.

McDUFFIE, Saskatoon Yes. That's a valid point. In our system on the reruns we have not rigorously observed this, I must admit, because our limitations have been that for all comparative studies we use one concentration. On the rerun we've used what we've had available because we oftentimes can't meet those concentration requirements.

KRAEMER, Los Alamos I understand that both Dr. Silbert and Dr. Horner have utilized ascorbic acid degradation and wonder if one of them could answer the following question? As I understand it, the original work with ascorbic acid degradation utilizing hyaluronate, indicated that these oxidoreductive cleavages were essentially random, since hyaluronate is an homogeneous polymer this followed from the fact that degradation occurred. Consequently one wonders what the purpose of using ascorbic acid degradation is since there may not be such a thing as a sensitive bond but that the material of any polymer could be cleaved in a few places randomly using this reagent including...possibly the peptide moiety?

HORNER, Toronto The use of ascorbate was serendipitous. It is certainly something that has not been done in my laboratory for many years precisely because it's mode of action is not known. It was used purely because my feeling when we first discovered macromolecular heparin was that it had to be a proteoglycan and that we were doing something wrong - so we went on, and on, hitting it with papain. As you know papain requires reducing conditions, we found that if we left the papain out and still used the buffer providing the reducing conditions we still got slow depolymerization of macromolecular heparin. Therefore I proceeded to try ascorbic acid, which seemed to be more efficient in this kind of oxidative-reductive depolymerization and got some dramatic effects. They have no physiological significance they just helped us to surmise that the thing must be multichained. I do not agree that it's random in the case of macromolecular heparin, gel filtration of the products gives two distinct separable species, furthermore, gel filtration patterns of products taken at different times would very much look like the graphs I showed today for the action of an enzyme - so I don't agree that it's random. Ascorbate produces something in the same molecular size range as pig mucosal heparin. What I think we may do some day is look at our enzymic products to see if the enzymes have attacked the same linkage regions as ascorbate. However, I once read an attempt by Rodin *et al.* to define the regions attacked by ascorbate in hyaluronic acid and I realized the enormity of the problem and never attempted it with rat skin heparin. It was useful in giving us an idea of the possible physiological significance because we showed that you could degrade the macromolecule without losing biological activity and that was one stimulus to look for enzymes that would do the same thing. Certainly it wasn't a stringent organic reagent used because it attacked a known specific bond. In defense of Dr. Silbert, I don't think that he has ever used ascorbate, have you, Dr. Silbert?

SILBERT, Boston We used it, but did not publish.

LINDAHL, Uppsala I think it would be very interesting now to discuss the possible mechanism of proteoglycan assembly on the basis of the model proposed by Dr. Silbert or the two alternative models that were left by Dr. Silbert on the basis of his labeling experiments. If I recall your previous data correctly you showed that polymerization and sulfation of heparin (as of chondroitin sulfate) are both extremely rapid processes. We also found this in our mastocytomal system, yet the two models that you presented here seem to involve change of one molecule over a long period of time. Can you reconcile these two views?

SILBERT, Boston Yes, in the work with chondroitin sulfate we were talking about the synthesis of an individual polysaccharide chain and that occurs very rapidly, but we don't know whether that represents addition of more chains onto a single proteoglycan molecule that has fewer chains or whether that means the entire proteoglycan molecule. We have not addressed that problem. In this case (heparin) it would appear that more chains are being added, that probably the core is intact and more chains are added with time. The two don't conflict, the same thing could very well be happening in the chondroitin sulfate proteoglycan biosynthesis as well. What we are saying is that in chondroitin sulfate a chain is formed in total and in the heparin proteoglycan model the same thing is occurring. We don't find different polysaccharides chains, they are all approximately the same, the early or the late, so that the polysaccharide chain is formed in total, but the individual chains could be added over a period of time. The thing that disturbs me about the heparin model is the length of time required (hours). If it were 5-10 minutes I would feel happier with it. We've repeated these experiments, we don't always find this phenomenon. At times material incubated for two hours looks very similar to material incubated for eight hours. There still was a very great polydispersity in terms of size of the proteoglycan. Variations in sulfation occur, there was a smaller amount of sulfate in small proteoglycan than in the larger size. The question of this change with time is not quite so clear but the polydispersity of size still holds.

LINDAHL, Uppsala There is a difference between this system and the chondroitin sulfate in that when you isolate the product by use of proteolytic enzymes you really get single chains, whereas in this case you would isolate the whole macromolecule. Or don't you even use proteolytic enzymes?

SILBERT, Boston Whether we use them or don't use them, we get the same thing. The whole molecule is obtained. The only thing that this molecule has seen is one molar sodium chloride. Aside from that we could call it native. It's just extracted from the cells by freezing and thawing without use of any other agent.

LINDAHL, Uppsala So your view would then be that there is one polypeptide core and then polysaccharide chains grow out from this same core over a very prolonged period of time but by very rapid growth of the individual polysaccharide chains.

SILBERT, Boston Yes, I would say that's what's happening.

McDUFFIE, Saskatoon Is there a critical length of polypeptide chain that is reached, or does the chain of polypeptide continue to grow as well?

SILBERT, Boston I don't know.

McDUFFIE, Saskatoon The reason I asked is that in a similar but not identical system using canine mastocytoma, in terms of the electrofocusing pattern, we were surprised that we found very little low molecular weight material. This would seem to be at variance with your comments of random growth. It would seem that there must be some critical point that's reached in time at which the chains just elongate and there is no further change.

SILBERT, Boston I think we're getting a little confusion here. Are you talking about the polysaccharide chains or the peptide chains?

McDUFFIE, Saskatoon Both, if it were a question of new polypeptide chains growing as well, then there would be little branches coming off beyond the critical size, but if polypeptide chain growth stops, the only place for polysaccharide growth is out from that. This would reduce the amount of low molecular weight material.

SILBERT, Boston Or add more chains. Now when we looked at the material that had been removed from the proteoglycan by alkali whether it was small proteoglycan or large proteoglycan, the average size of the chain was the same. However, this was very polydisperse so there were small chains and large chains - I have my own pet theory as to why you get this variation in size of the polysaccharide. I visualize the synthetic site as something of a cup. A fold in a membrane - like a cup with the protein core in the center and the enzymes for polymerization, sulfation, etc., distributed around the sides of that cup, and that protein core can move back and forth slightly, and the synthesis goes on very rapidly on that individual protein core as those enzymes attach. When the cup is filled, the polysaccharide chain stops growing. Depending upon the configuration of that cup, some chains are going to be longer than others and there is going to be a great random distribution in the size of the chains. This is the way I visualize it and I would think that the same thing could be occurring in the case of heparin. Why would you get fewer chains? Perhaps it's a limitation in the amount of substrate that is presented to the enzyme at the time. The synthesis occurs on one chain at a time, once the end of that chain attaches to the enzyme on the surface of that cup then that chain would be rapidly built. If one hasn't enough substrate, then there wouldn't be as many chains. It's conceivable that in the case of the mast cell the material could sit at the synthetic site for hours before being transported to the granules and could grow with time as more substrate is presented to it.

LINDAHL, Uppsala It is quite striking I think that there is such a marked difference between the neoplastic mast cell of the mouse mastocytoma and the peritoneal mast cells that you have. You find slow continued growth of the molecule to reach maximal size after a long time, we find that the newly synthesized material, after *in vivo* labelling has a very large molecular weight and then rapidly decreases in molecular size. The reason for the decrease is the endoglycosidase degradation and perhaps these enzymes are not present in your system. If you isolate the microsomal polysaccharide that is formed after very brief incubation with labeled nucleotide sugars; isolate it carefully by guanidine extraction, it is excluded from a sepharose 2B column. It seems to have a molecular weight of a million.

SILBERT, Boston This is the newly synthesized material of the microsomal fraction? I'm not surprised at that. We are talking about two different factors. We're talking about the polysaccharide size as opposed to the proteoglycan. I think the polysaccharide size in the rat mast cell system is probably similar to what you see in your mouse system except that the endoglycosidase is not present. When we looked at the Dunn and Potter mastocytomas we found there was no proteoglycan, just single polysaccharide chains. I wonder if these endoglycosidases are functional in the system, if they are, why don't they cleave the newly synthesized material that's synthesized *in vitro* and separate it from its protein core or separate it from the microsomal preparation. They don't. The material remains bound to a membrane fraction and can be separated by standard proteolytic enzymes, e.g., pancreatin.

LINDAHL, Uppsala It may be that these two events, degradation and biosynthesis, take place in two different compartments which are united only in a living cell. But going back to your question, how do you know the microsomal product is not proteoglycan, it would be resistant to proteolytic digestion?

SILBERT, Boston No, I think the microsomal product is proteoglycan because it is sensitive to proteolytic digestion but it is different from rat mast cell proteoglycan which is resistant to proteolytic digestion.

LINDAHL, Uppsala What do you mean when you say it is suceptible to proteolytic digestion?

SILBERT, Boston With the mouse tumor material a polysaccharide with a molecular weight of about 40,000 is released. Yours is the same length isn't it?

LINDAHL, Uppsala Yes, but we make the mistake of isolating things with papain digestion which causes nonspecific degradation.

SILBERT, Boston This is pancreatin digestion, or alkali, the same size fragment is obtained whether it's liberated with alkali or with pancreatin approximately 30,000 to 40,000 molecular weight. It's larger than commercial heparin.

PADAWER, New York I'd like to come back to the cytology again. Proteins are assembled in the rough endoplasmic reticulum, polysaccharide material is added to the protein in the golgi apparatus and sulfation also takes place in the golgi apparatus, yet the granules themselves are in neither of these two organelles as we understand them, certainly not in the rough E.R. and possibly in an extension of the golgi but not in the traditional golgi. If we look at mast cells by certain staining methods, whether it is the sequential Alcian Blue-Saffranin method or by another method that I use which is a mixture of two basic dyes, different granules within the mast cells stain differently, mixtures of blue stained granules and red stained granules appear. Indeed, the mast cells change as a function of age over a rather long period of time, at least 14 days (a time span that Dr. Silbert mentioned). So we have this continuation of a maturation of the granules in terms of their dye binding capacity which I intuitively feel is related to the chemical questions addressed here. How would Dr. Silbert fit his scheme to the assembly according to the chart that you showed since obviously the protein core would have to be made up in the rough E.R. and the polysaccharide added at some distance and sulfation perhaps also, and still further along in the granules we have continuing maturation, which must involve the difference between highly sulfated and less sulfated granules. This is the generally accepted argument in terms of the dye binding, that the Alcian Blue binds to carboxyl groups whereas the Saffranin binds to the more acidic sulfates?

SILBERT, Boston I can conceive of two possibilities. One is that with time the molecule is made with more chains on it. This doesn't mean that the same molecule is having more chains added to it. It's conceivable that with time in this *in vitro* system for some reason a different molecule is formed. It would suggest that after two hours incubation the material is packaged up and put into granules and it only has X amount of polysaccharide chains on it. After four hours for some reason the mast cell is changed in its metabolic scheme - it's not producing the same way and now it's making more highly polysaccharide substituted proteoglycan. This is one possibility.

I should comment on some work from Dr. Austen's laboratory. They released granules by various methods, e.g., by calcium iontophore, and showed a linear release of histamine with proteoglycan heparin but in addition, when they looked at the material that had been labeled after two hours, the material that was released tended to be the older, larger heparin, and the newly formed radioactive heparin was not released to as great an extent. This would suggest that either this newly synthesized heparin had not gotten to the granules, or if it had gotten to the granules, these granules were immature and were not releasing their heparin to the same extent as the material that had been formed there before.

CONRAD, Urbana I don't know whether you gave the conditions of your incubation but these are whole mast cells that you've got in culture and you are labeling - is that correct?

SILBERT, Boston That's correct. The culture medium is Tyrode's.

CONRAD, Urbana Does it have serine in it? Does it have any cold sulfate in it?

SILBERT, Boston Yes, well when we add the hot sulfate we add a known amount of cold sulfate to have a specific concentration so that we know its specific activity exactly.

CONRAD, Urbana The reason I'm asking is because we have recently done some work with labeling of chondrocytes with glucosamine and found that the specific activity of the nucleoside diphosphate N-acetyl hexosamine varied with the glucose concentration in the medium, so that these both fed into the same pool and changed the specific activity as the glucose was consumed. I'm wondering if the specific activity of your serine pool is changing during the labeling periods so that accounts for the dilution of the amount of label from serine going into your final product.

SILBERT, Boston Well, two answers to that - number 1, I don't see how that's possible really in the sense that so little is being incorporated in terms of actual total amount that I don't think that we are depleting the pool. We have no idea of what the specific activity of the serine is just for the same reason that you mentioned about the glucosamine. We do know as far as the sulfate is concerned, but the other thing is that we can look at material which is formed in two hours and we get small and large heparin which mimics the situation of a long term incubation.

UVNÄS, Stockholm Dr. Linker mentioned very briefly that one function of heparin should be to activate chymotrypsin and I would like you to comment a little more on that statement and its significance.

LINKER, Salt Lake City There was a recent paper that showed that heparin activated chymotrypsin similar to heparin activation of antithrombin. The comment in the paper was, as chymotrypsin is also present in mast cells one of the functions of heparin may be the activation of chymotrypsin. I have the reference if you'd like.

UVNÄS, Stockholm No, I don't need it. Rat peritoneal mast cell granules are insoluble in water and have a very high chymotrypsin activity. Most of the protein in the granule may be chymotrypsin. Heparin is not necessary for its activation. I have another question or comment that is, when Dr. Horner mentioned the possible activation of the lipoprotein lipase by heparin - this I think must be then different in different animals. In rats and other animals where the granules are insoluble, heparin doesn't leave the granules. It is difficult to understand how the heparin in these granules can activate any lipase in blood.

HORNER, Toronto Dr. Uvnäs, I entirely agree that the heparin in the mast cells does not activate lipoprotein lipase. I presented data showing that heparin in the molecular size range of that in the mast cell granules inhibits lipoprotein lipase. I believe that the mast cell exports some of its heparin in a low molecular weight form which can activate lipoprotein lipase whether it contains the depolymerases to release that physiologically active low molecular weight form or that these depolymerases are waiting to seize granules released containing the macromolecular form. I don't know but I intend to pursue that.

UVNÄS, Stockholm What animals do you use?

HORNER, Toronto We worked with rats too.

UVNÄS, Stockholm Have you any experimental evidence that low molecular weight heparin is released from the mast cells or is this just a suggestion?

HORNER, Toronto Oh, it's a suggestion, the only thing we've done, I mentioned already, was unphysiological that was to cause the mast cells to degranulate with compound 48/80 and then the granules got out with depolymerization of the macromolecular heparin. Something is doing it, for instance the last data I gave you was on the presence of both high and low molecular weight endogeneous heparins in adipose tissues. Are those both inside the mast cell or is the high molecular weight inside and the low molecular outside, I don't know. It was a very stimulating but preliminary experiment, that does show that depolymerization can occur.

UVNÄS, Stockholm There are old experiments using rats with mast cell granules labeled with radioactive sulfur and challenging these cells with 48/80, if I recall correctly, yields no release of radioactivity from the granules, at least very, very, little, so the question becomes *is any heparin released from these granules?*

PADAWER, New York Tomorrow I will propose that mast cells take things in from the environment in one direction, carry it over the granules and then dump it, much like chromatography columns. Use of degranulating agents, e.g., 48/80, causes the back door to be forced open and materials from the extracellular fluid can enter. Things like sodium and other cations are incompatible with maintaining the histamine association with the protein-polysaccharide of the granules and the cell flies to pieces. This is an unnatural situation. The normal function of the mast cell is to take things in and to do something to what it has taken in and that's where the mast cell granule begins to play a role. As far as Dr. Silbert's argument that the old material comes out first, this would be perfectly understandable, first in first out. Mast cell granules labeled with thorium dioxide may be observed in the electron-microscope. After flash labeling, mast cells still show the same number of granules labeled with the thorotrast for periods up to ten months suggesting that these granules were not released under the normal life of the rat in an animal room in a medical school. Hence we must reconcile the morphological and chemical studies.

LINDAHL, Uppsala In the rat the mast cell does not degranulate. Is there any situation under physiological conditions in any animal in which the mast cell is known to degranulate?

PADAWER, New York It depends upon what you mean by physiological conditions. If for instance you create a situation with a lot of IgE available and the antigen is presented after the IgE has become bound to the mast cell, degranulation will occur. I'm working on the supposition that that is not what the mast cell is present for. It is there for something different, for some everyday need that the body has and this can be derailed by some unusual circumstances such as a severe allergy and presentation of a large amount of antigen or by other things such as 48/80 or other basic cation, or polycation, that's in fact what causes it in wasp bite. So normally I would say offhand no. To the extent that the mast cell becomes degranulated, it is nonfunctional. If you degranulated it a little bit, it is less than fully operational. If you degranulate it completely, it ceases to function in its normal natural way, then yes, otherwise no.

SILBERT, Boston I'm not sure that I understand why Dr. Padawer feels that hypersensitivity is not a normal function of mast cells. They certainly do seem to function and in all sorts of sensitivity reactions and why do you feel that's not what mast cells are supposed to be doing?

PADAWER, New York Well for one thing the moment degranulation occurs nothing is left. I's a sort of all or none reaction which I find difficult to accept. It takes so long to replace the granule, approximately 50 days, while we are really left with our mast cells down, I can't imagine a system that is there to protect us that will react and then be finished and unable to respond for us for another 50 days. There is something about the physiological aspects of this as a protecting system in the immune area which is not convincing. I think that mast cells probably play a role in the immune area and my guess at the moment, and it's a very wild guess, might be that it has to do with self-nonself recognition. Now, probably, some other immune globulin including IgE can somehow trick the system and cause degranulation. I will touch upon that a little bit tomorrow. I think we are just in the beginning of trying to look at that, but the idea that mast cells release either heparin or histamine, I think should be put in the past. It has been something that has stimulated us to do a lot of very good studies, but I don't think that they are really to the mark. I think that it is very much something that is an accident of fate. What we should really look at is what do mast cells do when they don't degranulate? Once they degranulate they have had it.

BECK, Bern I think it's a very dangerous argument for basic research to look for a sense of a given system because we have many things that are rather more harmful than useful in our body even under the most physiological circumstances, such as the way our coagulation system functions. I think the mast cell may be a very old ancestor that doesn't necessarily lead to many great things in our body but may be very disagreeable in given circumstances.

UVNÄS, Stockholm I think we will come back to this problem tomorrow, but I just would like to make a comment on what Dr. Padawer has said. He said that the response of a mast cell to antigen in a hypersensitivity reaction is an all or none phenomenon. That is not true because you can challenge mast cells with various concentrations of antigens and you can see anything from one granule coming out, to all of them. So there is a graded response of a mast to the concentration of the antigen or the challenging agent. Theoretically, you might very well think that one releasing agent, a polypeptide or a molecule of a toxin, when it hits the mast cell surface causes a local reaction, and out will come one or two or more granules or contents of granules. We have to be, I think, a little more flexible about the action of a mast cell and its response to challenging agents and such challenging agents can exist under physiological conditions.

HIGGENBOTHAM, Louisville I would like to add to that. About six months ago we spent an afternoon counting granules in mast cells and it seems there are something like 700 granules per mast cell. I think it is very difficult for a mast cell to be watching all of its granules all of the time, as might be suggested by Dr. Padawer. It is difficult to believe that it keeps them intact, particularly, in terms of the large number of mast cells that do exist in the body. It's probably quite reasonable to suggest that a single mast cell granule or a few of them are being released all of the time as suggested by the work on IgG_1 (anaphylactic antibody). This is a very modest type of degranulating agent as compared to the IgE which gives an explosive type of degranulation in which the heparin and histamine are being released concomitantly. There is no problem either in suggesting the possibility that a macroheparin form is released that is subsequently degraded by an adjacent cell that picks it up and begins to digest it with its lysosomal capacity, such as the macrophage or even the fibroblast. I don't think that we have to consider the mast cell is existing in a vacuum in the laboratory, in all animals or in all species. This might be if we were examining just peritoneal mast cells.

HORNER, Toronto In listening to Dr. Padawer, it brought back to memory one report that I read on mast cells as having a physiological function which seemed perfectly reasonable to me. If you cannulate the bile duct of rats and then proceed to give them a high lipid diet you find mast cell granules in the bile. I don't see what is so unphysiological about that.

LINDAHL, Uppsala I think that if we go on with this discussion there will be nothing left to discuss tomorrow. Are any more questions specifically related to the lectures given today?

COLEMAN, Kalamazoo Can any one comment on the linkages in the heparins, are these all alpha or beta or is there a definite ratio between these two different types of linkages?

LINKER, Salt Lake City It is possible that there are a few other linkages that we are not aware of, but in general I think everyone, at least has agreed that all of the hexosamine linkages are alpha, that the glucuronidic linkages, which are a minor uronic linkage, are beta D and the iduronidic linkages are all alpha L. But with all the work done, even including Dr. Perlin's NMR, one cannot be completely certain that one may not miss some different linkage. It is extremely unlikely, I would say, that you have an additional linkage type in heparin, of course, it isn't that long ago, that Wolfrom very definitely showed that all the uronidic linkages were alpha D, so one should not make any very positive statements as I have just done.

DIETRICH, São Paulo I disagree, partially, with Professor Linker, about the type of linkages that are in heparitin sulfate for instance or even in heparin with alpha D glucuronic acid, versus beta D glucuronic acid. We have two lines of evidence, both indirect unfortunately, so that it is open for discussion but I think I have a tendency to agree with Wolfrom. The reasons are as follows: If you have a very purified heparitin sulfate B the measured optical rotation is greater than 100, positive. The second line of evidence is the specificity of glycuronidase. This enzyme is able to degrade all of the disaccharides that are produced either from heparin or from heparitin sulfate. This fact suggests either that all of those linkages are beta D type or alpha D type, and with this strong positive optical rotation I think it would favor an alpha D type linkage for glucuronic acid. The enzymes that are also present in *Fl. heparinum* are glycuronidases which degrade disaccharides from chondroitin sulfates. These enzymes are specific for disaccharides produced from chondroitin sulfates which we all agree are beta D-glucuronic acid type linkages. So I still hold the position that most of the linkages in heparitin sulfate and heparin are the alpha D type.

LINDAHL, Uppsala Would Dr. Perlin care to comment on that?

PERLIN, Montreal Well, I don't think one can be categorical. We have several pieces of spectroscopic evidence. We do use enzymes occadionally but we aren't very expert at handling them so I wouldn't want to comment on our enzymatic results.

Certainly the NMR spectra are helpful in giving configurational assignments. One has to be careful about the quality of the spectra, and the fragments that we have isolated from mucosal heparin, tetrasaccharide for example, in my opinion are definitely beta. The rotation is a little hard to relate because one is dealing with a fairly big fragment and one has to then be able to add up all of the contributions to the overall molecular rotation, but certainly the NMR spectrum is consistent with the beta and not with alpha at all. The same applies to the major fractions that we find from heparan sulfate or heparatin, the glucuronic acid residues both in terms of chemical shift in the carbon 13 NMR's and the proton NMR's, the coupling constants in the proton NMR's, the coupling constants in the carbon 13 NMR's are all consistent with the beta D configuration and not an alpha configuration. The one piece of evidence which suggested an alpha D configuration, Peter (Dr. Dietrich), was the material which as you remember I told you didn't give a good enough spectrum to rely on suggested an alpha gluco configuration perhaps on an unsaturated disaccharide but that's the one piece of evidence contrary to the others. So that I have no evidence from any of the fractions that we have looked at that glucuronic acid residues either in heparitin or in heparin indeed have an alpha configuration.

WEISSMANN, Chicago I wouldn't like to go into great detail at this point because we're not ready to report this work in completion, but we have been in the process of accounting for beef lung heparin in terms of its nitrous acid products quite completely. All that can be said is that all of the disaccharides one gets, and these are separable, which contain glucuronic acid are substrates for beta glucuronidase, from rat prepucial gland which is a fairly pure preparation not like commercial preparations and with which no action can be shown on synthetic alpha glucuronides. As far as beef lung heparin goes, I would be rather doubtful that anyone will ever find any alpha glucuronidic linkages in it.

LINDAHL, Uppsala I think we could add to this from the biosynthetic studies that the heparin precursor contains only glucuronic acid linkages when this is degraded with nitrous acid you get oligosaccharides and all of the nonreducing terminals can be completely released with beta glucuronidase a commercial preparation but it was shown not to attack alpha glucuronides.

WEST, Birmingham I can't say much about which kind of linkage you have, but I would like to present a little bit of evidence that we have been getting which indicates perhaps some cautions that should be observed. We have been studying the interaction of acridine orange with heparin and the rate at which the fading of this fluorescence takes place. The evidence we have experimentally indicates that only a small number of the dye molecules which are bound actually fluoresce, and it appears to us that after a photon is absorbed there is an excitatory migration of this energy down the heparin molecule until some anomaly is reached. Something is encountered which is different and therefore permits either a photochemical reaction or fluorescence to occur. We do have these anomalies down the length of the chains and it may be that blanket statements and most of the data generally based upon averages of large numbers should be treated a little bit cautiously.

LINDAHL, Uppsala Thank you, I think it is certainly true that a number of statements here are based on preconceived notions and this may be particularly true not so much perhaps for the glycosidic linkage but for the position of the sulfate groups where we all assume that they are located at *C6* of the glucosamine and *C2* of the iduronic acid. It has been suggested by Danishefsky for instance, on methylation data, that a portion of the glucosamine residues are sulfated at *C3* although it is probably a minor constituent, it could be very significant in relation to the specific binding of proteins or to conformational changes.

DIETRICH, São Paulo With regard to sulfate, even if another position is sulfated I think the percentage would be very low. I think that Danishefsky's work has shown that these would be around three or four percent if I'm not mistaken. Some *C3* sulfates might be found on the hexosamine of the heparin molecule but again you have to discuss that in terms of biological purity. Perhaps that could be still another molecule as we have seen in the heparitin sulfate; 95% of the sulfate at least is at the *6C* position.

STRUCTURE AND PHARMACODYNAMICS

SOME STRUCTURE-FUNCTION RELATIONSHIPS OF HEPARINS AND THEIR COMPONENT FRACTIONS

Sigmund E. Lasker

Department of Medicine
New York Medical College

Several active factors involved cooperatively in blood coagulation, both *in vivo* and *in vitro*, interact with high specificity with a family of structurally similar, naturally occurring sulfated polysaccharides called heparins. Dermatan sulfate, chondroitin sulfate, and heparan sulfate have little or no activity in this system or are active only at high concentrations.

Considerable effort has been expended exploring structural factors associated with activity using heparins prepared commercially or isolated in the laboratory (1). The commercial heparins are derived from different species, fed different dietary supplements, and isolated by modified techniques. It is not known if these variables influence the structural or biological parameters that are generally measured. The N-acetyl content and molecular weight of random commercial samples of heparin bear no relationship to biological activity measured by the USP technique (2-5). It has not been possible to correlated variations in chemical or functional group analysis of random samples of heparin with biological activity. An operational definition of the substance isolated or available commercially is that it possesses a high specific anticoagulant activity.

Heparin may act at several sites throughout the coagulation cascade (6,7) by combining with naturally occurring inhibitors and thereby accelerate the rate of inhibition of all the coagulation factors that have serine esterase sites. The interaction between antithrombin III and heparin appears to be highly specific and apparently no other polyelectrolyte can substitute for heparin at equivalent concentrations (8).

Some other biological activities of heparin, mediated through various mechanisms, may have some specificity or may be properties exclusively of its polyelectrolyte character. Other *in vivo* activities of heparin include protective action in endotoxin shock (9), diuretic action by inhibition of aldosterone production (10,11), interaction with platelets (12), and the display of carcino embryonic antigen activity (13). Heparins also have varying effects on cell proliferation that are unrelated to anticoagulant activity (14). The

ISBN 0-12-484850-8

structural requirements of lipoprotein lipase activation have not been defined.

I. ASSAYS BY DIFFERENT METHODS

Jaques (15) had demonstrated that a wide range of values can be obtained when a series of heparins are examined by a variety of indices of anticoagulant potency including *in vivo* tests. Anderson (16) also demonstrated that anticoagulant activities were markedly different when assayed by activated partial thromboplastic time or by anti-Xa activity.

The various methods for assaying heparin including whole blood clotting time (WBCT), activated partial thromboplastin time (APTT), *in vivo* assays, lipoprotein lipase activation, metachromatic methods, protamine neutralization, thrombin time, and recalcification time reveal differences between preparations of a single species. (20)

II. MOLECULAR WEIGHT MEASUREMENTS

Studies of physicochemical properties including molecular weight of fractionated polyelectrolytes and particularly heparin and heparin-like mixtures have been performed (3,18,19,26,27,28). The values obtained are sensitive to the conditions under which the measurements are made. At low pH the apparent molecular weight and partial specific volume are influenced at high ionic strength between 0.5 *M* and 1.0 *M* (28). At an ionic strength of 0.5 *M* both apparent molecular weight and partial specific volume are pH sensitive.

Gel permeation column estimates of molecular weight are dependent on a series of standards, preferable also polyelectrolytes, and are also sensitive to the ionic strength and composition of the mobile phase (29).

III. SOME STRUCTURAL REQUIREMENTS FOR ANTICOAGULANT ACTIVITY

Desulfation and resulfation of heparin (17) have demonstrated the importance of the sulfamino group for anticoagulant activity. The relationship of molecular weight to anticoagulant activity has been suggested by a number of investigators who have fractionated heparins by a variety of techniques (18,19,21,22,23,24,25). As many as 22 fractions have been prepared from a single source. A variety of techniques were used for fractionation. Polyacrylamide-agarose gel column fractionation (16) produced five heparin fractions, molecular weights were estimated by viscometry using the Mark-Houwink relationship and the biological activity was estimated by the partial thromboplastic time.

McDuffie (23) used electrofocusing to separate commerical heparin. Molecular weights were estimated on the basis of movement of fractions on gel slabs compared to chondroitin sulfate B, heparitin sulfate C, and a hexasaccharide obtained by enzymatic degradation. Anticoagulant activity was determined by USP assay. Laurent (18) fractionated heparin by cetyl pyridinium chloride precipitation and was able to separate a commercial preparation into four fractions of varying molecular weight and anticoagulant activity. Molecular weights were determined by an ultracentrifuge approach to equilibrium method and anticoagulant activity was measured by the method of Studer and Winterstein.

Lasker and Stivala (19) were able to prepare 11 fractions by nonsolvent-solvent elution of commercial heparins at low concentration of solute, while five fractions were obtained from an ECTEOLA Column. Molecular weights were estimated by equilibrium ultracentrifugation in a three-component system. Anticoagulant activity was measured by the USP method.

Up to eight fractions of heparin were recovered by use of solvent-nonsolvent precipitation with either ethanol or dioxane as the nonsolvents (25). Molecular weight was estimated by equilibrium ultracentrifugation. USP assay provided an index of anticoagulant activity. Cifonelli (21) was able to prepare up to five fractions by gel filtration. Molecular weights were estimated by use of a gel-filtration diagram established with heparin and heparin sulfate fractions of known molecular weight. Viscosity data were used to determine molecular weights. Anderson (16) showed a molecular size dependency for eight fractions prepared by gel filtration on Ultro gel column. Anticoagulant activity was estimated by the activated partial thromboplastic time and by the anti-Xa assay.

Figure 2 shows a composite of the above data where the molecular weight and anticoagulant activity for six preparations by different authors has been plotted. The data reveal a region of linearity in the low molecular weight range. The region of linearity for the preparations included in this survey spans the range 4000 to 14,000 daltons. There is considerable scatter of points in the upper molecular weight range. The data suggest that some critical portion of the molecule of appreciable molecular weight, i.e., the order of an octamer, as well as steric and conformational factors within this sequence could contribute to the unique biological properties of heparin.

Whether biological activity is confined to a component of the polymer admixture and to a particular sequence within a single chain, or whether several functional groups from more than a single chain, acting in concert, provide this activity

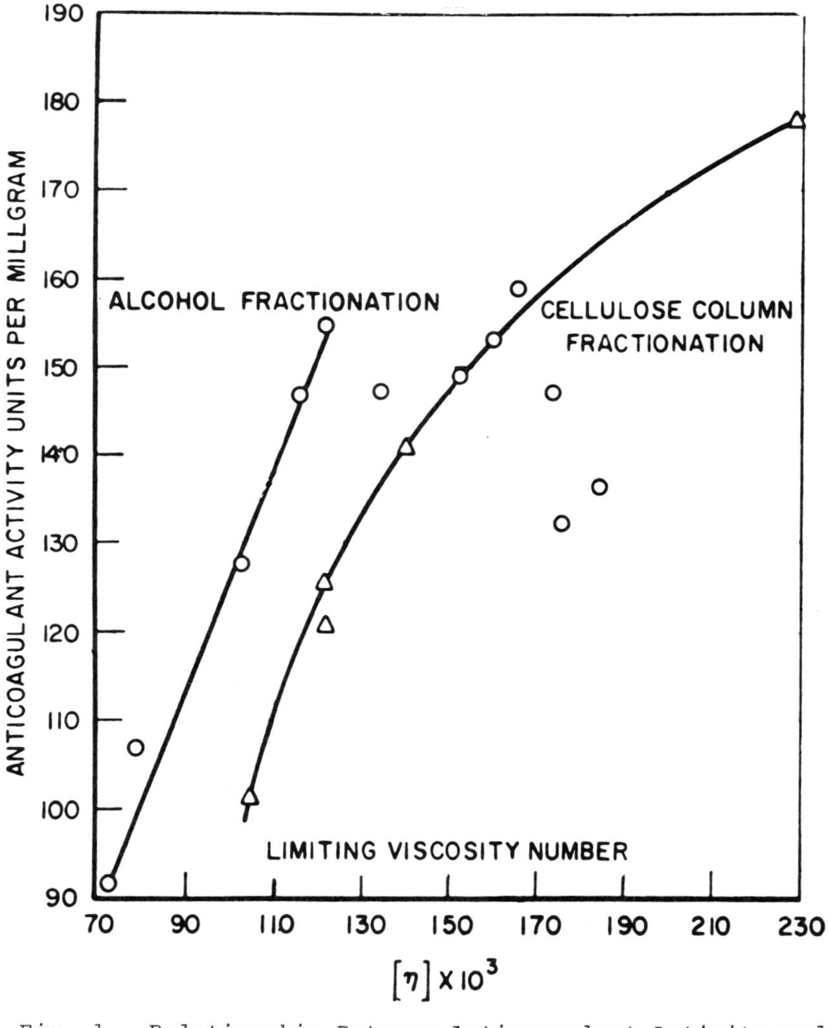

Fig. 1. Relationship Between Anticoagulant Activity and Viscosity for Heparin Fractions. Alcohol fractionation was accomplished in a dilute solution of heparin with increasing concentrations of ethanol from 41% to 65% (1a). Cellulose column fractionation yielded four fractions at NaCl concentrations of 0.3 M to 0.6 M. The relation of anticoagulant activity measured by USP assay to molecular weight in terms of limiting viscosity number is shown. The cellulose fractionation yielded the fraction of highest activity. At high molecular weight there is considerable scatter of values with some reduction in anticoagulant activity for fractions having the highest molecular weight.

has not been established. It appears however there is a minimum molecular weight requirement for biological activity, and there appears to be some critical maximum length for maximum activity.

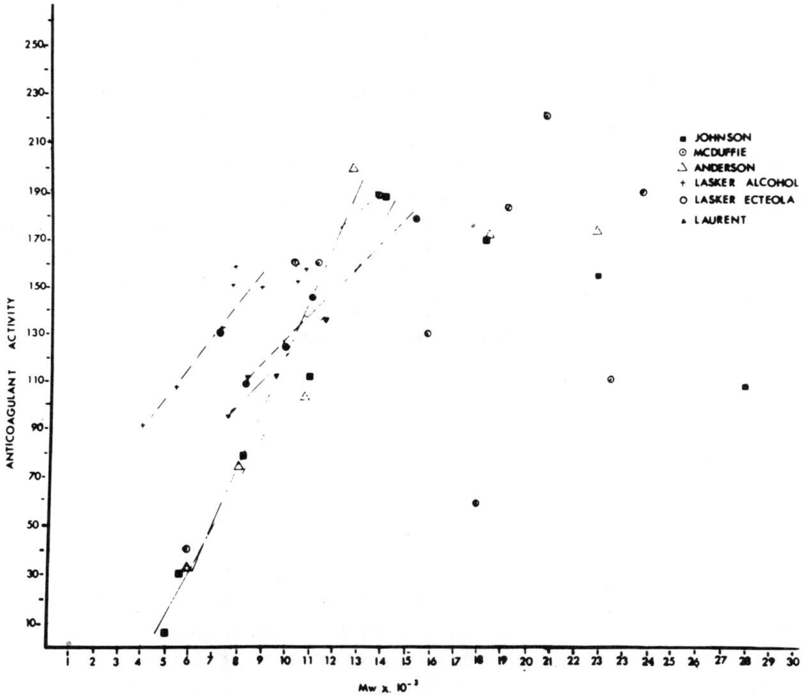

Fig. 2. A Comparison of Anticoagulant Activity Versus Molecular Weight Data from Literature. Molecular weights were estimated by Gel permeation or by the ultracentrifuge. Anticoagulant activity was measured by various methods cited in the text. Where large numbers of fractions have been obtained (McDuffie, Lasker, Johnson, Anderson). The high molecular weight range of the MW-activity curve shows scatter. For alcohol fractions, the nonlinear scatter occurs at MW 7000, for isoelectric focusing the linearity ceases at 14,000 Daltons.

IV. DISPLACEMENT OF MOLECULAR WEIGHT DISTRIBUTION BY DEPOLYMERIZATION

By controlled depolymerization of commercial heparin, either by heparinase or by a free radical method, low molecular fragments with appreciable activity can be isolated (Table I). The depolymerized products can be separated into a series of fractions of varying molecular weight and anticoagulant activity with no detectable alteration in the molecule (31). Proton magnetic spectra of the larger fragments that retain appreciable anticoagulant activity are essentially similar (31). The displacement of the distribution curve with no overlap toward the lower molecular weight suggests that all the polysaccharide chains have experienced cleavage at at least one site.

TABLE I. Molecular Weight Dispersion of Fractionated Commercial and Depolymerized Heparins

Preparation		*Molecular Weight*	*Anticoagulant Activity I.U./mg*
Heparin		*11,600*	*139*
Fraction	*A*	*15,800*	*170*
	B	*13,200*	*150*
	C	*9,000*	*100*
	D	*6,680*	*70*
Depolymerized		*5,300*	*70*
Fraction	*A*	*5,900*	*95*
	B	*4,880*	*80*
	C	*4,920*	*60*
	D	*3,260*	*45*

Heparin used was undecolorized. Molecular weight was measured by equilibrium ultracentrifugation and anticoagulant activity by the USP method. Controlled depolymerization was accomplished with heparinase and fractionation by sephadex column chromatography (31).

V. STRUCTURAL SIMILARITY OF PARTIALLY DEPOLYMERIZED AND COMMERCIAL HEPARINS

Proton nmr studies of an admixture of partially depolymerized heparins showing no significant differences from their high molecular weight components or from the depolymerized starting material are shown in Fig. 3. When the ascorbate peroxide depolymerized heparin mixture was subjected to ethanol fractionation, four well defined precipitates appeared between 30% and 60% and over 60% alcohol. The lowest molecular weight fraction reveals profound proton shifts and resolution of the spectrum but a broadening of the N-acetyl protons. This low molecular weight fraction on the order of an octamer was inactive as an anticoagulant. Spectrum C, while mostly resolved, also shows spectral broadening of the N-acetyl peak at 2 ppm and some evidence of the major broad peaks of the anomeric protons of active preparations. This preparation had a molecular weight of 3100 daltons and an anticoagulant activity of 20 u/mg.

VI. EFFECT OF IONIC STRENGTH ON REACTIVE SITE

Because of electrostatic effects in solution, the heparin polyelectrolyte appears extended when viscosity measurements are made in water. A decrease in viscosity (and other colligative properties) accompanies increasing salt concentration with a limiting value approached when the solution is approximately isotonic (25,32,33). At higher concentrations the apparent molecular volume is not further reduced by an increase in ionic strength. (Interactions of heparin with cations that are dissociated at low ionic strength may be sensitive to both conformational changes as well as electrostatic shielding phenomena.)

In an effort to examine the sensitivity of the heparin interaction with components of the whole coagulation system to the ionic environment, we measured the apparent anticoagulant activity of heparins in varying concentrations of sodium chloride. The USP assay was used as a test system.

Both high molecular weight and high activity (7-6A) and low MW, low activity heparin (7-3A) are relatively insensitive to increasing ionic strength up to 1.0 *M*. At higher concentrations of salt, the apparent activity of 7-6A decreases and that of 7-3A increases. Normal unfractionated commercial heparin is insensitive to increasing ionic strength up to 0.4 *M*. At higher concentrations there is a progressive decrease in activity. At 1.0 *M*, 30% of the apparent activity is lost.

The salt effect on activity of the two major components of OH2, 7-6A and 7-3A, does not appear to be additive. On the contrary, between 0.8 *M* and 1.0 *M* the activity of OH2 decreases more than 20 units, while for the corresponding salt concentration in 7-6A and 7-3A there is no change in activity. These differential responses to salt suggest that components of the heparin admixture do not act independently in the coagulation cascade but may inhance or reduce interactions with reactive components of the system.

Alcohol fraction 47B with molecular weight of 11,340 and 61B with molecular weight of 13,060 decrease in activity with increasing ionic strength up to 1.2 *M*. The low molecular weight fraction 43B is less sensitive to salt.

When commerical heparin is *inactivated* with acid reducing the activity from 145 u/mg to 130 (sample 1) and to 80 (sample 6) with no significant change in molecular weight, the more active preparation (sample 1) is more sensitive to ionic strength increases when compared to the lower activity preparation (sample 6).

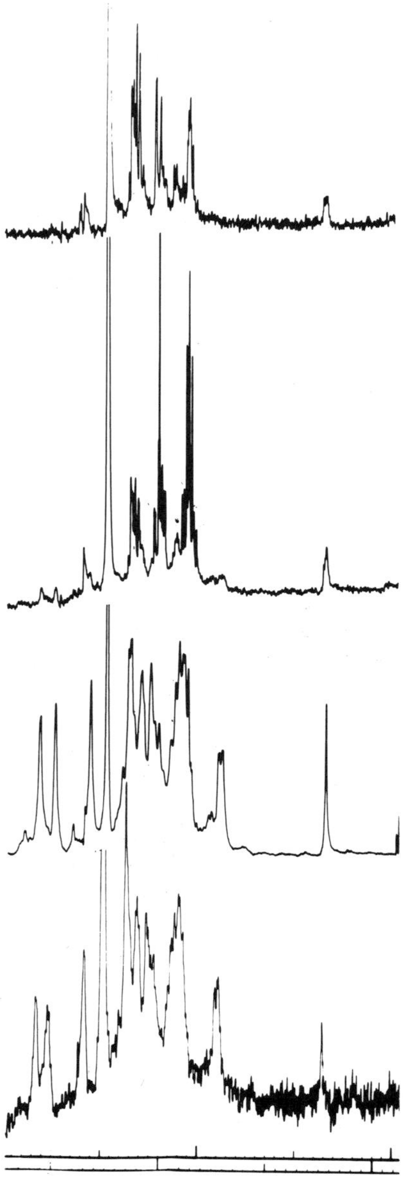

Fig. 3d. Precipitated at greater than 60% ethanol molecular weight 2100 and inactive as an anticoagulant.

Fig. 3c. Precipitated at 60% ethanol, molecular weight 3100 anticoagulant activity 21 u/mg.

Fig. 3b. Precipitated at 40% ethanol, molecular weight 5100 anticoagulant activity 63 u/mg.

Fig. 3a. Precipitated at 30% ethanol, molecular weight 5500 anticoagulant activity of 140 u/mg.

The data suggest that different components of the heparin complex, prepared by either fractionation, depolymerization, or partial inactivation interact with antithrombin and other reactants with different binding constants, and that these complexes are susceptible to the ionic environment and to the presence of other polyelectrolytes. The activity of high-affinity and low-affinity heparins, however, does not contribute to increased activity beyond the calculated sum of their activities (30).

Because the range of ionic strength in which the changes in apparent activity is observed occurs above 0.5 *M*, it is not expected that the ionic atmosphere or the configuration of heparin can play a major role in some of the effects observed. Electrostatic effects at specific binding sites could account for the observed effects. Thrombin inactivation by antithrombin in the presence of heparin is significantly different between 0.03 *M* and 0.1 *M* NaCl (34).

Fig. 3. Proton Magnetic Resonance Spectra of Depolymerized and Fractionated Heparin. Undecolorized commercially prepared heparin was depolymerized with ascorbic acid and hydrogen peroxide and then fractionated from dilute solution with increasing concentrations of ethanol. The spectrum of the fraction precipitated at 30% ethanol (Fig. 3a) is identical to the original undepolymerized unfractionated heparin. Fig. 3b also shows similar structural characteristics. Fig. 3c reveals a resolve spectrum for most of the hexosaminyl and uronosyl reside protons. The intensity of hexosaminyl 2 proton has been reduced as are the uronosyl and hexosaminyl 1 protons. The methyl protons of the N-acetyl group have been broadened suggesting that the environment of the acetyl has been altered. Fig. 3d shows a shift of the peaks assigned to the 1 protons of the uronosyl and hexosaminyl residues and broad N-acetyl peaks that are partially resolved. The original preparation had a molecular weight of 13,200 and an USP anticoagulant activity of 147 u/mg.

Spectra a and b are not significantly different from the original spectrum of commercial heparin. The molecular weights were 4200 and 5100 daltons and the biological activities 40 and 63 u/mg. The original crude undecolorized heparin from which these preparations were derived had a molecular weight of 13,700 and an anticoagulant activity of 147 u/mg. These preliminary data suggest that some residual anticoagulant activity will survive significant structural and molecular weight change. I would appear that there is some minimal structural unit with residual biological activity.

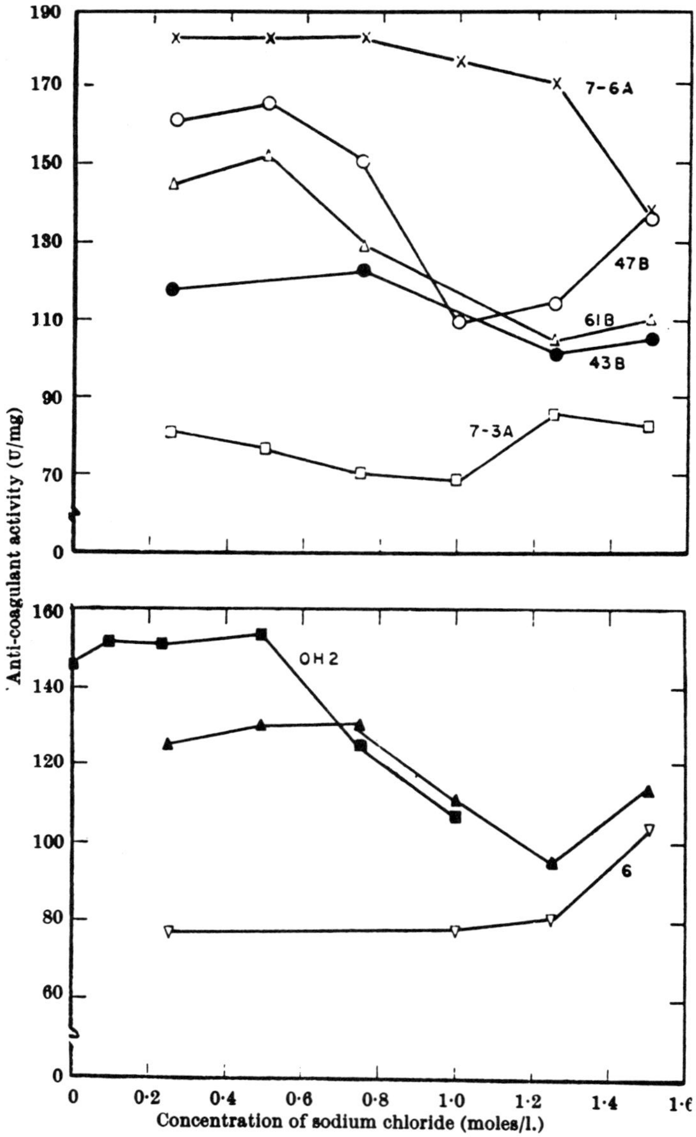

Fig. 4. Effect of Ionic Strength on Apparent USP Anticoagulant Activity. Molecular weight of preparations were 0H2, 8940; 7-6a, 15,680; 47B, 11, 340; 61B, 5540; 43B, 13,060; 7-3a, 8460. Samples 7-6A and 7-3A were prepared by elution from a cellulose column and fractions 43B, 47B, and 61B were alcohol fractions of the commercial preparation 0H2. Samples 1 and 6 had reduced anticoagulant activity by treatment with acid (34).

VII. EFFECTS OF DIVALENT CATIONS

Interactions of divalent ions with polysaccharides (36-38) and with heparin (39,40), have been studied by various methods. An extensive study by Dunstone (41), who measured ion distributions between mucopolysaccharides in solution and cations present in solution, demonstrated that the potassium ion has a greater affinity than the sodium ion and that calcium has the greatest affinity of the ions studied. The second virial coefficient, a measure of the interactions in solution, is significantly decreased in the presence of calcium ions when compared to sodium ions. Further indicating that the divalent ion is selectively associated with the polyelectrolyte (40). It is of interest to examine whether ions of different size and charge distort the heparin molecule in solution.

Figure 5 shows the proton magnetic resonance spectrum of a preparation of heparin in which sodium has been replaced by calcium. The spectrum of calcium heparin has been broadened, and the resonances assigned to H-1 of uronic acid (4) has been shifted downfield. Magnesium and zinc, other divalent ions studied, also show evidence of ionic association. Heparin salts of the monovalent ions ammonium, lithium, potassium, and sodium do not show these spectral shifts.

The interactions of heparin with divalent ion is a non-specific electrostatic association. At the low concentrations of heparin examined there is no evidence of intermolecular interactions with divalent ions. Molecular weight measurements did not show evidence of dimers.

Some evidence is available suggesting that the kinetics of interactions of calcium and sodium salts of heparin *in vivo* are significantly different (42).

VIII. CONCLUSIONS

Fractionation of commercial heparin by a variety of methods yields a dispersion of molecular weights as well as fractions with differing anticoagulant activities. For a limited molecular weight range there appears to be a linear relationship between activity and molecular weight. With controlled depolymerization of heparin, a displaced dispersion curve can be achieved. High resolution proton nuclear magnetic resonance spectroscopy of depolymerized fractionated heparins reveal that the fractions with highest molecular weight (greater than 3000 daltons) and activity have similar nmr spectra. High salt concentrations from 0.2 to 1.5 *M* affect the apparent anticoagulant activity of heparin fractions of low and high anticoagulant activity differently.

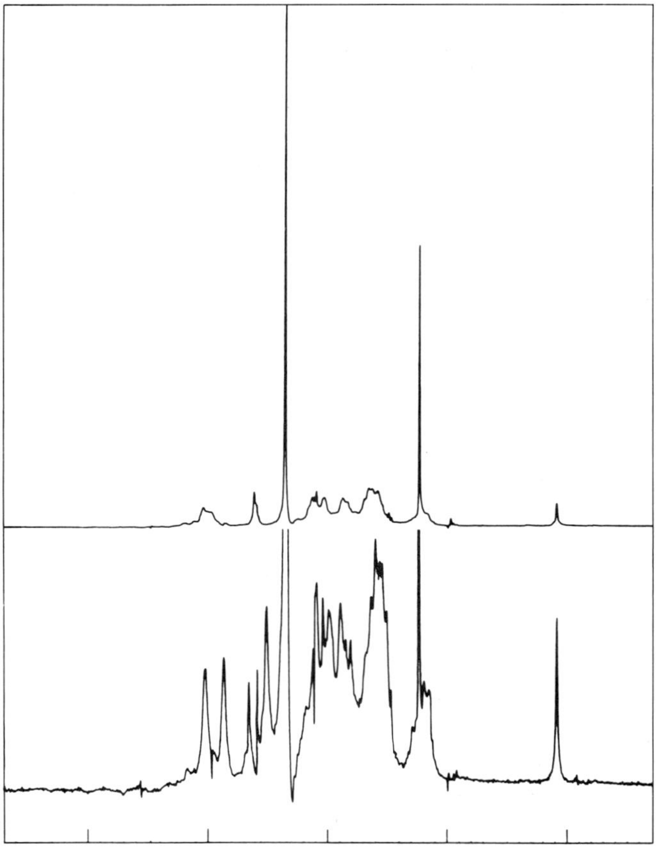

Fig. 5. Comparison of Calcium and Sodium Heparin Proton Magnetic Spectra.

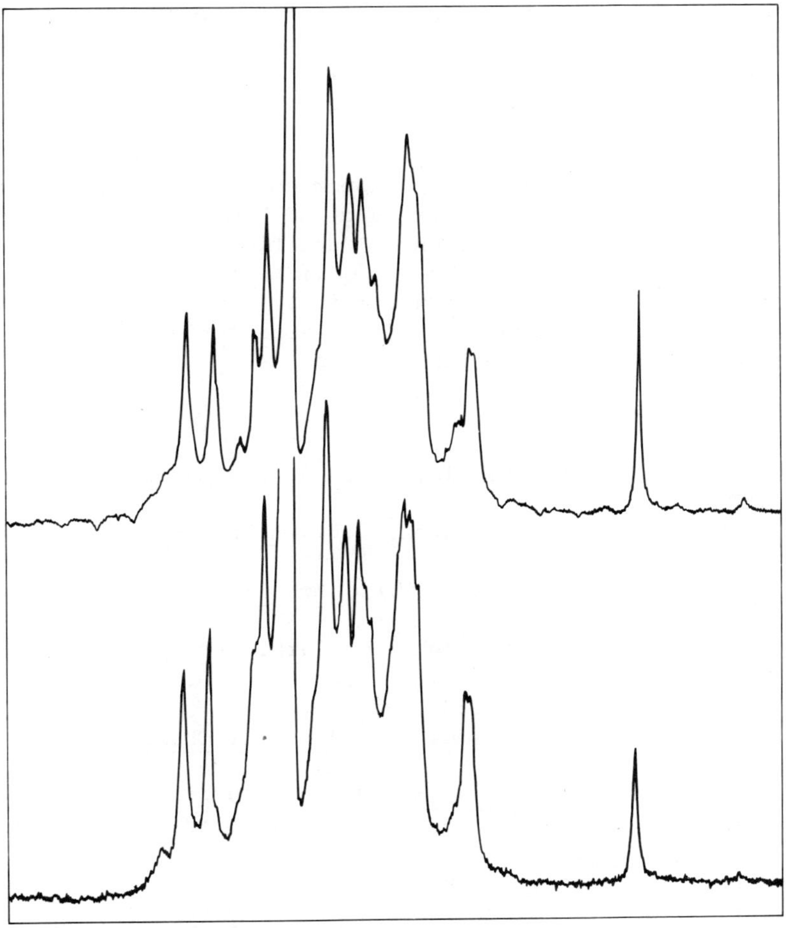

Fig. 6. Proton nmr of High Activity and Low Activity Heparins Prepared by AT III - Sepharose Fractionation. Proton spectrum of high activity heparin shown in Fig. 6 with an anticoagulant activity of 300 u/mg and low anticoagulant activity - 25 u/mg appear to be not significantly different. The well-defined peaks in high activity heparin are equivalent to the shoulders in the spectrum of the low activity preparation. The spectral similarities suggest that there are no major detectable structural differences between these preparations (30).

When measured by the USP method, divalent cations, particularly calcium, magnesium, and zinc bind heparin, broaden the nmr spectrum and produce a spectral shift associated with the uronic acid HI proton. Monovalent cations lithium, ammonium, and potassium provide nmr spectra similar to that of sodium.

ACKNOWLEDGEMENTS

These investigations were supported by an NIH Grant Hl 18068, from the National Heart Lung and Blood Institute and by grants from the National Science Foundation, Research Corporation, and Sloan Foundation to a Nuclear Magnetic Resonance Facility at the Rockefeller University. Heparins were supplied by Mr. E. Coyne, Cohelfred Laboratories. Dr. G. Van Dedem provided the high affinity heparins.

REFERENCES

1. Ehrlich, J., and Stivala, S.S., J. Pharmacol. Sci. *62*, 517 (1973).
2. Kavanagh, L.W., and Jaques, L.B., Arzneim-Forsch. *23*, 605 (1973).
3. Barlow, G.H., Sanderson, N.D., McNeil, P.D., Arch. Biochem. Biophys. *84*, 518 (1961).
4. Perlin, A.S., and Mazurek, M., Carb. Res. *7*, 369 (1968).
5. Taylor, R.L., Shively, J.E., Conrad, H.E., Cifonelli, J.A., Biochem. *12*, 3633 (1973).
6. Rosenberg, R., and Damus, P., J. Biol. Chem. *248*, 6490 (1973).
7. Rosenberg, R., Circulation *44*, 603 (1974).
8. Reisenfeld, J., Hook, M., Björk, I., Lindahl, U., Ajxon, B., Fed. Proc. *36*, 39 (1977).
9. Gans, H., Surgery *77*, 602 (1975).
10. Bailey, R.E., and Ford, H.C., Acta Endocrinologica *60*, 249 (1969).
11. Majoor, C.H., Schlatmann, R., Jansen, A.P., Prenen, H., Clin. Chem. Acta *5*, 591 (1960).
12. Fratantoni, J.D., Pollet, R., Gralnick, H.R., Blood *45*, 395 (1975).
13. Wu, J.T., Wu, L.H., Herbst, J.J., Fed. Proc. *37*, 693 (1977).
14. Lippman, M.M., and Mathews, M.B., Fed. Proc. *36*, 55 (1977).
15. Jaques, L.B., Kavanagh, L.W., Kuo, S.H., Thrombosis Research *3*, 295 (1973).
16. Anderson, L.O., Barrocliffe, J.W., Holmer, E., Johnson, E. A., Thrombosis Research *9*, 575 (1976).

17. Levy, L., and Petracek, F.J., Proc. Soc. Exp. Biol. Med. *109*, 901 (1962).
18. Laurent, T., Arch Biochem. Biophys. *92*, 224 (1961).
19. Lasker, S.E., and Stivala, S.S., Arch. Biochem. Biophys. *115*, 360 (1966).
20. Brozovic, M., and Bangham, D.R., *in* "Heparin Chemistry and Clinical Usage" (V.V. Kakkar, and D.P. Thomas, eds.) 49, (1976).
21. Cifonelli, J.A., Carb. Res. *37*, 145 (1974).
22. Johnson, E.A., and Mulloy, B., Carb. Res. *51*, 119 (1976).
23. McDuffie, N.M., Dietrich, C.P., and Nader, H.B., Biopolymers *14*, 1473 (1975).
24. Nader, H.B., McDuffie, N.B., and Dietrich, C.P., Biochem. Biophys. Res. Comm. *57*, 488 (1974).
25. Liberti, P., and Stivala, S.S., Arch Biochem. Biophys. *119*, 510 (1967).
26. Braswell, E., Biochem. Biophys. Acta *158*, 103 (1968).
27. Wasteson, A., Biochem. J. *122*, 477 (1971).
28. Ehrlich, J., and Stivala, S.S., Polymer *15*, 204 (1974).
29. Sugisaka, N., and Petracek, F.J., Fed. Proc. *36*, 89 (1977).
30. Höök, M.M., Björk, T., Hopwood, J., and Lindahl, U., FEBS Letters *66*, 90 (1976).
31. Lasker, S.E., *in* "Advances in Experimental Medicine and Biology" (R.A. Bradshaw, and S. Wessler, eds.) Vol. 52. p. 119. Academic Press, New York, 1974.
32. Lasker, S.E., and Danishefsky, I., Proceedings American Chemical Society, Boston, 1959.
33. Lasker, S., Stivala, S.S., Danishefsky, I., and Eiber, H., Fed. Proc. *21*, No. 2 (1962).
34. Lasker, S.E., and Stivala, S.S., Nature (London) *213*, 804 (1967).
35. Machovich, R., Blasko, G., Himer, A., and Szikla, K., Thrombosis Research *7*, 305 (1975).
36. Hall, L.D., Preson, C.M., and Stevers, J.D., Carb. Res. *41*, 41 (1975).
37. Czarniecki, M.F., and Thornton, E.R., Biochem. Biophys. Res. Comm. *74*, 553 (1977).
38. Stivala, S.S., Fed. Proc. *36*, 83 (1977).
39. Casu, B., Gatti, G., Cyk, N., and Perlin, A.S., Carb. Res. *41*, 66 (1975).
40. Loucas, S.P. Yeh, K.C., and Haddad, H.M., J. Pharm. Sci. *60*, 1109 (1971).
41. Dunstone, J.R., Biochem. J. *85*, 336 (1962).
42. Thomas, D.D., Safar, J., Stamatakis, J.D., Maffei, F.H.A., Erdi, A., and Kakkar, V.V., Thrombosis Research *9*, 241 (1976).

HEPARIN: PHYSICAL AND BIOLOGICAL FACTORS IN ABSORPTION

T.K. Sue

Department of Physiology
University of Saskatchewan

Absorption of a drug is usually defined as the transfer of the drug from the site of administration (e.g., the alimentary tract, subcutaneous tissue, or other depots) to the general circulation or its target organ. Heparin is unique in this very aspect. Traditionally heparin is introduced directly into the blood circulation, which is also its target organ. Thus, it can be regarded as being absorbed instantly on both bases, when heparin is administered intravenously.

In the first report in the literature regarding administration of heparin other than by intravenous injection, Fisher and Astrup (1) administered heparin into the gastrointestinal tract by intubation, and found no heparin activity in the blood but recovered its activity in the feces. Since then, it has been believed that heparin is not absorbed from the intestine. However, it was not a quantitative study. Many other possibilities can be suggested for the failure to obtain an anticoagulant effect after oral administration. For example, hydrolysis by gastric acid may be one explanation. Heparinase activity in rabbit liver was reported 37 years ago (2), so heparin may be inactivated in liver or elsewhere before reaching the blood circulation. Indeed, Kokot (3) reported that after placing heparin in the intestine, anticoagulant activity was detected in the portal blood but not in the general circulation. We administered ^{35}S-labeled heparin into the duodenum of mice. The small intestine was then tied with surgical thread at the upper end of the duodenum as well as at the lower end of the ileum. The entire intestine remained inside the abdomen of the animal with the vascular supply intact. After 2 hr the animals were killed and the radioactivity measured (Table I). We found 98% of the radioactivity remained in the small intestine. This indicated that poor absorption from the intestine was responsible for the failure to obtain an anticoagulant effect when heparin was administered into the gastrointestinal tract.

ISBN 0-12-484850-8

TABLE I Distribution of Radioactivity after Placing ^{35}S-Heparin (2,050,000 DPM) in Small Intestine of Mice

		Radioactivity (DPM)				
Animal	Intestinal content	Intestine	Liver	Plasma (per ml)	Kidney	Urine
#1	1,864,392	170,062	11,115	9430	3700	4712
#2	1,799,382	174,340	10,492	7746	2084	8491

The lack of absorption may be related to the high ionization of the sodium salt of heparin, which is the common form of commercially available heparins. After studies on a large number of drugs, Schanker and co-workers (4) concluded that the degree of ionization of an organic electrolyte in solution appears to be one of the most important factors determining its absorption from the rat small intestine. High ionization causes lower lipid solubility and this will make it difficult for the drug to pass through a membrane which is lipoidal in nature. Loomis (5) instilled sodium heparin into dog duodenal loops in buffers of pH 4 and 8 and found that a systemic anticoagulant effect was obtained in the presence of acidic buffer (pH 4) but not with the alkaline buffer (pH 8). Koh and Bharucha (6) reported that increased blood clotting time was obtained after placing heparin complexes with weak nitrogenous bases or amino acids into the jejunum of rabbits, and the anticoagulant effect was related to the ionization constant of the base or amino acid.

We compared directly the effects of placing heparin in the stomach and the small intestine of mice (Table II). A

TABLE II Anticoagulant Activity Resulting from Administration of Sodium Heparin in Gastrointestinal Tract

		Heparin activity in circulation[a]			
Administration site	Dosage (mg/kg)	F.X. Inhibition (sec)[b]	(n)	W.B.C.T.[c] (min)	(n)
Control animal	-	49.5±1.1	(20)	4.42 (1.05)	(6)
Stomach	(water)	49.3±0.9	(12)	4.58 (1.06)	(5)
Stomach	240	80.0±6.6	(12)	9.67 (1.05)	(8)
Small Intestine	260	56.7±4.3	(14)	6.64 (1.08)	(8)

[a] *Heparin activity was measured 1 hr after the administration of heparin.*
[b] *Values are means ± SE.*
[c] *Because of the logarithmic relationship between blood level of heparin and blood clotting time, the blood clotting times of each group is expressed as the geometric mean and algorism of SE of the geometric mean in parentheses.*

TABLE III Anticoagulant Effect on Administration of Heparin with Acids into Mouse Duodenum

Solvent	Whole blood clotting time (min)[a]				
	Control	Na-hep.	Ca-hep.	NH_4-hep.	K-hep.
Distilled water	4.88(1.02)	5.25(1.09)	6.06(1.11)	5.07(1.07)	4.94(1.03)
0.1 N HCl	4.46(1.06)	21.93(1.38)	22.93(1.37)	15.17(1.35)	13.16(1.37)
Citric acid[b]	4.88(1.05)	15.91(1.33)	17.55(1.30)	19.73(1.47)	9.01(1.20)
Tartaric acid	5.15(1.05)	24.31(1.34)	17.05(1.32)	13.54(1.14)	8.72(1.06)

[a] W.B.C.T. was determined 1 hr after the administration of heparin (40 mg/kg). Values reported are geometric and algorism of SE of the geometric mean in parentheses; n = 6 for each experimental group; n = 4 for each control group (solvent only or heparin in water).

[b] The concentration of citric acid and tartaric acid was 30 mg/ml.

ligature was placed just below the pylorus. A high dose of sodium heparin was placed in the stomach or the small intestine. Heparin activity in the circulation was determined 1 hr later by Factor X inhibition method (7) as well as whole blood clotting time. In contrast to other substances, the absorption of heparin from the stomach was higher than that from the small intestine, an area anatomically constructed for absorption.

This result is in line with Loomis' experiment. One of the significant differences between stomach and small intestine is the pH value. It is known that acidic environment decreases the ionization of an acidic compound such as heparin. Better absorption from the stomach suggests that ionization of heparin is an important factor in interfering with its absorption from the gastro-intestinal tract. This idea is supported by the improvement of heparin absorption from the small intestine by administering acids simultaneously (Table III). When Na-, Ca-, NH_4-, or K-heparin were introduced into the small intestine of mice with 0.1 *N* HCl, citric acid, or tartaric acid, in all cases an increased anticoagulant effect was obtained. This indicates the acidic environment not a specific ion increased the absorption of heparin.

For the passive transport of a drug of low lipid solubility such as heparin through a membrane, molecular size should have great effect. Naturally the smaller the molecule, the easier it is to pass the membrane. The heterogeneity of heparin has been reported by different investigators. At this conference Dr. McDuffie has clearly demonstrated to us that there are more than 20 different molecular species in commercial heparins. Lasker (8) placed a low molecular weight heparin obtained by depolymerization of commercial heparin in the buccal cavity of mice and obtained prolonged blood clotting times. We fractionated a commerical heparin preparation into five different molecular weight fractions (Table IV). Each was introduced into the duodenum of mice with the same concentration of citric acid (Table V). From fraction I to fraction IV, despite the lower anticoagulant potency *in vitro*, decrease in molecular weight resulted in increased anticoagulant activity in the blood. These results demonstrated that the decrease in molecular size facilitated the absorption of heparin.

The absorption of heparin is probably complicated by its polyanionic nature. We administered heparin to mice through a stomach tube. The animals were killed the next day. The small intestines were removed, washed with saline (5 x 5 ml), stained with toluidine blue, and compared to the control. We still found exogenous heparin present on the intestinal mucosal surface. Since heparin can complex with proteins readily,

TABLE IV Alcoholic Fractionation of Heparin

Fraction no.	% Ethanol	M.W.	In vitro anti-coagulant activity (unit/mg)
I	< 45	17,000	112
II	45-50	13,200	105
III	50-55	10,800	103
IV	55-60	8,700	84
V	60-65	6,700	67

TABLE V Anticoagulant Effect on Administering Heparin Fractions into Small Intestine[a]

Heparin fraction	Solvent	W.B.C.T. (min)[b]
control	water	4.89(1.03)
nonfractionated	3% citric acid	13.61(1.36)
I	"	8.34(1.21)
II	"	10.94(1.20)
III	"	29.70(1.34)
IV	"	38.68(1.27)
V	"	10.29(1.14)
IV	water	5.69(1.03)

[a] W.B.C.T. was determined 1 hr after introducing heparin (40 mg/kg) into mouse duodenum.
[b] Geometric means and algorism of SE of the geometric mean in parentheses.

it may be bound to mucosal proteins and not be available for absorption. Engel and co-workers (9,10) reported that heparin-oil emulsion or sulfated and sulfonated surfactants improved the absorption of heparin from the small intestine. The mechanism is not known, It may be due to a change in surface tension resulting in decreased binding of heparin to mucosa. Sulfated and sulfonated surfactants have been shown to bind to proteins such as serum albumin, it is possible that surfactants bind to mucosal proteins to permit the passive diffusion of heparin across the mucosa.

Although there is no evidence of active transport of heparin in the gastrointestinal tract, cellular uptake of heparin has been shown at other places. Oh and co-workers (11) demonstrated the uptake of heparin by macrophages in tissue culture. When heparin was administered intrapulmonarily, Mahadoo demonstrated that there is cellular uptake of heparin

TABLE VI Comparison of Anticoagulant Effect of Heparin in Swiss Mice and C3H Mice

Strain	Whole blood clotting time (min)[a]					
	Subcutaneous (600 units/kg)[b]					
	0 hr	1 hr	2 hr	3 hr	6 hr	8 hr
Swiss	4.5	17.0	76.0	20.2	14.9	7.6
C3H	4.7	76.5	90.0	90.0	24.7	5.5
	[c] $p<0.3$	$p<0.001$	$p<0.01$	$p<0.001$	$p<0.001$	$p<0.05$

Strain	in vitro (0.4 μ/ml) (n)	I.V. (85 μ/kg) 15 min (n)	I.V. (85 μ/kg) 1 hr (n)	small intestine (40 mg/kg)[d]
Swiss	12.0 (4)	27.3 (6)	20.5 (8)	13.6
C3H	11.5 (4)	25.1 (5)	18.7 (6)	71.1
	$p<0.7$	$p<0.7$	$p<0.7$	$p<0.01$

[a] Clotting time longer than 90 min was calculated as 90 min.
[b] $n = 8$.
[c] Student t test for significance of difference between two strains. If $p<0.05$ the difference is significant.
[d] Heparin was dissolved in 3% citric acid.

in the lung. This would be a different picture of transport. Mr. Mahadoo will discuss the cellular uptake of heparin later at this conference.

It is usual to find a difference in response to a drug between species. We discovered that there is even an inter-strain variation in the absorption of heparin between two strains of mice: Albino Swiss mice, and Agouti C3H mice. After injection of the same dose of heparin subcutaneously, C3H mice had a much greater anticoagulant response than the Swiss mice (Table VI). The anticoagulant effects of adding heparin to the blood in the test tube, and after intravenous injection, were similar in these two strains ($P<0.6$). This indicates that there was no difference in response to heparin in the blood system of these two strains. The similar changes in anticoagulant effect between 15 min and 1 hr after intravenous injection suggest the rates of heparin removal from the blood stream were similar in these two strains (Table VI). Hence, the possibility for the different responses after subcutaneous injection appears to be a difference in absorption of heparin from the injection site to the blood circulation. We injected ^{35}S-heparin into the foot pads of these two strains of mice subcutaneously and determined radioactivities in the feet at different time intervals and found that the removal of radioactivity from the foot pad was faster in C3H mice than Swiss mice.

The difference in response after subcutaneous injection of heparin can be obtained from different sites of injection: the dorsal side of the neck, foot pad, posterior axilla. When heparin was placed in the small intestine together with citric acid, the blood clotting time obtained from C3H mice was also longer than that of the Swiss mice (Table VI). These indicate that the difference in transport of heparin to the general circulation following local administration is not limited to one area of the body but probably represents a general difference. These mice may provide a useful model for studying factors in absorption of heparin.

ACKNOWLEDGEMENT

This work was supported by the Canadian Heart Foundation and Saskatchewan Heart Foundation.

REFERENCES

1. Fischer, A., and Astrup, T., Proc. Soc. Exp. Biol. Med. *42*, 81 (1939).
2. Jaques, L.B., J. Biol. Chem. *133*, 445 (1940).
3. Kokot, B., Thromb. Diathes. Haemorrh. *30*, 284 (1973).

4. Schanker, L.S., Tocco, D.J., Brodie, B.B., and Hogben, C.A.M., J. Pharm. Exp. Ther. *123*, 81 (1958).
5. Loomis, T.A., Proc. Soc. Exp. Biol. Med. *101*, 447 (1959).
6. Kohn, T.Y., and Bharucha, K.R., J. Lab. Clin. Med. *80*, 47 (1972).
7. Yin, E.T., Wessler, S., and Butler, J.V., J. Lab. Clin. Med. *80*, 298 (1973).
8. Lasker, S.E., *in* "Advances in Experimental Medicine and Biology" (R.A. Bradshaw and S. Wessler, eds.). Vol. 52, p. 119. Plenum Press, New York, 1975.
9. Engel, R.H., and Fahrenbach, M.J., Proc. Soc. Exp. Biol. Med. *129*, 772 (1968).
10. Engel, R.H., and Riggi, S.J., Proc. Soc. Exp. Biol. Med. *130*, 879 (1969).
11. Oh, T.H., Naidoo, S.S., and Jaques, L.B., J. Reticul. Soc. *13*, 134 (1973).

STRUCTURAL BASIS FOR THE BIOLOGICAL EFFECTS OF HEPARIN

Ulf Lindahl

The Swedish University of Agricultural Sciences

The biosynthesis of heparin is initiated by formation of a monosulfated polysaccharide consisting of alternating D-glucuronic and N-acetyl-D-glucosamine residues. This polymer is modified in a stepwise manner by a series of reactions, including deacetylation of N-acetylglucosamine units, formation of N-sulfate groups, formation of L-iduronic acid residues by C5-epimerization of D-glucuronic acid units, and incorporation of O-sulfate groups. Since most of the polymer-modification reactions are incomplete, the final product has a complex structure, involving a number of different disaccharide units. Possible regulatory mechanisms determining the sequence of these units are discussed.

The significance of such mechanisms becomes apparent in relation to the anticoagulant properties of heparin. The anticoagulant activity depends on the ability of the polysaccharide to bind with high affinity to antithrombin; only a fraction of the molecules in heparin preparations is capable of such interaction. These molecules possess an antithrombin-binding site composed of about six disaccharide units. Structural analysis of oligosaccharide fractions assumed to represent this binding site revealed the presence of several different disaccharide units. The same disaccharide units were present in heparin incapable of high-affinity binding to antithrombin, although in slightly different proportions. It is suggested that binding of heparin to antithrombin may require a specific sequence of different disaccharide units. This conclusion provides a partial explanation for the molecular-weight dependence of the anticoagulant activity of heparin.

The structural requirements for the interaction of heparin with lipoporotein lipase are discussed. These requirements appear to be less exacting than those pertaining to the interaction with antithrombin.

I. INTRODUCTION

Heparin impedes the coagulation of blood by accelerating the reaction between antithrombin (a protease inhibitor in plasma) and a number, possibly all, of the serine proteases participating in the coagulation mechanism (13). Recent evidence suggests that heparin exerts its anticoagulant effect by

ISBN 0-12-484850-8

inducing a conformational change of the antithrombin molecule, resulting in a more favourable topography of its active site (4,5; I. Björk and B. Nordenman, personal communication). While the physical-chemical aspects of this interaction begin to unfold, the relationship between the structure of heparin and its antithrombin-stimulating properties remain poorly understood. Similar uncertainty applies to another important biological property of heparin, namely the ability to increase the rate of triglyceride clearance from plasma on administration *in vivo*. This effect is due to the heparin-induced release of lipases (lipoprotein lipase and hepatic lipase) from tissue sites into the circulating blood, presumably by formation of heparin-lipase complexes (6). The present report attempts to summarize our current knowledge regarding the structure-function relationships pertaining to the interactions of heparin with antithrombin and lipoprotein-lipase, respectively. The structure of heparin is summarized in Fig. 1 (for recent review see (7)). It is a polysaccharide composed of alternating glucosamine (N-sulfated or N-acetylated) and uronic acid (IdUA[a] or GlcUA) residues. Some of these residues are O-sulfated in the positions indicated;

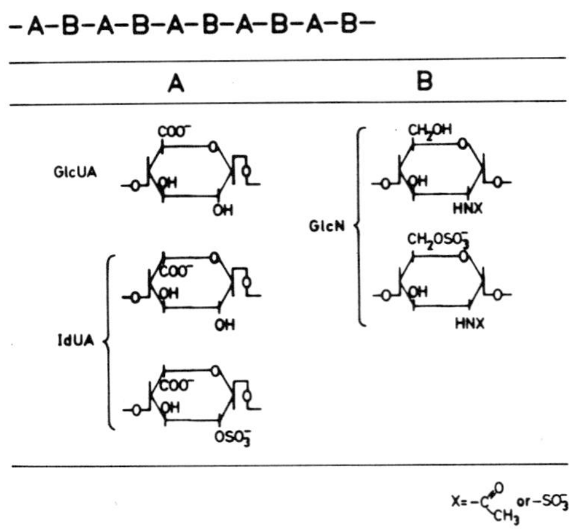

Fig. 1. Structure of heparin.

---

[a] *Abbreviations: GlcUA, D-glucuronic acid; IdUA, L-iduronic acid; GlcNAc, 2-deoxy-2-acetamido-D-glucose; GlcNSO$_3$, 2-deoxy-2-sulfamino-D-glucose; N-sulfate group, sulfamino group; O-sulfate group, ester sulfate group; PAPS, 3'-phosphoadenylyl-sulfate.*

the total sulfate content of heparin generally ranges between 1.8 and 3.0 sulfate groups per disaccharide unit. By combining the various uronic acid and glucosamine residues shown in Fig. 1 a large number of different disaccharide units may be obtained; although the number of combinations is limited by restrictions imposed during biosynthesis, considerable variability is retained and expressed in the marked heterogeneity observed for heparin and, in particular, for heparan sulfate (a structurally related polysaccharide that essentially lacks anticoagulant activity).

Recent results (see Section III) indicate that the interaction of heparin with antithrombin is highly specific and depends on the sequence of variously substituted disaccharide units in the polysaccharide molecule. It therefore seems appropriate to combine a discussion of structure-function relationship with a survey of heparin biosynthesis, particular consideration being given to possible regulatory mechanisms determining the fine structure of the polysaccharide molecule.

II. BIOSYNTHESIS OF HEPARIN

The biosynthesis of heparin has been studied using microsomal fractions from mouse mastocytoma tissue (7-9). Incubation of such fractions with UDP-GlcUA, UDP-GlcNAc and PAPS yielded a series of polymers that could be separated into distinct components by chromatography on DEAE-cellulose (Fig. 2). These components were shown to be intermediates in the biosynthetic process, formed by stepwise modification of an initial polymerization product composed of alternating GlcUA and GlcNAc residues. A scheme for the overall modification process has been postulated on the basis of the structures of these intermediates (Fig. 2), and has been verified by studies of the individual reactions involved (7,8,10).[b] The concerted action of these reactions will be described and followed by a discussion of possible control mechanisms.

A. Polymer-Modification Reactions

1. *Deacetylation of GlcNAc Residues*

The extent of N-deacetylation may be estimated in either of two ways (Riesenfeld et al. in manuscript): (a) by the

---

[b] *Preliminary studies on the biosynthesis of heparan sulfate in rat liver tissue point to a polymer-modification process similar to that implicated in heparin biosynthesis (Riensenfeld et al. unpublished observations).*

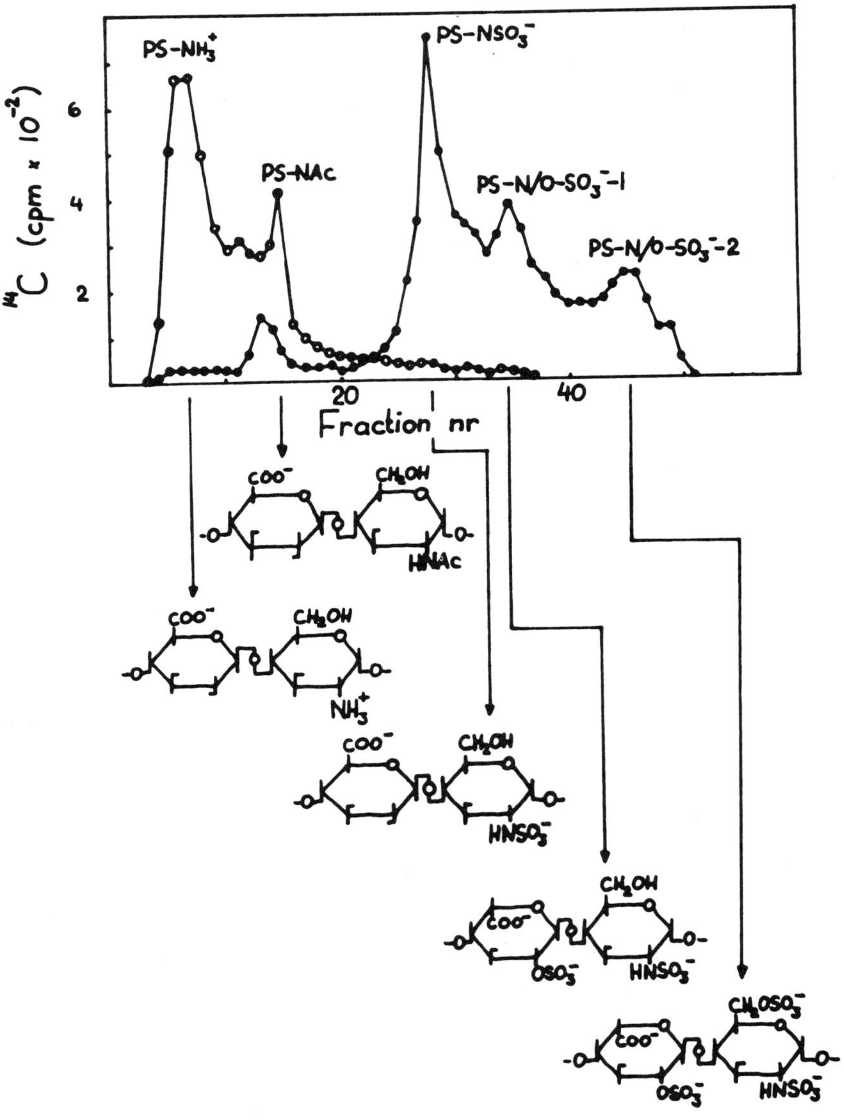

Fig. 2. Chromatography of ^{14}C-labeled polysaccharide obtained by incubating mouse mastocytoma microsomal fraction with UDP-[^{14}C]GlcUA and UDP-GlcNAc in the absence (O) and presence (●), respectively, of PAPS (for further experimental details, see (10) and (11)). Each peak represents an intermediate in the series of reactions leading from the initial polymerization product (PS-NAc) to the fully modified polysaccharide (PS-N/O-SO_3^--2). The various reactions are indicated by the structures of the resulting disaccharide

size-distribution of fragments obtained after treatment of partially N-deacetylated polysaccharide with nitrous acid; (b) by the amount of [^{3}H] acetate liberated from a polymer substrate having ^{3}H-labeled N-acetyl groups. An assay method based on (b) has been developed and used to determine the basic kinetic properties of the microsomal N-deacetylase from mouse mastocytoma. N-deacetylation of the natural substrate

($\xrightarrow{1,4\alpha}$ GlcUA $\xrightarrow{1,4\beta}$ GlcNAc $\xrightarrow{1,4\alpha}$ n); PS-NAc in Fig. 2 occurs in a random fashion and yields a product (PS-NH_3^+) retaining about half of the original N-acetyl groups. Further N-deacetylation may occur after sulfation of the exposed free amino groups. The specificity of the N-deacetylase has not been examined in detail; however, it may be noted that hyaluronic acid

($\xrightarrow{1,4\beta}$ GlcUA $\xrightarrow{1,3\beta}$ GlcNAc $\xrightarrow{1,4\beta}$ n) does not appear to be attacked by the enzyme.

2. Formation of N-sulfate Groups

The free amino groups formed in the preceding reaction are substituted with sulfate groups, yielding the intermediate. PS-NSO_3^- (Fig. 2) (10,11). The corresponding N-sulfotransferase may be assayed by a procedure involving transfer of labeled sulfate groups from [^{35}S] PAPS to N-desulfated heparin (12). N-Sulfation initiates further deacetylation of remaining GlcNAc residues, thus providing sites for further N-sulfation (Riesenfeld et al. in manuscript; see also (9)). N-Sulfation appears to be completed before any O-sulfate groups are introduced into the polysaccharide molecule (10).

3. Uronosyl C5-Epimerization

GlcUA residues are converted to IdUA units on the polymer level, in a reaction that is strongly promoted by concomitant introduction of O-sulfate groups (10,13; see intermediate PS-N/O-SO_3^- -1 in Fig. 2). An assay method has been devised using the N-sulfated polymer intermediate, PS-NSO_3^-, specifically ^{3}H-labeled at C5 of the GlcUA residues, as a substrate; epimerase

---

units, listed downwards in chronological order of formation. It should be noted that the polymer-modification reactions are generally incomplete; in addition to the disaccharide units shown the intermediates thus contain other units remaining at a lower level of modification (see the text).

activity is proportional to the amount of ^{3}H-labeled water formed during incubation (8; Jacobsson et al. in manuscript). The enzyme requires N-sulfate (but no O-sulfate) groups in the polysaccharide substrate and, contrary to the other polymer-modifying enzymes, shows no requirement for divalent cations. The epimerization process is freely reversible; by selective O-sulfation IdUA residues may be withdrawn from the reaction and thus accumulate in certain regions along the polysaccharide chain.

4. *Formation of O-Sulfate Groups*

The O-sulfation reactions conclude the polymer-modification reactions (Fig. 2), yielding a product (PS-N/O-SO_3^--2) with the diverse structural features typical of heparin. Sulfate groups are introduced in two positions, at C2 of IdUA and at C6 of glucosamine units. Total O-sulfotransferase activity may be assayed by using a low-sulfated heparin sulfate as acceptor for labeled sulfate groups, with [^{35}S] PAPS as sulfate donor (12); this procedure does not distinguish between different O-sulfotransferases. Recent observations (K. Jacobsson, M. Höök, and U. Lindahl, unpublished) provide some insight into the mechanisms of O-sulfation. Studies on the substrate specificity of mastocytoma O-sulfotransferases thus indicated that O-sulfate groups are preferentially incorporated into N-sulfated rather than into N-acetylated regions of a heparin precursor polysaccharide. Furthermore, a partially O-sulfated intermediate (PS-N/O-SO_3^--1 in Fig. 2) was detected, containing mono-O-sulfated but no significant amounts of di-O-sulfated disaccharide units. Identification of the mono-O-sulfated disaccharide units in this intermediate polysaccharide, as well as in the final product (PS-N/O-SO_3^--2), clearly indicated that sulfation at C2 of the IdUA residues precedes sulfation at C6 of GlcNSO_3^- units. Since formation of the intermediate, PS-N/O-SO_3^--1, also involves uronosyl C5-epimerization, these findings support the postulated link between formation and sulfation of IdUA residues.

B. Regulation of Polymer-Modification Process

Due to incomplete polymer modification virtually all heparin and heparan sulfate preparations contain more than one type of disaccharide unit; the resulting structural complexity may indeed form the basis for specificity in biological interactions involving these polysaccharides. While the extensively modified disaccharide unit consists of IdUA, GlcNSO_3^-, and two O-sulfate groups (Fig. 2), incomplete modification manifests itself by the presence of GlcUA and

GlcNAc residues and by a relative lack of O-sulfate in the final product. The mechanisms controlling the polymer-modification process are only vaguely understood; however, it seems evident that the substrate specificities of the enzymes involved should be of major important. In each step of the

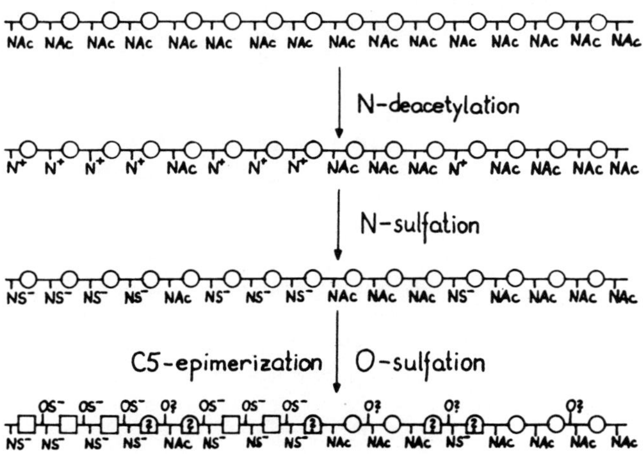

Fig. 3. Schematic representation of polymer-modification reactions in heparin biosynthesis, illustrating a possible regulatory role of the initial N-deacetylation reaction. This reaction leads to the formation of D-glucosamine residues with free amino groups (-N+) that subsequently become sulfated (-NS⁻). GlcUA (-O-) residues in the vicinity of N-sulfated glucosamine units are converted to IdUA (-■-) residues, along with or prior to the introduction of O-sulfate (-OS⁻) groups. The -OS⁻) symbols do not specify the number of O-sulfate groups incorporated. There is some uncertainty as to the distribution of uronic acid residues and O-sulfate groups (indicated by -?- and by -O?, respectively) at isolated GlcNAc residues in N-sulfated sections as well as at isolated $GlcNSO_3^-$ residues in N-acetylated sections of the polysaccharide. Also, while O-sulfate groups locate preferentially in N-sulfated sections (7), the occurrence of some O-sulfate groups in extended N-acetylated regions cannot be excluded. The scheme conveys the impression that the N-sulfated sections, amenable to further polymer modification, are invariably modified to the endpoint of the process. This is evidently not true, as demonstrated by structural analysis of heparin (see the text). Sites indicated by -□- may thus be occupied by either IdUA- or GlcUA-containing disaccharide units, whereas -O- denotes GlcUA-containing units exclusively.

modification process, the corresponding enzyme (or enzymes) is presented with the product from the preceding step; in most or all of the reactions the modifications introduced appear to be essential for substrate recognition by the enzyme next in turn. Considering the series of modification reactions following the initial polymerization process, it is apparent that N-deacetylation represents a key regulatory step; polysaccharide segments escaping N-deacetylation will presumably be withdrawn from the series of reactions which leads to the fully modified, final product (Fig. 3). A polysaccharide intermediate largely consisting of such N-acetylated, inert sequences will ultimately convert into a product that by current criteria of classification should be designated as heparan sulfate. The mode of regulation of N-deacetylation is unknown and should be investigated; the observed promotion of N-deacetylation by concomitant N-sulfation of the substrate (see A. 2) is of obvious interest in this context.

Heparin and heparan sulfate generally do not contain any significant amounts of N-unsubstituted glucosamine residues, indicating that the sulfation of free amino groups proceeds essentially to completion. All other polymer-modification reactions are characteristically incomplete, thus leading to progressively increasing structural complexity as the process proceeds. In Figs. 2 and 3 this property has been neglected, since N-sulfation is depicted as being not only prerequisite to, but invarably followed by uronosyl C5-epimerization and O-sulfation. In reality a considerable number of different N-sulfated disachcharide units have been identified, not only in the final products of cell-free heparin biosynthesis (Fig. 4), but also in preparations of heparin and heparan sulfate from various tissues (14-16). The amounts of "undersulfated" disaccharide units (including N-acetylated species, in addition to the N-sulfated units identified (Fig. 4) in heparin and, particularly, in heparan sulfate may be considerable; polymer sequences composed of such units along with di-O-sulfated disaccharide units may obviously have highly complex structures. Information regarding the fine structure of such sequences is scarce and will have to be acquired (e.g. expressed as nearest-neighbor frequencies) before any detailed concepts of biosynthetic control mechanisms or specific structure-function relationships can be formulated.

III. INTERACTION BETWEEN HEPARIN AND ANTITHROMBIN

The anticoagulant activity of heparin has generally been determined by measuring the effect on clot formation in various whole-blood assays (17). Interpretation of such data in terms of interaction between heparin and antithrombin is hampered by the complexity of the assay systems, which include a multitude of components capable of binding to heparin. More

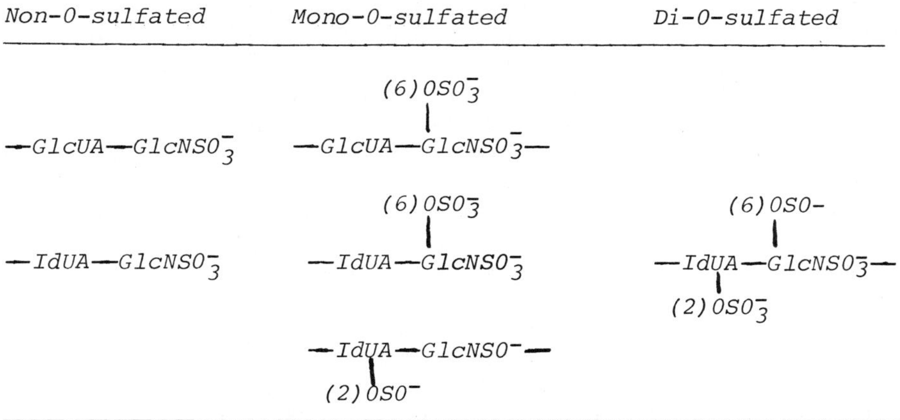

Fig. 4. N-Sulfated disaccharide units identified in heparin obtained by cell-free biosynthesis (analogous to PS-N/O-SO_3-2 in Fig. 2). The labeled polysaccharide (containing [^{14}C] uronic acid and 6-[^3H] glucosamine residues) was deaminated with nitrous acid and the resulting uronosyl-anhydromannose disaccharides were reduced and separated by paper electrophoresis and paper chromatography. They were identified by uronic acid analysis, periodate oxidation (Smith degradation) and digestion with β-D-glucuronidase and α-L-iduronidase (Jacobson et al. unpublished results).

direct measurements of the effect of heparin on antithrombin may be performed by a photometric method (18) based on the heparin cofactor assay of Ødegard *et al.* (19); this procedure is based on the release of *p*-nitroaniline from a synthetic chromogenic thrombin substrate. Both clotting (20) and photometric (21) assay methods have been used in attempts to define the structural features of the heparin molecule that are essential to its anticoagulant activity. N-desulfation thus resulted in loss of activity that could be restored by re-N-sulfation but not by N-acetylation. Modifications at the carboxyl groups of the uronic acid residues likewise impeded anticoagulant action (22). Also the influence of molecular weight has been studied using these methods (see below).

Recently, additional information was obtained by a different approach, involving fractionation of heparin with regard to affinity for antithrombin. Separations accomplished by either sucrose density-gradient centrifugation of heparin mixed with antithrombin (23) or affinity chromatography of heparin on immobilized antithrombin (23,24) showed, unexpectedly, that only about one-third of the heparin molecules were able to bind strongly to antithrombin. This high-affinity fraction (HA-heparin) had an exceedingly high anticoagulant activity whereas the remaining, low-affinity material (LA-heparin) had little or no activity. An oligosaccharide fragment thought to represent the antithrombin-binding site of heparin was isolated after digestion of the HA-heparin-antithrombin complex with bacterial heparinase (25). No corresponding fragment could be derived from LA-heparin. The molecular weight of the HA-heparin fragment was about 4×10^3, indicating that the antithrombin binding site would correspond to approximately a dodecasaccharide segment of the heparin molecule.

While a preliminary characterization of HA- and LA-heparin failed to reveal any gross structural differences (23,25), recent studies on isolated antithrombin-binding site (obtained by heparinase digestion of HA-heparin-antithrombin complex) proved to be somewhat more informative (Lindahl *et al.* unpublished observations). Digestion with bacterial heparinase in the *absence* of antithrombin thus showed a higher proportion of enzyme-resistant linkages in binding-site oligosaccharide (derived from mouse mastocytomal heparin) than in LA-heparin obtained from the same starting material. This finding indicates a relative lack of sulfate groups in the binding site (26). Furthermore, a "fingerprint" investigation (using the procedures generally outlined in the legend to Fig. 4) of binding-site oligosaccharide isolated from bovine lung HA-heparin showed the presence of all the four N- and O-sulfated disaccharide units indicated in Fig. 4 and, in addition, significant amounts of N-acetylated units. However, only one of these components, the di-O-sulfated, N-sulfated disaccharide unit, occurred in amounts equivalent to or exceeding one mole per mole of antithrombin-binding site. The binding-site oligosaccharide fraction must therefore have been heterogeneous, suggesting that more than one sequence of disaccharide units may be involved in the binding of HA-heparin to antithrombin.

The mechanisms determining the sequence of disaccharide units in heparin are only partly understood (see Section IIB). Apparently, the substrate specificities of the polymer-modification enzymes is one of the factors involved; however, since most of the corresponding reactions do not proceed to completion (at each step of polymer modification a fraction of the potential substrate residues remains unchanged) it seems reasonable to imply, in addition, a certain element of randomness. In view of this randomness and the appreciable size of the antithrombin-binding site (a dodecasaccharide sequence) in heparin, it is not surprising that only a fraction of the molecules, i.e., HA-heparin, has the structure required for binding to antithrombin.

These considerations have recently been extended to partially explain the relationship between the anticoagulant activity and the degree of polymerization for heparin preparations (Laurent *et al.*,in manuscript). When polydisperse heparin preparations are fractionated according to molecular weight the anticoagulant activity of the fractions generally increases with the degree of polymerization (20,21,24,27,28, 29). It was proposed that the anticoagulant activity of heparin is a function of the probability of finding, in a polymer of randomly distributed different disaccharide units, a dodecasaccharide sequence which binds to antithrombin. This probability was shown to be a function of the degree of polymerization of heparin. The hypothesis was tested by subjecting a series of essentially monodisperse heparin fractions (separated by gel chromatography) to affinity chromatography on immobilized antithrombin. For all fractions tested, up to a molecular weight of 18×10^3, the ratio of HA- to LA-heparin increased with increasing molecular weight, according to the predicted probability relationship. This finding would seem to explain the relationship between the molecular weight and the anticoagulant activity of heparin; however, the problem is apparently more complex, as the activity of HA-heparin remained correlated to molecular weight. The anticoagulant activity therefore cannot solely depend on the availability of binding sites for antithrombin.

IV. INTERACTION BETWEEN HEPARIN AND LIPOPROTEIN LIPASE

The effect of heparin on lipoprotein lipase may be studied *in vivo* by determining lipase activities in post-heparin plasma. Recently, the interaction between lipoprotein lipase and various glycosaminoglycans has been more directly demonstrated by affinity binding of the enzyme to polysaccharide-substituted agarose gels (Bengtsson *et al.*, in manuscript; see also (6)). In either system the ability of heparin to interact with lipoprotein lipase (isolated from bovine milk) was eliminated by N-desulation; however, this ability was restored not only by re-N-sulfation but also by N-acetylation of the polysaccharide. Furthermore, the lipase-releasing activity was shown to be less affected by modification of the carboxyl groups than was the anticoagulant activity (3). These observations indicate that lipoprotein lipase binds polysaccharides less specifically than does antithrombin (see Section III). In agreement with this conclusion dermatan sulfate, which does not activate antithrombin (31), was found to have appreciable binding capacity for lipoprotein lipase (6). It was also noted, however, that chondroitin sulfate had a significantly lower binding capacity than dermatan sulfate. Chondroitin sulfate has the same negative charge density as dermatan sulfate but differs from the latter in lacking IdUA residues; the interaction between lipoprotein lipase and glycosaminoglycans is apparently not entirely non-specific.

It was considered of interest from a functional point of view to test the affinity for lipoprotein lipase of HA- and LA-heparin, separated with regard to affinity for antithrombin (see Section III). Three types of experiments were conducted (32): (a) release of lipases *in vivo*; (b) release of lipoprotein lipase from immobilized heparin with free HA- or LA-heparin; and (c) affinity chromatography of heparin on immobilized lipoprotein lipase. As expected, HA- and LA-heparin invariably showed equal ability to interact with lipoprotein lipase. The (LA-heparin) that affects lipoprotein lipase but lacks effect on blood coagulation may have important physiological and therapeutic implications.

REFERENCES

1. Damus, P.S., Hicks, M., and Rosenberg, R.D., Nature *245*, 355 (1973).
2. Björk, I., and Nordenman, B., Eur. J. Biochem. *68*, 507 (1976).
3. Chan, J.Y.C., Burrowes, C.E., Habal, F.M., and Movat, H.Z., Biochem. Biophys. Res. Comm. *74*, 150 (1977).
4. Li, E.H.H., Fenton II, J.W., and Feinman, R.D., Arch. Biochem. Biophys. *175*, 153 (1976).
5. Villanueva, G.B., and Danishefsky, I., Biochem. Biophys. Res. Comm. *74*, 803 (1977).
6. Olivecrona, T., Bengtsson, G., Marklund, S.-E., Lindahl, U., and Höök, M., Fed. Proc. *36*, 60 (1977).
7. Lindahl, U., *in* "International Review of Science" (G.O. Aspinall, ed.), Organic Chemistry Series Two, Vol. 7, p. 283. Butterworths, London, 1976.
8. Lindahl, U., Höök, M., Backström, G., Jackbsson, I., Riesenfeld, J., Malmstrom, A., Roden, L., and Feingold, D.S., Fed. Proc. *36*, 19 (1977).
9. Silbert, J.E., Kleinman, H.K., and Silbert, C.K., Adv. Exp. Med. Biol. *52*, 51 (1975).
10. Höök, M., Lindahl, U., Hallen, A., and Backström, G., J. Biol. Chem. *250*, 6065 (1975).
11. Lindahl, U., Backström, G., Jansson, L., and Hallen, A., J. Biol. Chem. *248*, 7234 (1973).
12. Jansson, L., Höök, M., Wasteson, A., and Lindahl, U., Biochem. J. *149*, 49 (1975).
13. Höök, M., Lindahl, U., Backström, G., Malmstrom, A., and Fransson, L.-A., J. Biol. Chem. *249*, 3908 (1974).

14. Höök, M., Lindahl, U., and Iverius, P.-H., Biochem. J. *137*, 33 (1974).
15. Shively, J.E., and Conrad, H.E., Biochemistry *15*, 3943 (1976).
16. Linker, A., and Hovingh, P., Fed. Proc. *36*, 43 (1977).
17. Brozovic, M., and Bangham, D.R., Adv. Exp. Med. Biol. *52*, 163 (1975).
18. Björk, I., and Nordenman, B., Eur. J. Biochem. *68*, 507 (1976).
19. Odegard, O.R., Lie, M., and Abildgaard, U., Thromb. Res. *6*, 287 (1975).
20. Cifonelli, J.A., Carbohyd. Res. *34*, 145 (1974).
21. Risenfeld, J., Höök, M., Björk, I., Lindahl, U., and Ajaxon, B., Fed. Proc. *36*, 39 (1977).
22. Danishefsky, I., Fed. Proc. *36*, 33 (1977).
23. Lam, L.H., Silbert, J.E., and Rosenberg, R.D., Biochem. Biophys. Res. Comm. *69*, 570 (1976).
24. Höök, M., Björk, I., Hopwood, J., and Lindahl, U., FEBS Lett. *66*, 90 (1976).
25. Andersson, L.-O., Barrowcliffe, T.W., Holmer, E., Johnson, E.A., and Sims, G.E.C., Thromb. Res. *9*, 575 (1976).
26. Linker, A., Fed. Proc. *36*, 43 (1977).
27. Hopwood, J., Höök, M., Linker, A., and Lindahl, U., FEBS Lett. *69*, 51 (1976).
28. Laurent, T.C., Arch. Biochem. Biophys. *92*, 224 (1961).
29. McDuffie, N.M., Dietrich, C.P., and Nader, H.B., Biopolymers *14*, 1473 (1975).
30. Danishefsky, I., Adv. Exp. Med. Biol. *52*, 105 (1974).
31. Teien, A.U., Abildgaard, U., and Höök, M., Thromb. Res. (1976).
32. Bengtsson, G., Olivecrona, T., Höök, M., and Lindahl, U., FEBS Lett., *79*, 59 (1977).

EVIDENCE FOR A CELLULAR POOL FOR EXOGENOUS HEPARIN

J. Mahadoo

Department of Physiology
University of Saskatchewan

In an attempt to improve on the existing modes of administering heparin to patients, we have successfully developed a new procedure: heparin administration by aerosol. Our studies on the mechanism involved in the absorption of heparin when administered via the lung have produced certain data that may throw some light on the way the body deals with administered heparin. Mice and rats were given heparin by tracheal instillation. The mice were sacrificed after 15 min and the rats after 24 hr. One-micron sections of epon-embedded lung tissue from the mice revealed the involvement of macrophages in the uptake of the administered heparin. These cells storing the heparin were also observed in subcutaneous tissue indicating a possible mode of storage and transport of the drug. It has already been shown that vascular endothelium can take up and accumulate exogenous heparin. Our present findings on lung histology and arterio-venous differences in heparin concentrations after intrapulmonary administration of the drug support the idea of endothelial sequestration of heparin. The redistribution phase of the elimination curve for intravenous heparin, the longer duration of action of heparin administered via indirect routes, the observations on the uptake and storage of exogenous heparin by macrophages and endothelial tissue are evidence supporting the concept of a cellular pool that modulates heparin concentration in the blood following the administration of the drug by either intravenous, intramuscular, subcutaneous, or intrapulmonary route.

I. INTRODUCTION

It is usually assumed that the changes in coagulation test values following administration of heparin provide an insight into the distribution of the drug between blood plasma and organs. Heparin administered by a single intravenous injection in the usual therapeutic dose range (10,000 to 20,000 units/70 kg of B.W.) has an anticoagulnt effect lasting up to 2 to 4 hr. When administered subcutaneously the same dose of heparin shows a lower grade of hypocoagulation lasting up to 8 hr. Heparin administered by the intrapulmonary route

ISBN 0-12-484850-8

does not show any significant degree of hypocoagulation at this dosage, but at higher dosages (10 to 50 mg/kg of B. Wt.) a moderate but more prolonged degree of hypocoagulation occurs, somewhat reminiscent of the effect following subcutaneous administration of the drug. The anticoagulant effect of heparin administered intravenously appears to be similar to the *in vitro* effect following mixing of blood and heparin, while the effect observed following subcutaneous and intrapulmonary administration seems to be due to a slow release of the drug into the blood circulation. This slow release of heparin into the circulation would normally mean a slow degree of absorption from the site of administration. However, our findings from intrapulmonary administration of ^3H heparin (1) indicate just the opposite. This is a rapid disappearance of radioactivity from the site of administration. Therefore, an examination of blood and lung tissue following intrapulmonary administration of heparin was undertaken. These observations call for the postulation of a cellular pool, in which exogenous heparin may be sequestered and released gradually into the circulation.

If such a pool exists, why then does the intravenously administered heparin escape it? Or does it? With large intravenous doses of heparin, Solandt and Best (2) observed that the effect of heparin on platelets persisted long after the hypocoagulability has subsided. There have been similar reports on the effect of heparin on antithrombin III activity.

II. METHODS, MATERIALS, AND PROCEDURES

Sodium heparin from pig intestinal mucosa, Lot #31733 was a gift from Fine Chemicals Division, Canada Packers Ltd., USP activity as determined by the manufacturer was 157 units/ mg. Heparin was administered to C_3H inbred mice (n=12) and Sprague Dawley rats (n=6) by tracheal instillation. The animals were anesthetized with pentobarbital and then a tracheotomy was performed. A fine polyethylene catheter was introduced into the trachea and the heparin solution (25 mg/ ml) instilled slowly. The mice each recieved 2 mg while the rats each received 10 mg of heparin. The wound was then closed in layers and the skin stitched. Control mice (n=10) and control rats (n=5) received a volume of saline similar to the volume of heparin solution, by tracheal instillation. All other procedures were similar.

The mice were sacrificed after 15 min. Lung samples were taken and fixed in osmium tetroxide 4% and sodium bicarbonate buffer pH 7.2. Embedding was done in epon and one-micron thick sections were cut and stained in 1% toluidine blue in sodium tetraborate. The rats were used for the observation of migrating macrophages. These cells were obtained from a subcutaneous inflammatory area caused by the insertion of a glass micro coverslip under the skin through an incision. The rats were sacrificed 24 hr after receiving intrapulmonary heparin. The coverslips were removed and stained in 1% toluidine blue. For the examination of heparin in blood, four rats were given each 2000 units of sodium heparin by tracheal instillation. After 15 min simultaneous arterial and venous blood samples were collected from the aorta and inferior vena cava, respectively. These samples were centrifuged, and the plasma concentration of heparin was determined by the *inhibition of Factor Xa* procedure (3). Another rat was given 50 units of ^{3}H-heparin by tracheal instillation. Arterial and venous plasma samples were obtained as above, and the radioactivity was measured by liquid scintillation. Endothelium was obtained from aorta and vena cava by the Hautchen technique (4). Samples of the endothelial tissue from each vessel were counted for radioactivity. The fluor used was Aquasol, and the liquid scintillation counter was an Isocap 300 from Searle Co.

III. RESULTS AND DISCUSSION

An examination of the lung tissue of mice was done at the light microscopy level. This revealed the uptake of heparin by macrophages, the fixation of heparin to the endothelial tissue, and the presence of heparin in the pulmonary blood vessels and small lymphatics. Figures *1a* and *1b* show alveolar macrophages from control and experimental mice. The macrophages from the heparinized mouse show red-purple granules (dense dark spots on the black and white print) in their cytoplasm as well as around them. They show evidence of pinocytosis. The red-purple particles are heparin-toluidine blue particles. They are also found in the alveolar space. After tracheal instillation of the heparin solution the animal was put in a vertical position to facilitate the flow of the heparin down to the smaller bronchioles. The respiratory air flow probably helps to move the heparin down to the alveolar spaces By the time the heparin reaches the alveoli it is probably well mixed with mucus and the alveolar surfactant. This mixture when stained with toluidine blue appears as red-purple particles. Figures *1c* and *1d* show macrophages obtained from skin windows in control and experimental rats. The macrophages from the experimental rats show the presence of red-purple particulate material in the cytoplasm. Figures *1e* and *1f* show pulmonary blood vessels. The blood vessels from the heparinized mice show the presence of red-purple particulate material attached to the endothelium.

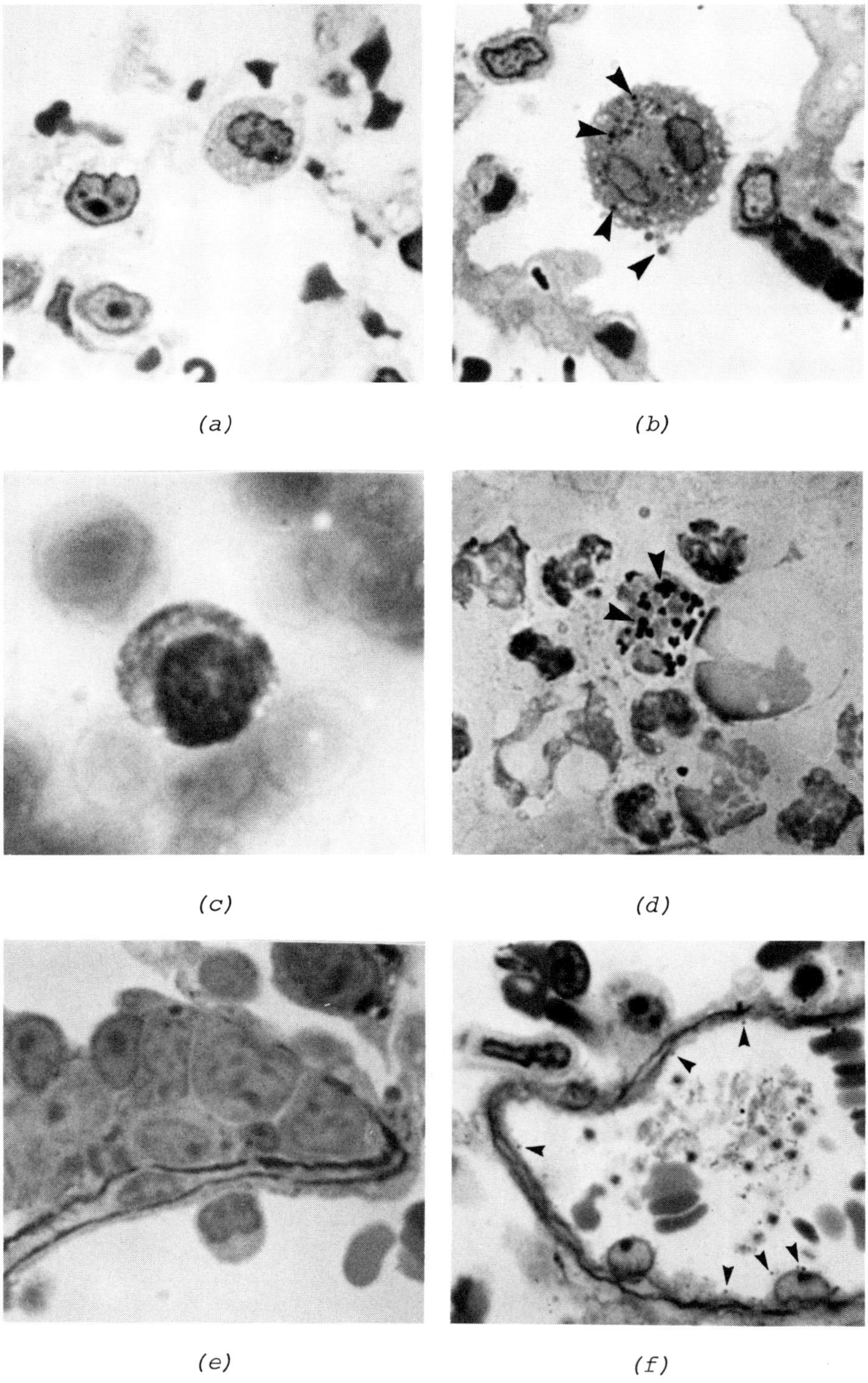

Fig. 1. Cellular uptake of heparin (x 3600).

Further evidence for the sequestration of administered heparin by the endothelial tissue is obtained by analyzing the arterial and venous blood for heparin content (Table I). Also shown in this table is the amount of radioactivity in arterial and venous plasma from the ^{3}H-heparin administered.

TABLE I Heparin Concentration in Plasma

	Arterial units/ml	*Venous units/ml*
Rat #1	*0.72*	*0.58*
Rat #2	*1.50*	*1.10*
Rat #3	*0.36*	*0.18*
Rat #4	*1.00*	*0.88*
Rat #5	*17,384 cpm*	*11,614 cpm*

Dose administered by tracheal instillation: 547 units/100 gm B.Wt.

The venous plasma shows a concentration of heparin consistently lower than is present in arterial plasma. The radioactivity in the venous plasma is also lower than is present in arterial plasma. The concentration of heparin in the plasma is below the level at which heparin extravasates into tissue fluid or is excreted by the kidney. Hence the plausible explanation for this arterio-venous difference is sequestration by the endothelial tissue. This represents a tremendous uptake by the endothelium. The heparin absorbed from the lungs enters the blood stream and is continually taken up by the endothelial tissue along the vascular tree. The pinocytic activity of the endothelial tissues varies with the size of the vessel and the location of the vessel. By the time the blood laden with the absorbed heparin reaches the venous side of the circulation a great proportion of it (25 to 30%) is already taken up by the endothelial surface. Endothelium from the aorta and vena cava was also examined for radioactivity. The amount of radioactivity observed on the aortic endothelium per square centimeter of tissue was higher than was present on the corresponding surface area of vena caval endothelium. This lends additional support to the idea of sequestration of plasma heparin by the endothelial tissue. After heparin administration, the macrophages show abundant metachromatic material. It has already been demonstrated (8) that peritoneal macrophages can migrate out of the peritoneal cavity and distribute themselves all over the body. The present study suggests that pulmonary macrophages may also migrate out of the lungs. In fact, this illustrates a probable means of transport and storage of heparin administered by the pulmonary route. As pointed out in a previous publication (6), mast cells are not involved to any significant extent in the absorption or storage of exogenous heparin. In the present study the pleural membrane from both normal control and heparinized rats was examined by light microscopy. The large number of mast cells in the pleural membrane did not show any evidence of accumulation of exogenous heparin. Until recently it has been casually reported in the literature that some cells are capable of taking up heparin. As early as 1939, Asplund and co-workers (7) reported the location of injected heparin in cells of the R.E.S. In 1955, Fawcett (8) and in 1958, Smith and co-workers (9) reported the location of injected heparin in fibrocytes. More recently in our own laboratory, Oh and co-workers (10) have shown the uptake of ^{35}S-heparin by peritoneal macrophages and Hiebert (11) has demonstrated the fixation of heparin to endothelial tissue. All of these observations lend support to the concept of a cellular pool for exogenous heparin. Endogenous heparin when liberated from mast cells as granules is taken up and is probably degraded by macrophages (12). The dissimilarity of the effect of intravenous heparin compared to the in vitro effect, the longer low grade hypocoagulability obtained from subcutaneous heparin and the very long duration of action of intrapulmonary heparin all suggest that exogenous heparin is treated differently *in vivo* from endogenous heparin. The administration of a certain dose of heparin by the subcutaneous route produces a longer duration of effect than when the same dose is given by the intravenous route. The peak effect in blood, however, is lower when the drug is given by the subcutaneous route. Moreover the peak concentration of heparin reached in the blood is less than 5% of that obtained after intravenous administration. With intrapulmonary heparin, the effective dose is in a much higher range (above 8 mg/kg of B.Wt.) but here again we observe an even more prolonged duration of effect with a low peak effect. These features (lower peak effect and prolonged duration of action) are characteristic of indirect routes of administering heparin. One distinct and common feature of these indirect routes (subcutaneous, intramuscular, intraperitoneal, intrapulmonary) is that of exposure to a population of macrophages. Exogenous heparin may, by virtue of its foreign character attract macrophages to the site of administration. This has been observed in the lungs after intrapulmonary heparin. These cells would take up the heparin and store them. The prolonged duration of effect observed when heparin is administered by the indirect routes suggests that the drug is somehow released into the blood circulation; thus, a release function for the cellular pool. It is possible that the heparin sequestered by the cellular pool is released as the cells die. Cellular death normally occurs as a wear and tear process, the older population disintegrating first.

IV. CONCLUSION

The histological studies on mice and rats, and heparin determination on blood from rats that had received heparin by the pulmonary route, have provided evidence for the sequestration and storage functions of macrophages and endothelial tissue in dealing with exogenous heparin. Migrating macrophages, containing heparin, indicate one of the possible modes of transport of administered heparin. Release of the sequestered or stored heparin is evidenced by the prolonged duration of action obtained when heparin is introduced into the circulation by indirect routes. Thus a cellular pool composed mainly of macrophages and endothelial tissue may operate to modulate the duration of action and the concentration of heparin in systemic blood.

V. ACKNOWLEDGEMENT

This research was supported by a grant from the Saskatchewan Heart Foundation. Additional financial assistance and donation of generous quantities of heparin were received from Canada Packers Ltd., Toronto, Ontario, Canada.

REFERENCES

1. Jaques, L.B., Mahadoo, J., Kavanagh, L.W., The Lancet, p. 1157, 27 November (1976).
2. Solandt, D.Y. and Best, C.H., The Lancet, p. 1042, June 8 (1940).
3. Yin, E.T., Wessler, S., Butler, J.V., J. Lab. Clin. Med. *81*, 298 (1973).
4. Pugatch, E.M.J., Saunders, A.M., J. Ather. Res. *8*, 735 (1968).
5. Vernons-Roberts, B., Nature *222*, 1286, June 28 (1969).
6. Jaques, L.B., Mahadoo, J., Riley, J.F., The Lancet, p. 411, February 19 (1977).
7. Asplund, J., Holmgren, H., Borell, U., Z. mikrosk-anat. Forsch. *46*, 16 (1939).
8. Fawcett, D.W., Anat. Rec. *121*, 29 (1955).
9. Smith, D.E., Lewis, Y.S., Anat. Rec. *132*, 93 (1958).
10. Oh, T.H., Naidoo, S.S., Jaques, L.B., J. R.E.S. *13*, 134 (1973).
11. Hiebert, L.M., Jaques, L.B., Thromb. Res. *8*, 195, (1976).
12. Riley, J.F., Ann. N.Y. Acad. Sci. *103*, 151 (1963).

HEPARIN AND FACTOR VIII

E.A. Beck

Hamatologisches Zentrallabor Inselspital

Factor VIII comprises two biological functions which are essential for normal hemostasis, i.e., the classical antihemophilic or coagulant and the so-called von Willebrand activities. Factor VIII related protein appears to be normal in classical hemophilia but qualitatively and/or quantitatively deficient in von Willebrand's disease (1). *In vitro* this protein is found as a macromolecular complex with an estimated size well in excess of 10^6 daltons. Following treatment with reducing agents subunits with a molecular weight of about 250,000 are found. Intact factor VIII subunits are homogenous on SDS-polyacrylamide electrophoresis (2).

Following prolonged dialysis of factor VIII-related protein at low ionic strength, a decrease of the size of non-reduced protein complex was found on SDS-polyacrylamide electrophoresis. Since the size of reduced subunit chains remained unaltered, a non-proteolytic degradation and/or dissociation was postulated (3). We found that activity responsible for this type of dissociation was variable in factor VIII preparations obtained from different blood donors and possible in the same person. In search of enzymes with similar properties we investigated several types of glucosidases as well as lipases. None of them dissociated factor VIII, with the notable exception of a mold (Rhizopus arrhizus) triglyceride lipase (4). In recent unpublished experiments we also found that rat adipose tissue contains enzyme(s) with dissociating properties.

Factor VIII is not thought to be a typical lipoprotein (2). However, relatively small amounts of associated lipids could favor hydrophobic interactions and thus promote formation of larger aggregates. If triglyceride lipase indeed dissociates factor VIII, a disulfide-type of subunit linkage seems rather improbable.

In view of these preliminary results we were interested to study effects of heparin-induced lipoprotein lipases on

ISBN 0-12-484850-8

factor VIII. Following injection of 10,000 units of commercial heparin (Liquemine, Roche) in man, we were, however, unable to detect significant alterations of isolated factor VIII complex. In this same experiment we confirmed the previous observation that high concentrations of heparin interfere with von Willebrand activity as tested by ristocetin-induced platelet aggregation (5,6).

In conclusion, heparin may interfere with hemostatic properties of factor VIII at the level of von Willebrand activity/platelet interactions. Whether or not molecular properties of factor VIII are influenced by lipase-like activity in man remains to be shown.

REFERENCES

1. Firkin, B.G., and Howard, M.A., Brit. J. Haemat. *32*, 151 (1976).
2. Hershgold, E.J., *in* "Progress in Hemostasis and Thrombosis" (T.H. Spaet, ed.), Vol. *2*, p. 99. Grune and Stratton, New York and London, 1974.
3. Furlan, M., and Beck, E.A., Thrombos. Res. *10*, 153 (1977).
4. Furlan, M., Jakab, T., and Beck, E.A., Thrombos. Res. *10*, 431 (1977).
5. Pekcelen, Y., and Inceman, S., Thromb. Haemost. (Stuttg.) *35*, 485 (1976).
6. Beck, E.A., Thromb. Haemost. (Stuttg.) in press.

FUNDAMENTAL RELATIONS OF HEPARIN TO FIBRINOGEN AND TO OTHER LIVING PROTEINS

Herbert L. Davis and Nora L. Davis

Departments of Surgery and Biochemistry
University of Nebraska College of Medicine, Omaha

In these days there are many searches for improved concepts and comprehension of the composition and properties of the sulfated mucopolysaccharides, with special reference to the heparins. This applies also to interactions of these substances with proteins involved in life processes of humans and animals. Probably the most important of these is fibrinogen as it determines the coagulability of flowing blood, and thus controls perfusion and nutrition of all living tissues. It is desirable to consider general relations and the maintenance of fibrinogen and other living proteins in states of healthy functioning.

Fifty years ago it was widely recognized that all living systems are colloidal in their form and function, and that life depends on the maintenance of many proteins in an optimum intermediate state. Deviations from this condition result in discomfort, disease, and disaster. The task of medicine is to prevent such deviations and to restore the optimum state. Many more sophisticated techniques and procedures have been developed but the fundamental relations still govern. Many mysteries will be clarified by reference to colloidal concepts and principles (1,2,3).

The form and function of all living proteins depend on the relative excess of one charge over the other, and upon sufficient hydration (bound water) on both the negative and positive sites. The hydrophilic nature of the polar sites is opposed by the hydrophobic (water repellent) nature of the nonpolar sites. Reduction in the charge and/or hydration on a dispersed protein, such as fibrinogen in plasma, results in relative shift toward hydrophobic character, resulting in colloidal dispersion destabilization. Cationics and/or dehydrants may thus destabilize fibrinogen (or other proteins) to the intermediate gel state, and higher concentrations of the same reagents may then produce precipitation of the protein.

Plasma proteins fall into the following classes when examined by electrophoresis: Globulin (gamma, fibrinogen, beta, $alpha_2$, $alpha_1$) albumins. In this series there is progressive fall in molecular weight, rise in charge (electrokinetic, zeta potential), etc. Salting out by ammonium sulfate brings a similar progression, fibrinogen being pre-

ISBN 0-12-484850-8

cipitated first at 12% concentration. These facts mean that albumin is the smallest of these major proteins, with maximum charge and hydration and with maximum binding sites for both positive and negative ions, etc. Fibrinogen is at the other end of the scale, with maximum molecular weight, moderate negative charge, and minimal hydration. Indeed, the natural state of fibrinogen is one of metastability - just ready to be destabilized to the gel (clot) state by reduction in its charge and/or hydration. Further additions of procoagulants retard or prevent gel formation, and finally precipitate fibrinogen. These U-curves of clot times vs. procoagulant additions are clear indications of the colloidal nature of the gel formation. The orthodox action of thrombin is to split from fibrinogen two tiny, very negative fragments. This reduction in its overall negative charge causes the "fibrin" residue to polymerize into a gel structure. This is only one of the ways in which the flowing blood can be changed to a clot. Identical gels are formed from pure fibrinogen plus thrombin, *or* protamine, *or* ethanol, and similar substances produce many cases of hypercoagulability (14).

I. THE CONTROL OF FIBRINOGEN DISPERSION STABILITY

Four classes of substances modify and control the charge and/or hydration of fibrinogen and thus determine blood coagulability. *Procoagulants* lower the negative charge and/or reduce the hydration on polar sites. In general, charge and hydration are interdependent. All charged sites are hydrated and all hydrated sites carry some charge. Adsorption of calcium ion on a negative site lowers the overall negative charge *and* prevents both participants from binding water molecules. *Cationics* are adsorbed on negative sites, and thus lower the charge and hydration. A few examples are calcium, hydrogen ion (acidosis), histamine, serotonin, local anesthetics, catecholamines, protamine, basic dyes, heroin, and many others. *Dehydrants* are negative, surfactants, bound on positive sites. Their chief effect is to displace water by attachment of their hydrophilic ends, while exposing hydrophobic ends to the water phase. With fibrinogen, this marked increase in hydrophobic surface results in increased tendency to gel formation. Further addition of alcohol, for example, is adsorbed on the same site, and exposes new hydrophilic groups. Some examples are alcohols, lipids (especially free fatty acids as soaps at pH 7.4), thromboplastins, steroids, aspirin, x-ray opaque dyes, general anesthetics, and many other (6).

Irregular series are ubiquitous in physiology. Low to moderate concentrations of these substances are procoagulant-lower clot times, increase tendency to thromboembolic episodes, etc. Higher plasma levels retard and prevent coagulation and are anticoagulant, even to the point of hemorrhagic tendencies. Relevant U-curves of clot times vs. substance concentration can be shown in citrated plasma plus calcium, in fibrinogen plus thrombin, in animals and in human beings.

The two classes of procoagulants are major factors in clotting to death. Opposing their influence are the two *anti*-coagulant classes. *Anionics* are highly negative substances, bound on the positive sites of fibrinogen to increase the negative charge overall and the hydration. Heparin and heparinoids are prime examples; citrates and phosphates function by abstracting calcium and thus indirectly increasing the negative charge. *Hydrants* are substances that increase (water dilution) or preserve the hydration of fibrinogen (dextrans, albumins, gelatins). Irregular series effects are observed also with anticoagulants. Note that excess cationics and/or dehydrants exert anticoagulant effects.

In addition to the four classes of substances listed above, blood coagulation can be induced or prevented by *electrical* currents. Yoshida (17) formed standard thrombi in the carotid artery of the dog by making a platinum wire the anode (positive). Negative fibrinogen formed thereon a gel that could best be dispersed by streptokinase plus heparin. Schwartz (15) showed that a clamped-off segment of the femoral vein did not clot if it was surrounded by a negative electrode - even if thrombin was injected. Putting a positive charge on the electrode caused rapid clotting. *Osmotic* effects are significant in coagulation. Merely altering the sodium chloride concentration of the blood results in a U-curve, with elevated times at low and high salt concentration. Electrolytes alter ionic strength to control the zeta potential, but nonelectrolytes have similar effects on hydration.

Several alternate or supplementary "anticoagulants" can reduce the need for heparin in the common hypercoagulable episodes. *Glucose* provides living energy and minimizes mobilization of free fatty acids, the most common procoagulant in human stress. *Steroids* in high doses are anticoagulant - among other effects. *Aspirin* in high doses prevents destabilization of fibrinogen, and thus prevents general adhesiveness of all plasma components. Bicarbonates reduce the hydrogen ion concentration with their procoagulant effects. *Glycerol* or *ethanol* act somewhat as glucose in furnishing calories, but the drunk on a binge is markedly hypercoagulable. *Dextran* 40 is mostly a plasma expander, but *Dextran* 70 is definitely an anticoagulant.

II. THE CLINICAL SIGNIFICANCE OF HYPERCOAGULABILITY

Gradually, it is becoming clear that most people clot to death. Many years ago, MacFarlane (13) said, "For every patient who dies because of the failure of his blood to clot, many thousands of people die because of the failure of their blood to remain fluid in vital parts of their circulation". Increasingly, books and papers shift emphasis from hypocoagulability to hypercoagulability, disseminated intravascular coagulation, and the need to prevent and correct the latter. Dr. Tullis's book, "CLOT" (16), includes three excellent chapters on hypercoagulability, and he estimates the relative hazard at one to one hundred. After many years of investigating blood sludging, Knisely (12) summarized it in the title "Blood Must Circulate", listing 160 diagnoses in over 8000 patients with accelerated erythrocyte sedimentation, and this appears due to coating of the cells with the sticky destabilized fibrinogen (7).

This destabilization causes fibrinogen to be driven from the aqueous phase onto all surfaces in or exposed to plasma. This results in aggregation of *platelets* and their adhesion to vascular walls, entrapment of *leucocytes* in capillaries, rouleaux formation of *erythrocytes* and their settling, and increase in *viscosity* as the gel state is approached (4,9,11).

The changes in blood flow and perfusion lead to corresponding clinical manifestations depending on stressor agents, individual susceptibility, vascular anomalies, deposits, injuries. With many overlaps and coincidences, the following clinical observations are made: deep vein thrombosis, mesenteric thrombosis with ulcers and necrosis, kidney impairment with elevated blood pressure and shut-down, pulmonary embolism, transient ischemic attacks and stroke, coronary arrhythmias, infarcts, and arrest. Countless discussions of these clinical catastrophes start with ischemia and include thromboemboli, but rarely get to underlying mechanisms. Each of these states have important hypercoagulable aspects, and can be treated with anticoagulants.

In the recognition and treatment of DIC appropriate assays of whole blood seem most relevant. Generally, the standard clot factor tests employ large excesses of potent procoagulants to obtain gels in short times. These tests are relevant to hypocoagulable states. The single exception is the activated partial thromboplastin time test depending on the surfaces of clay particles and the potent thromboplastins to give gels with plasma in 40-60 sec. (10). Low times in this test are associated with thromboembolic hazards and have been so used.

More convenient and promising appears the activated clot time (ACT) test of Bull and associates (5). Whole blood is drawn into an evacuated tube containing 12 mg of celite clay. Their use of this test is to titrate each patient's resistance to heparin, to be injected for extracorporeal surgery procedures. They find linear relations between the units of heparin and the ACT times for protection, but they find a three-fold difference between patients in the amount of heparin required to reach the desired 480 sec and they report that subjects without operation taken to this 480 sec level show a four-fold difference in the rate of heparin loss from plasma. Any attempt to standardize heparin must still deal with the impossibility of standardizing the patient or his coagulability state. Individual titration appears inevitable.

Experience with these ACT tubes shows that control values for subjects or for patients before surgery range from 70 to 120 sec. It appears likely that low values in this test, or some improvement thereof, may provide a convenient index of coagulability states. This would recall deTakats' repeated suggestions of a heparin tolerance test (8).

III. GENERAL EFFECTS ON LIVING PROTEINS

In the sections above, the colloidal dispersion stability of fibrinogen has been the primary consideration. This stability is continually changing as the plasma environment responds to a variety of stresses (physical, chemical, psychic). Such changes control the nutrition and health of all living organs and tissues. Further study reveals that all other

TABLE I Substances Controlling Living Proteins

Agglomerating agents		*Dispersing agents*	
Reduce charge Class A	*Hydration Class B*	*Increase charge Class C*	*Hydration Class D*
Cationics	*Dehydrants (surfactants)*	*Anionics*	*Hydrants*
			Water dilution
Histamine	*Alcohols*	*Heparin*	*Albumins*
Calcium	*Lipids - free fatty acids*	*Heparinoids*	*Dextrans*
Acidosis (H+)	*Anesthetics (General)*	*Citrates*	*Gelatins*
Anesthetics (Local)	*Steroids*	*Phosphates*	*Excess - dehydrants*
AMP, ADP, ATP	*Hydrocarbons*	*Excess - cationics*	
Catecholamines	*X-ray opaques*		
Protamine	*Acid Dyes*		
Basic Dyes			

living proteins are also subject to similar alterations in their form and function. No drug does only what it is used for. Table I lists a few members of the four classes affecting fibrinogen. These are listed under the terms "Agglomerating" and "Dispersing Agents" to connote their procoagulant and anticoagulant influences in the blood. Members of each class act cumulatively with each other. Members of each class of cationics and dehydrants cooperate synergistically with each other, and antagonisms against the anticoagulants are predictable and useful.

Table II shows how the members of the four classes alter the form and function of other living proteins. The proteins of nerves control neural sensitivity, the proteins of cell membrane pores govern permeability, and protein enzymes are modified in their activity by various concentrations of these same chemicals. Only rarely are the total effect vs. concentration curves run, so that any single concentration may lie anywhere on the curve. Irregular series are ubiquitous in physiology.

TABLE II Physiological Effects

	Agglomerating agents		*Dispersing agents*	
	Low concs.	*High concs.*	*Low concs.*	*High concs.*
Fibrinogen coagulability	*Pro-coag.*	*Anti-coag.*	*Anti-coag.*	*Pro-coag.*
Neural sensitivity	*Increased*	*Decreased*	*Increased*	*Decreased*
Membrane permeability	*Increased*	*Decreased*	*Decreased*	*Increased*
Enzyme activity	*Increased*	*Decreased*	*Decreased*	*Increased*

In summary, the great majority of stressors in human beings involve accentuation of cationic and/or dehydrant substances. Their principle effect is to decrease the colloidal stability of fibrinogen, and thus to conduce to hypercoagulability. Heparin is the most convenient and effective agent to increase both the negative charge and the minimal hydration on polar sites of fibrinogen. It is thus able to restore the natural equilibrium of the flowing blood sol. Both procoagulant and anticoagulant substances produce associated effects on other living proteins, comparable to those effected on fibrinogen. Suitable administrations can thus maintain all living proteins in the optimum intermediate state for healthy functioning.

REFERENCES

1. Alexander, J., "Colloid Chemistry, Vol. II, Biology and Medicine". Chemical Catalog Co., 1928.
2. Bancroft, W.D., "Applied Colloid Chemistry". McGraw-Hill New York, 1929.
3. Bechhold, H., (trans. by J.G.G. Bullowa), "Colloids in Biology and Medicine". D. van Nostrand, 1919.
4. Bicher, H.I., "Blood Cell Aggregation in Thromboembotic Processes". Thomas, Springfield, 1972.
5. Bull, B.S., *et al.*, Heparin Therapy During Extracorporeal Circulation, J. Thorac. and Cardiovasc, Surgery *69*, 674-84, 685-9 (1975).
6. Davis, H.L., "Heparin is an Anionic Hydrated Anticoagulant, Heparin," (R.A. Bradshaw and S. Wessler, eds.) p. 31-71. Plenum New York, 1975.
7. Davis, H.L., and Musselman, M.D., The Mechanism and Significance of Increased Erythrocyte Sedimentation Rate, J. Trauma *14*, 963-6 (1974).
8. DeTakats, G., Heparin: The Need for a Flexible Protocol, Editorial. Am. J. Surg. *132*, 1-3 (1976).
9. Dintenfass, L., "Rheology of Blood in Diagnostic and Preventive Medicine". Butterworth, Boston, 1976.
10. Hirsh, J., Experimental Basis for Heparin Therapy in Venous Thrombosis and Pulmonary Embolism, this symposium.
11. Kakkar, V.V., and Thomas, D.P., eds., "Heparin Chemistry and Clinical Usage". Academic Press, New York, 1976.
12. Knisely, M.H., Blood Must Circulate, pp. 61-68, "Reversibility of Cellular Injury Due to Inadequate Perfusion", (T.L. Malone, etc., eds.). Thomas, Springfield, 1972.
13. MacFarlane, R.C., "Forward to the Contact Phase of Blood Coagulation". H.L. Nossel, F.A. Davis, Philadelphia, 1964.
14. Niewiarowski, S., Stewart, G.J., and Marder, V.J., Formation of Highly Ordered Polymers from Fibrinogen and Fibrin Degradation Products, Biochimica et Biophysica Acta *221*, 326-41 (1970).
15. Schwartz, S.L., Prevention and Production of Thromboses by Alterations in the Electrical Environment, Surg., Gyn., and Obstet. *108*, 333-6 (1959).
16. Tullis, J.L., "CLOT". Thomas, Springfield, 1976.
17. Yoshida, K., (with H. Handa), Experimental Studies on the Production and Treatment of Carotid Thrombosis in Dogs, Archiv fur Japanese Chirugie *33*, 502-25 (1964).

Thursday, July 7, 1977, 4:00 p.m.

VAN DEDEM, Oss Dr. Rosenberg, you showed a slide relating the initial rate of thrombin-antithrombin complexation to the heparin concentration. The heparin concentrations were from 10^{-8} to 10^{-6}, which were higher than the concentrations of thrombin or antithrombin. How do you reconcile this with the idea of this reaction being catalyzed by heparin rather than going through a ternary complex?

ROSENBERG, Boston If you take into account the concentrations of the proteins, it can be shown that where the maximal plateau is reached is indeed the point at which one to one complexing occurs. It may not be obvious but it really works. I think that it is necessary to obtain a value about 10-fold greater than the binding constant to reach a maximum at the concentrations that we are employing. I think it's not inconsistent.

VAN DEDEM, Oss But can you really compare it to an enzyme catalyzed reaction where the enzyme concentration is usually several orders of magnitude lower?

ROSENBERG, Boston No. It's just different kinetics. It is true that a maximum is reached at one to one complexing. Our fluorescent data when compared with the data that we get for plateau point shows coincidence remarkably well, given the errors of the analysis.

VAN DEDEM, Oss The number of reducing groups which you find, how do they relate to more or less accepted molecular weights that are now in existence for heparin?

ROSENBERG, Boston I wouldn't be prepared to say. We're in the midst of that kind of analysis and it would be premature for me to say. I think they are in reasonable accord but that estimate can be off by 30%, easily.

SILBERT, Boston You stated that the reducing groups were all uronic acids. Did you ever examine the entire active fragment to determine if there was any hexosamine reducing group at all?

ROSENBERG, Boston In the Wilson heparin, as near as we can tell, it's alluronic acid. That was by direct labeling of the end group and then degrading the molecule.

ISBN 0-12-484850-8

SILBERT, Boston Do you know how this material was prepared?

ROSENBERG, Boston Well, with the Wilson heparin there is no bleaching. It presumably is taken out at stage 14, whatever that is, and then we prepare it by CPC precipitation by Lindahl's method that was described in 1965.

SILBERT, Boston This structure would imply that the heparin that you are looking at had seen an endoglycuronidase.

ROSENBERG, Boston That's right. I think that most of the molecules have been clipped by an endoglycuronidase. I think that's in excellent accord with Lindahl's work on very similar material.

PADAWER, New York Dr. Lasker mentioned potassium, sodium, calcium, and lithium with respect to the association of certain cations with heparin. In the literature I have seen reference to copper and maybe iron, but I have never come across anything with zinc, and since there is a lot of zinc in mast cells I wonder whether anyone could comment on whether there is a special effect which zinc may have with heparin.

LASKER, New York I haven't looked at zinc, it might be worth the effort.

SHERRY, Philadelphia Since Dr. Rosenberg did enter into some speculation, let me ask him a question. In the antithrombin III system we consider a main regulator for the entire coagulation cascade, yet we're informed that this is a relatively slow inactivator alone, something which is very rapidly activated by heparin, yet no one has ever demonstrated significant quantities of endogenous heparin in the blood. How do you postulate that this system really works in terms of controlling or providing a defense mechanism against the problem of thrombosis in man? Specifically, do you assume that the antithrombin III molecules are homogeneous, and that heparin is heterogeneous? Is there heterogeneity with antithrombin III and particularly, is there a small fraction of antithrombin III in the circulation which is capable of immediately inactivating either thrombin or some of the early cascade components like activated factors IX, X or XI?

ROSENBERG, Boston I am strongly struck by the fact that the inhibitor-enzyme interactions are so slow at the concentrations at which they must occur *in vivo*, hence heparin or some heparin-like mucopolysaccharide has to be involved in the system if we are to explain antithrombin deficiency as a major thrombotic event. I can only conceive of a system in which heparin is intimately involved as a method of revving up antithrombin. With respect to antithrombin I think that the majority of the molecules, at least with respect to usual physical-chemical evidence are homogeneous. There are some minor components in human blood, I have some of them although we have never reported on this, they appear to behave similarly with respect to heparin. So my guess is that antithrombin isn't heterogeneous. In thinking about the coagulation mechanism in general I view the coagulation mechanism to be set up to capture rare events. It begins with a protein that is relatively inactive, there is a plentiful supply so that when a rare event occurs a very small quantity of the protein is converted to an active form and I really look upon the antithrombin mechanism in many ways as being identical to that - on the one hand very large amounts of any of the zymogens exist, only trivial amounts are converted to active enzyme. For antithrombin large amounts of bulk specie are present but there must be heparin-like material, introduced in only trivial amounts, that promote activation to deal with an initial insult. I think the question really comes down to how much activated antithrombin is required to function in a physiological fashion. That becomes a matter of gut reaction but it is really essential because if that can be decided then one may consider what characteristics the heparin-like material must possess. We're focusing on a high activity heparin as being physiologically very important. It may well be the low activity heparin that may be critical if indeed it is able to activate the antithrombin molecule, because the activation of the inhibitor may well depend upon how much is partitioned, given a ligand that has a lousy binding constant. I'm attracted to the idea that the stuff has to be on the vessel wall and on the platelet surfaces, because that's where coagulation takes place. I'd like to think that heparan sulfates serve some purpose but I think our present analytical tools with respect to structure or function are blunt and probably wouldn't allow us to dissect this kind of mechanism, but I really think the future may lie in the low activity components rather than the high activity ones, at least in the physiological sense.

SHERRY, Philadelphia Is it possible that by looking at antithrombin activity that we may be missing the fact that there is a small fraction of material which has been activated and that this may be more easily picked up if you look at activated factors IX, X, or XI?

ROSENBERG, Boston We're now in the midst of looking at all of the enzymes. My own gut reaction is, if you use a radioactive substrate working at enzyme concentrations that are roughly comparable, it's not a coagulation assay and I suspect that all of them will be pretty much the same, but I have no hard data to demonstrate if that's true. I think your idea that an occasional antithrombin molecule gets into the right activated state to act is an intriguing one, and it may even be true. We may be biasing a whole series of confirmations which have a real continuum. There may be one in a million antithrombin molecules in solvent, that is, in activated state and maybe that molecule is responsible for the residual antithrombin activity as we see it. Perhaps these ligands merely bias and pull confirmation in one or another direction, that would fit in very well with what is known of proteins and their confirmations in solutions, but I think that's too complex to even to begin to think about, although it may be the physiologically relevant way of considering this.

HURST, Birmingham This is addressed to either Dr. Rosenberg or Dr. Lindahl or both and it relates to heparin as an informational molecule or an information carrying molecule and the methods for the synthesis. Are specific sequences introduced in very specific ways into the heparin molecule or are the two heparins related, the inactive and active? Is one a precursor or is one converted into the other?

LINDAHL, Uppsala We know very little about the regulation of the sequence formation, one mechanism which I touched upon is that of the deacetylation. If you look at the deacetylation reaction, with an exogeneous substrate it's clearly random so this would not give rise to a specific sequence. The other factor that leads to the formation of different disaccharides and thus to different sequences is the incompleteness of the modification reactions. I find it very difficult to see any specific mechanism determining whether one potential disaccharide residue is selected for modification or not. My present inclination is to think of the whole thing very much as a random mechanism. It's difficult to see that there should be any specific regulatory formation of heparin binding site.

HURST, Birmingham Would it be possible that there is a specific enzyme which acts on the finished product to make some specific alteration which is somehow coded for in the structure of the protein by the nature of its binding site? This then might make specific alterations afterwards, in analogy with some of the specific DNA altering enzymes.

LINDAHL, Uppsala This possibility cannot be excluded, of course, but I think the element of randomness in the process is also reflected in the molecular weight dependence of the anticoagulant activity of the heparin.

HURST, Birmingham With regard to that, if, as Dr. Rosenberg points out, there are two sites required then there may be a minimum size of molecule which would incorporate both. Perhaps that would explain the nature of the molecular weight dependence.

LINDAHL, Uppsala Well, this is relevant to Dr. Lasker's paper explaining the molecular weight dependence on the anticoagulant activity. If you assume that the sequence is determined by random factors, and that it somehow has to end up with a binding site of the size of the dodecasaccharide, the anticoagulant activity of a given heparin preparation should be expressed by the probability of finding this specific dodecasaccharide sequence in a polymer made up of randomly distributed disaccharide units. This probability of finding this dodecasaccharide again is a function of the molecular weight of the polysaccharide. The number of possible dodecasaccharide sequences can be related to molecular weight, mathematically. In collaboration with T. Laurent in Uppsala, we derived an equation and then tested it on heparin preparations of different molecular weight. The proportion of high affinity molecules was determined because that would be a direct way of testing this hypothesis. We've taken pig mucosal heparin and separated it into a large number of fractions by gel chromatography and then we have passed each fraction over antithrombin-sepharose and determined the fraction of high affinity molecules. With the low molecular weight material (5,000 daltons) less than 1 out of 10 chains bind to antithrombin and these values have then been fitted to a hypothetical probability function based on the randomly assembled dodecasaccharide sequence. There is very good agreement up to a molecular weight of 18,000 actually including 95% of the entire heparin preparation. The one that deviated (higher molecular weight) differed from the other molecules by containing large amounts of the polypeptide core. The presence of these amino acids would lead one to expect them to deviate from the relationship, and this, I think, provides a partial explanation for the data shown by Dr. Lasker of the increased anticoagulant activity with molecular weight, although it's not the only explanation since the molecular weight of the high affinity heparin itself also increases with molecular weight.

MEYER, New York Dr. Lindahl, a question about the deacetylase.

Is it specific for the precursor of the heparin or is it nonspecific? Could this be a transacetylase which transfers the acetyl group to some other acceptor and, in this respect, one would be tempted to see if there is any effect of coenzyme A.

LINDAHL, Uppsala We have tested the specificity by using hyaluronic acid as an alternative substrate and it is completely inactive. This would be similar to the natural substrate for the deacetylase, containing both glucuronic acid and N-acetyl-glucosamine, in similar fashion although the linkages are different. A beta 1,3 linkage exists in hyaluronic acid.

MEYER, New York Did you try oligosaccharides from hyaluronic acid?

LINDAHL, Uppsala No, we didn't, but since it works on a very large polymer, the heparin precursor, I think you would be able to detect it acting also on hyaluronic acid if the action was nonspecific. There does not seem to be any need for an acceptor since the way we assay it is by introducing tritiated acetyl groups into the polymer and then quantitating these as free labeled acetic acids released by the enzymes.

WEISSMANN, Chicago I have two questions for Dr. Lindahl. One is, is there necessarily a correspondence between the region of the active heparin which is protected by complexing and the size of the essential binding piece? In other words, could the binding region not be considerably smaller than what you isolate after heparinase treatment? Secondly, could not the statistical treatment that you have applied to this apply equally well to, let us say, a segment the size of a hexasaccharide or you name it?

LINDAHL, Uppsala The first question, the answer is, of course, we don't know. It may be that the actual binding site is smaller and that the heparinase for steric reasons is not able to get closer. We have tested the statistical treatment by making the same curve assuming that the binding site is composed of either five or seven disaccharide units, or deviating even more, and these curves cannot be made to agree with the experimental data. That's indirect, of course, and backward proof for the dodecasaccharide's size or the binding site but it seems to fit.

LINKER, Salt Lake City I have some comments about Dr. Rosenberg's active site that I would like to bring up. Lung heparin, as has been pointed out here earlier, has very little if any N-acetyl but one could easily visualize that one of the chains, perhaps out of 6 or 7, would have an N-acetyl which we couldn't pick up easily. On the other hand whale heparin has a lot of N-acetyl and has even somewhat better activity so one must consider the N-acetyl in that light. With respect to the tetrasaccharide of glucuronic acid-acetyl glucosamine-iduronic acid-glucosamine N-sulfate, this is one that can be isolated fairly readily from nitrous acid degradation of heparan sulfate which indeed must contain this as a structural unit. Heparan sulfate has very little, if any, anticoagulant activity. However, Dr. Rosenberg did point out that more than this particular site is needed. Our enzymatic data agree very well with his idea that there is more glucuronic acid and, in general, somewhat less sulfation in the active area. In other words, the original idea that everyone had that the ideal heparin would be a heparin that is completely sulfated, with three sulfate groups per disaccharide, probably would not have any anticoagulant activity at all. Indeed, we find that if we degrade the somewhat less degradation by the heparinase which is probably due to the fact that there is less sulfate in the active area. We feel particularly that the uronic acids are lacking sulfate. We do find also iduronic acid that is free of sulfate, therefore, this in addition to the glucuronic could play a role in an active area.

ROSENBERG, Boston I'm not really saying that the acetyl group is necessarily essential for the function. The reason I chose porcine heparin is because I thought it was a good marker for such a sequence and it may well be that such sequences exist in beef lung and are just difficult to capture with nitrous acid because that acetyl marker is not there. With regard to biosynthesis, I find it still very difficult to believe that synthesis can be so random. I think that one has to be cautious about such a model given the heterogeneity of material within what's termed the high activity fraction. I think what is really needed is to determine the structure of some highly active molecule and its abundance and then determine if it could be synthesized by a wholly random process. Until we have such information it would be, I think, very risky to say that there is no information that's involved in heparin synthesis.

DAVIS, Omaha Dr. Rosenberg, the major purpose of this whole group here is to save people from clotting to death, not to do a lot of organic reactions. The only reason that they can clot to death is because fibrinogen is destabilized and the classical picture of destabilization involves thrombin and the splitting off of two small negative fragments. It is also true that if you take pure fibrinogen and add protamine to it in critical amounts you obtain a gel. If you take pure fibrinogen and add ethyl alcohol to it in critical amounts, you get a gel. If those three gels are observed in the electron microscope they show a spacing of cross-striations of 240 angstroms, hence they are not distinguishable. The gels formed by the action of thrombin or by a positively charged agent like protamine or a dehydrating agent like alcohol are similar. Dr. Rosenberg, do you think that each of those substances activate antithrombin? As far as we can tell there is no antithrombin present in these purified systems. How then can we protect the people against a procoagulant effect of many substances, e.g., dozens of cationic materials and many more of the surface active materials and dehydrating agents like alcohol?

ROSENBERG, Boston From my biased view, it depends on what you are thinking about as normal pathophysiology. Now, I wouldn't argue that it may be possible to form fibrinogen gels. I think it becomes a question of does it happen, is this reaction competitive with enzymatically driven reactions. My own feeling is that it isn't, but I can't argue that to some extent some such reactions may play a role in normal physiology.

LINDAHL, Uppsala I should make an additional comment on the specificity of the biosynthetic process. Obviously the process is not entirely random and this can be realized quite simply by doing backwards calculations from the ratios of high affinity fractions versus molecular weight. One can find that one out of forty dodecasaccharides has the right sequence for binding and that is a very high proportion considering a completely non-random assembly. I think there is some specificity or some information being brought out by this modification process because of the fact that it occurs in a stepwise way and that each modification that is introduced limits the frame within which further modifications can take place. Once you have one single N-acetyl group that limits the number of possibilities enormously and in this way you can obtain specificity.

ROSENBERG, Boston I understand that. I think, to my mind, as you well know, I feel there must be more specificity in systems and so I find it difficult to accept the apparent lack of fidelity. Now I agree with you, maybe this system has less fidelity than nucleic acids and proteins but I think it's dangerous not to stress that there indeed is information. Perhaps it's of the order that you suggest, perhaps it's even of a higher order.

LINKER, Salt Lake City But, of course, you are starting out with the assumption that heparin is an anticoagulant.

ROSENBERG, Boston I would find it difficult for me not to accept that, given what I know about antithrombin.

LINDAHL, Uppsala Let's put it this way, if you are looking for a template mechanism, we still haven't found it.

BECK, Bern A technical question to Dr. Rosenberg. I believe you mentioned earlier in your report that you prefer to work with your ligands in solution rather than on affinity chromatography. Since very many people are using affinity chromatography that is a very pertinent remark and I would like to know a little more about the reason for you saying so.

ROSENBERG, Boston I explored, for about a year or so, a variety of ways of attaching antithrombin to sepharose with a variety of arms and reacting groups on the proteins and I found it very difficult, indeed impossible, to mimic the kinds of separations that you can conduct in solution. We probably have heterogeneous columns which we make by binding antithrombin to sepharose. They might be quite reasonable in their abilities to make an active pool but I think the problem really lies in the fact that we may be losing discrimination because it is difficult to resolve heterogeneous species when your column is sufficiently heterogeneous. From the studies that I have performed I have not found a way of binding to the matrix, even if you protect the binding site before binding it, so that you actually don't do something to the antithrombin molecule. If you calculate what the differences in kilocalories are for the various active heparin pools, these are really exquisitely small. I would guess that the slightest conformational change in protein restricts its ability to bind to a ligand and will effect is ability to discriminate.

PADAWER, New York Dr. Mahadoo, I recall there were a couple of papers some 20 years ago in which it was found that the heparin became localized on the cement between endothelial cells on endothelium. You have been talking about endothelium and from your slides I couldn't quite be sure whether the granules seem to preferentially bind to the cement between cells or whether it was over the part which was actual plasmalemma.

MAHADOO, Saskatoon From my own observations at the light microscopy level and at the EM level I have not seen any heparin particles on the cement between the endothelial cells. I have seen them along the luminal surface of the cells.

CELLULAR FUNCTION

HEPARAN SULFATE: FUNCTIONAL ROLE AT THE CELLULAR LEVEL

Paul M. Kraemer

Los Alamos Scientific Laboratory
Los Alamos, New Mexico

Metabolic and structural characteristics of cellular heparan sulfate are used to formulate guidelines for the possible functional roles of the N-sulfated glycosaminoglycans.

I. INTRODUCTION

It should be conceded that there does not currently exist any compelling evidence regarding the natural function of heparan sulfate. However, it seems possible that heparan sulfate rather than heparin may turn out to have more important and more general functions. This follows from the widespread occurrence of heparan sulfate in tissues. For instance, in Dietrich's recent surveys of rat tissue (1), heparan sulfate was a constituent of every tissue and quite abundant in the highly cellular viscera. With the exception of skin (personal communication), heparin was not found at a level of sensitivity that was perfectly adequate for the general glycosaminoglycan survey.

The push to find a physiological role for heparan sulfate was stimulated by the recognition that this substance is not only a general constituent at the tissue level but also of individual cells. Many laboratories have now contributed to the proposition that all kinds of cells, including established cell lines, primary isolated cells, etc., can be shown to make heparan sulfate if adequate detection methods are used (2). The ubiquity of heparan sulfate in such a wide range of cellular types raises the following functional question: Does heparan sulfate serve some general function that is required for life at the level of single cells? If this were true, then any well characterized cell culture system might serve as a suitable study model. In particular, since the heparan sulfate isolated from tissues has always proven to be a wide spectrum of molecules in terms of size, sulfation, etc., a well behaved cell culture system, with its advantages of cellular homogeneity and versatile usage of radioactive precursors, might help distinguish the metabolic, functionally meaningful, and preparative sources of molecular heterogeneity.

ISBN 0-12-484850-8

II. MATERIALS AND METHODS

We discovered very early in our work with CHO cells that some of the cell-associated heparan sulfate could be removed from the cells by gentle trypsin treatment (3). However, it is important not to underestimate the problems associated with validating the conclusion that such trypsin-removable material represents material from the outer cell surface. Figure 1 illustrates, for one set of experiments, the type of ancillary

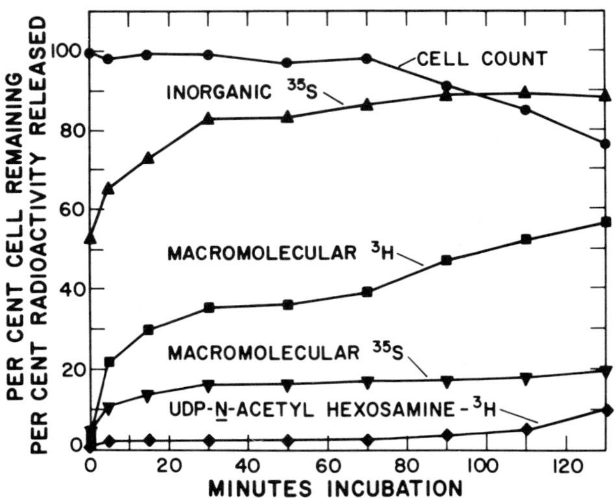

Fig. 1. Release of radioactivity from CHO cells during trypsin treatment (3).

data that contribute to this validation. It shows that the release of macromolecular material from washed cells labeled from ^{3}H-glucosamine and inorganic $^{35}SO_4$ reached a definite plateau well before significant loss of cells had occurred. At the same time, there was little escape of UDP-N-acetyl hexosamine from the cell sap, although inorganic SO_4 leached out. Without this type of data showing cell number accountability during trypsin treatment, as well as ascertaining normal exponential growth of the cells during the labeling period and freedom from *Mycoplasma* contamination of the cells, trypsinates from cultured cells, in our experience, will not yield reproducible data. Since trypsin rapidly lyses trypan blue-positive cells (4), the use of trypan blue to monitor cell loss is not an acceptable substitute for cell number accountability.

In addition to the trypsin-removable material, washed cells also yield an additional portion of the total cell-associated heparan sulfate as direct acid-soluble fragments from the cell sap (Fig. 2). Bio-Gel P-2 runs of this material quantitatively yielded the same excluded double-labeled

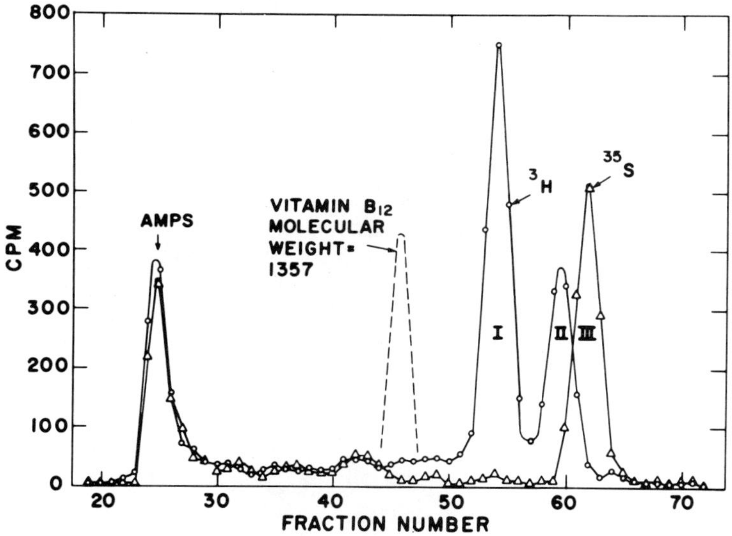

Fig. 2 Bio-Gel P-2 elution diagram of total acid-soluble fraction of CHO cells grown in medium containing ^{3}H-glucosamine and $Na_2{}^{35}SO_4$ (5).

fraction whether or not the cells had been trypsinized before trichloroacetic acid (TCA) precipitation or whether 105,000 x g supernatant fluids of broken cells were used in place of whole cells (5). The total protocol used in our laboratory, not considering at this time the culture medium, then consists of digesting the residual TCA precipitate from the cells with a protease such as papain, thereby rendering TCA-soluble almost all the remaining complex carbohydrate radioactivity. After Bio-Gel P-2 isolation of macromolecular material, the basic separations are done on DEAE-cellulose columns, an example of which is illustrated in Fig. 3.

Since radioactive glucosamine is a general label for all the complex carbohydrates, all of these DEAE-separated materials can be examined for heparan sulfate. As it happens, with CHO cells the material eluting in fractions denoted by the bars in Fig. 3 is the main portion containing heparan sulfate. Glycopeptides elute first, then hyaluronate (if present), and chondroitin sulfates follow the heparan sulfate. These put-

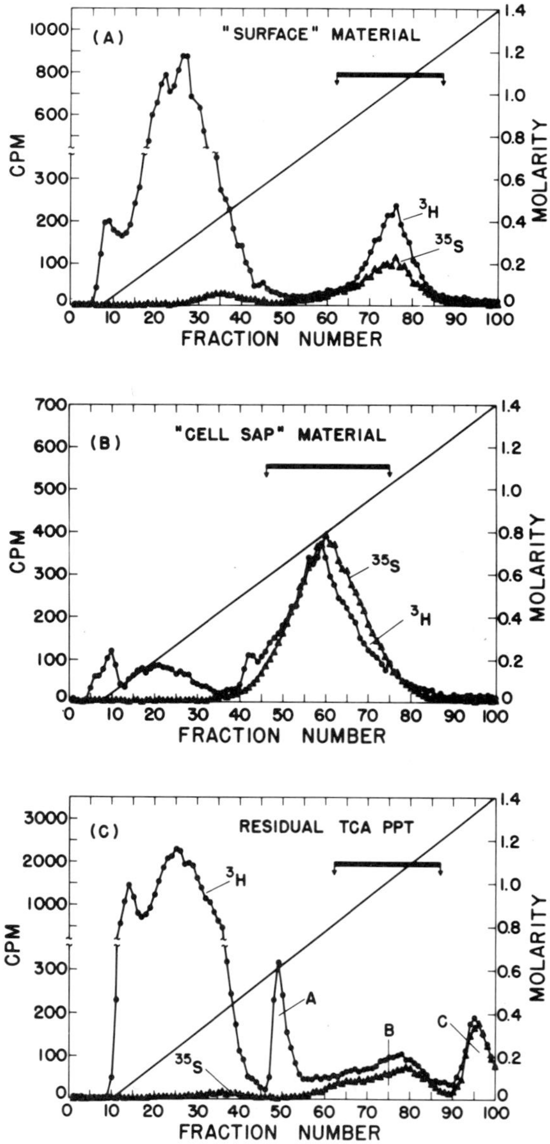

Fig. 3. DEAE-cellulose chromatography profiles of Bio-Gel P-2 excluded material from different cellular compartments (3).

atively identified fractions are then authenticated in a variety of ways.

Portions are rerun on Bio-Gel P-2 after chondroitinase-ABC digestion. For instance, in the particular experiment illustrated in Fig. 4, the purpose of which will not be discussed here, the putative heparan sulfate fractions were essentially free from degradable material; the putative

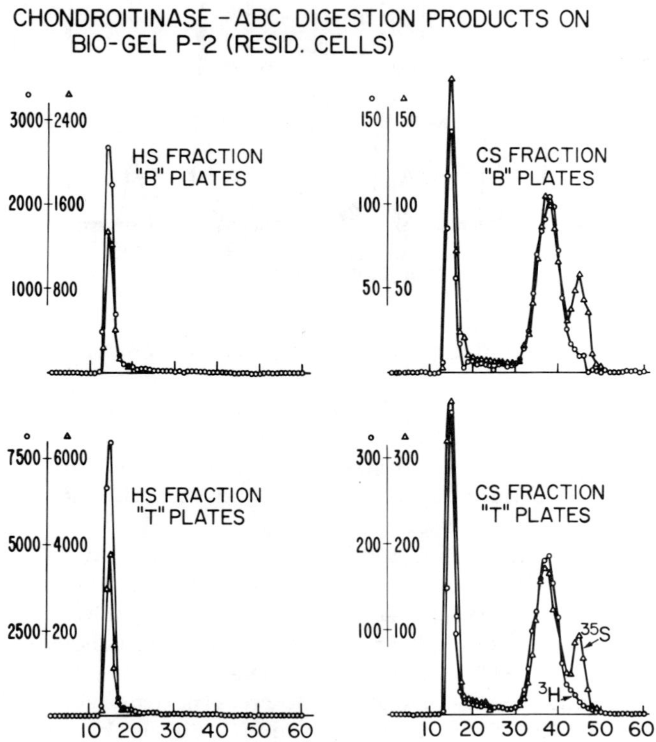

Fig. 4. Illustrative example of determining the purity of isolated mucopolysaccharide fractions.

chondroitin sulfate fractions contained some chondroitinase-ABC-resistant material. Re-isolation of all these resistant materials was done, and each proved to be nitrous acid-degradable.

As illustrated in Fig. 5, reruns of the three putative heparan sulfate fractions on Bio-Gel P-2 after mild acid (0.04 *N* HCl, 100°C, 90 min) did not change the elution of the ^{3}H.

However, a portion of the $^{35}SO_4$ was released, representing

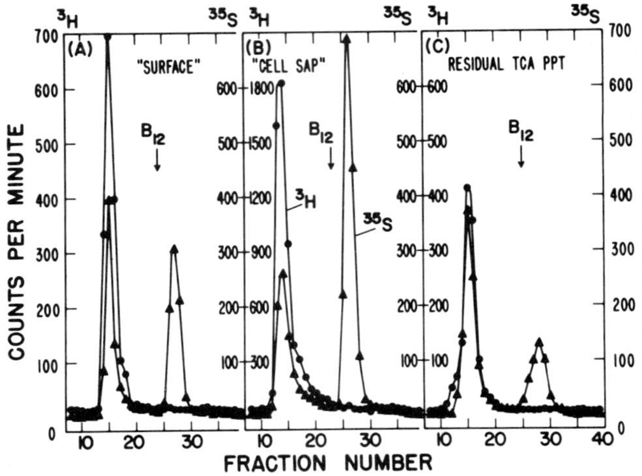

Fig. 5. Bio-Gel P-2 returns of Bio-Gel P-2 excluded heparan sulfate fractions after mild acid treatment (3).

mostly labile N-sulfates, although a little $O\text{-}SO_4$ may have been released also. We can see, however, that the proportion of total ^{35}S released is quite different in different cell fractions in that much more is released for the heparan sulfate from the cell sap.

The nitrous acid fragments were examined on Bio-Gel P-10 rather than on P-2. In this case, the interpretation is more complex because the range of size of the fragments produced by deaminative cleavage is quite broad. For instance, in Fig. 6 is illustrated a P-10 profile of untreated heparan sulfate from the residual cell precipitate papain digested and isolated from DEAE fractions. Figure 7 illustrates the same material after nitrous acid degradation. Essentially all ^{35}S has changed elution position, while the first portion of the ^3H-labeled material now elutes as if it were as large as the smallest of the untreated material. If the acid-labile sulfate had first been removed using the mild acid Bio-Gel P-2 technique illustrated in Fig. 5, the sharp prominent peak of ^{35}S would still elute past the vitamin B_{12} marker, but the ^3H profile would be completely unchanged. An idea can be obtained by this technique of the differences, if any, between surface, cell sap, and internal membrane-associated heparan sulfate in terms of frequency and size of clustered N-

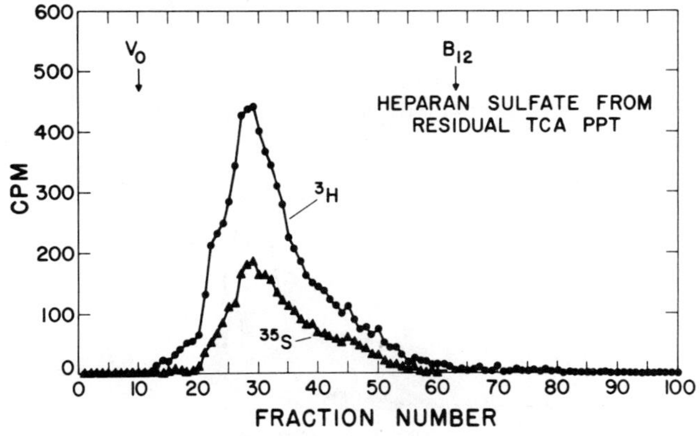

Fig. 6. Bio-Gel P-10 elution profile of heparan sulfate isolated from the papain digest of internal cellular membranes (3).

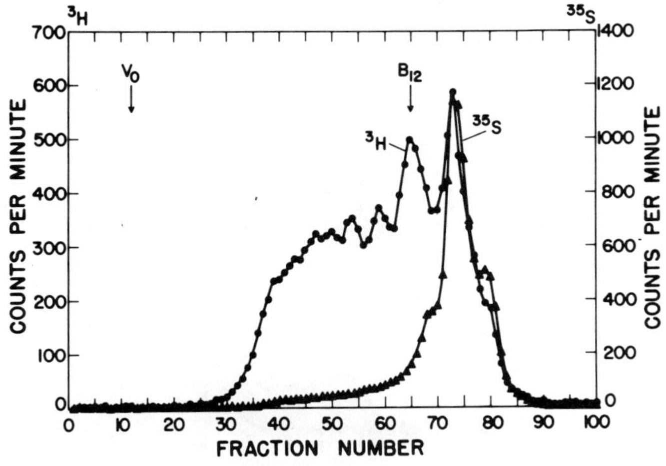

Fig. 7. Bio-Gel P-10 profile of material illustrated in Fig. 6 after HNO_2 treatment (3).

acetylated regions and the relation of these to O-sulfated regions of the sugar chains. For instance, one conclusion that seems paradoxical is that, despite the higher labile sulfate content of the cell sap heparan sulfate, this material still contains long regions that are N-acetylated (Fig. 8).

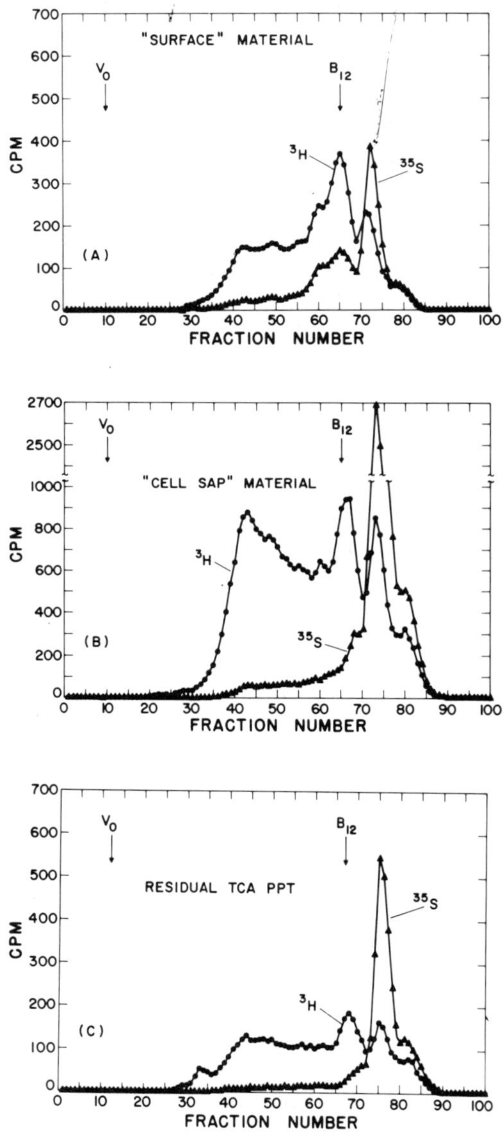

Fig. 8. Bio-Gel P-10 profiles of cellular heparan sulfate fractions after HNO_2 treatment (3).

We can also compare the enzymatically derived breakdown products of the three types of heparan sulfate. Table I (Silva and Kraemer, in preparation) compares the disaccharide composition of these materials after complete degradation with heparitinases I and II and heparinase (6). The data confirm the idea that cell sap heparan sulfate is much richer in N-sulfates than the other two. In addition, it appears that the

TABLE I Disaccharide Composition (%) of Heparan Sulfate from Different Cellular Compartments of CHO Cells.

	Total N-Ac	(O-Sulfates) (Zero	One)	Total $N\text{-}SO_4$	(O-Sulfates) (Zero	One	Two)
Cell surface	75	(62	13)	25	(15	5	5)
Cell sap	20	(16	4)	80	(64	8	8)
Internal membranes	75	(8	67)	25	(15	5	5)

internal membrane-associated material is surprisingly rich in N-acetyl-mono-O-sulfated material. The cell-surface material is quite sparsely sulfated, averaging overall about 0.6 sulfate per disaccharide; the others are slightly over 1.0.

Figure 6 shows that the heparan sulfate from papain-digested acid precipitates of internal membrane-associated material was all partially retained on Bio-Gel P-10. It turned out, however, that the cysteine hydrochloride of the papain buffer was breaking up a very interesting portion of this material. We now use Pronase and thus can demonstrate that this material also contains some larger fragments that are excluded from Bio-Gel P-10 and is much less highly sulfated. It is, in fact, very similar to the heparan sulfate of the cell surface.

III. RESULTS AND DISCUSSION

The metabolic relationships of these various heparan sulfate fractions have been examined by a tandem labeling method. In this type of experiment, the cells are labeled for three generations with ^{3}H-glucosamine and for a final 4 hr with ^{14}C-glucosamine (Table II). It is apparent that the large internal membrane-associated heparan sulfate is extremely active metabolically. The labeling ratio for it was very low when compared either to the other heparan sulfate fractions or to other complex carbohydrates. A very similar

TABLE II Radioactivity[a] of Isolated Fractions from Cells Tandem Labeled with Glucosamine-6-t and Glucosamine-1-^{14}C

Cell fraction	Total cpm - Column ^{3}H	Total cpm - Column ^{14}C	Column $^{3}H/^{14}C$	Electrophoretic $^{3}H/^{14}C$[b]
Surface glycopeptides[c]	228,840	70,100	3.26	
Surface heparan sulfate	58,300	36,120	1.61	1.52
Cell-sap UDP-N-acetyl hexosamine[d]	337,120	312,140	1.08	
Cell-sap heparan sulfate[c]	205,340	32,780	6.26	4.35
Residual precipitate -- glycopeptides[c]	1,054,040	327,880	3.21	
Residual precipitate -- hyaluronic acid[c]	14,880	2,730	5.45	
Residual precipitate -- heparan sulfate A[e]	30,440	20,240	1.50	1.48
Residual precipitate -- heparan sulfate B[e]	117,600	22,960	5.12	3.77
Residual precipitate -- chondroitin SO_4[c]	116,250	29,210	3.98	

[a]The cpm represent material isolated from approximately 5×10^9 cells after growth for three generations with 0.025 μCi/ml of glucosamine-6-t (specific activity 1300 cpm) and for the final 4 hr before harvest with additional 0.50 μCi/ml of glucosamine-1-^{14}C (specific activity 51.4).

[b]Aliquots of the heparan sulfates pooled from column fractions were run on cellulose acetate electrophoresis; the isolated spots were cut out and counted (from ref. 3).

[c]Pooled fractions from DEAE-cellulose chromatography.

[d]Pooled fractions from 1° Bio-Gel P-2 chromatography.

[e]The residual precipitate A fraction could be separated from the remainder of the residual precipitate fraction (precipitate B) since it eluted earlier on Bio-Gel P-10.

low ratio, however, was the heparan sulfate of the cell surface. Since many of the possible functions of heparan sulfate relate specifically to the cell-surface form of the molecule, we have focused our attention on this form.

The heparan sulfate of the cell surface is one of the most metabolically active constituents of this region of the cell. We have shown that a large portion of this material is released from cells just prior to mitosis and appears in the medium as acid-precipitable proteoglycan (7). If this cell surface heparan sulfate is physiologically important, then it should be noted that it represents only about 14% of the mass of total cell-associated heparan sulfate and is quite sparsely sulfated (see Table III). These facts emphasize the idea that the functions of heparan sulfate may continue to be elusive if rapid metabolic relationships are not clarified.

TABLE III Characteristics of Heparan Sulfates of Different Cellular Compartments

Cellular compartment	*Mass %*	*Relative "turnover"*
Cell surface	*14*	*0.62*
Cell sap	*50*	*0.16*
Internal membranes A	*7*	*0.67*
Internal membranes B	*29*	*0.20*

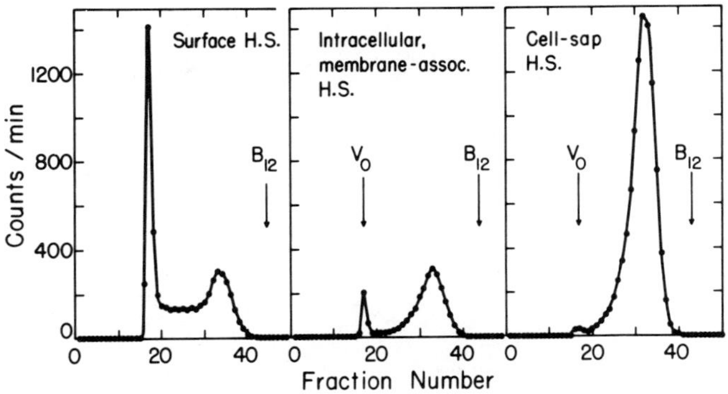

Fig. 9. Agarose A 0.5 M profiles of cellular heparan sulfate fractions (8).

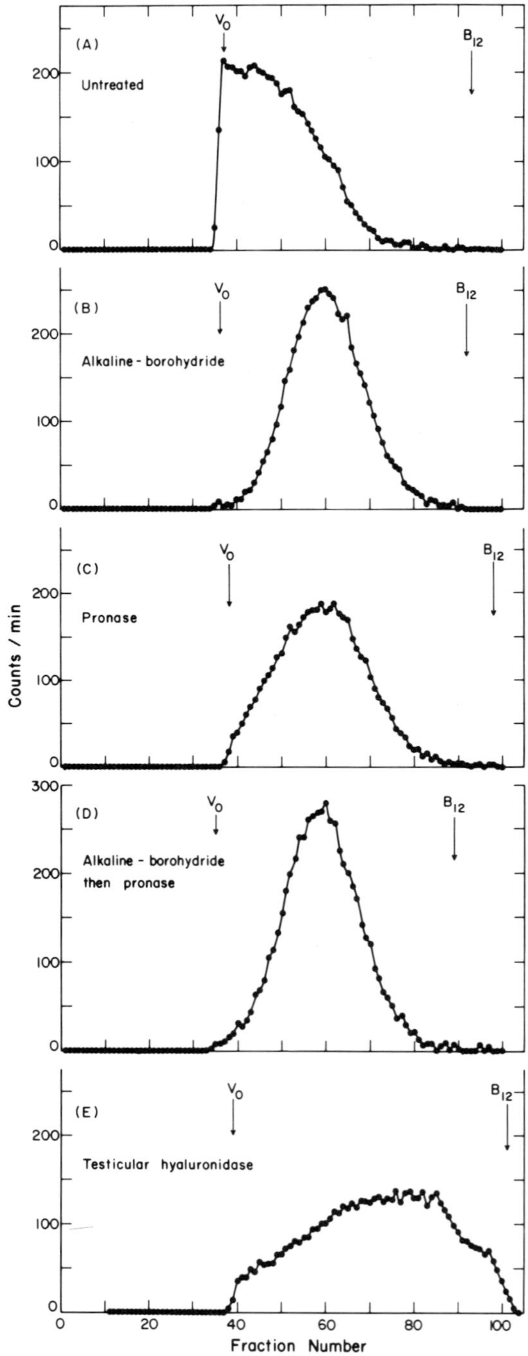

Fig. 10. Agarose A 5 M profiles of cell-surface heparan sulfate fraction excluded from agarose A 0.5 M, before and after various treatments (8).

The cell-surface heparan sulfate, after removal with trypsin, includes a distribution of sizes of molecules up to some rather large material. The profiles illustrated in Fig. 9 are gel filtration runs on agarose A 0.5 *M*. If the excluded material from the cell-surface heparan sulfate is rerun on agarose A 5 *M*, some of the material is again excluded as shown in the top frame of Fig. 10. Treatment with alkali and/or Pronase, shown below, indicates that it represents multichain proteoglycan. We have done sedimentation equilibrium analyses on a variety of cuts from these distributions and have shown that the individual sugar chains range up to about 50,000 daltons, while the while tryptic fragments go to about 150,000 daltons (8).

As a result of all these studies, we have tended to visualize the surface heparan sulfate as a multichain proteoglycan rooted in plasma membrane (Fig. 11) and have speculated

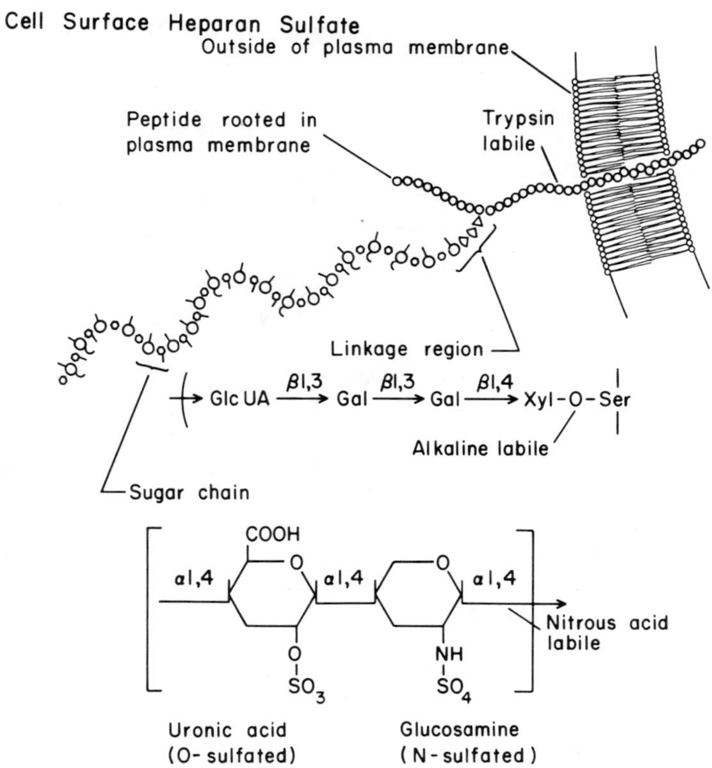

Fig. 11. Diagrammatic view of cell-surface heparan sulfate.

that its function may relate to providing an anionic screen controlling access to cell-specific receptors of one sort or another. We believe that the large internal membrane-associated species is the direct precursor of this surface material, while the other internal varieties represent degraded molecules. The cell sap material is totally lacking in either amino acids or linkage sugars, while the smaller internal membrane-associated material is proteoglycan, perhaps relating to the cell sap material as proximal residuals after a "pruning" process. If so, this might suggest that much of the complexity of the total sulfation process relates to keys for degradation rather than for specific function per se.

It should be mentioned that there is an important alternative to this visualization of cell-surface heparan sulfate. The recent work of Magnus Höök and his co-workers (9), which showed reversible and saturable binding sites for both heparin and heparan sulfate on freshly dissociated rat liver cells, has raised an extremely interesting alternative possibility. It now seems conceivable that not only surface localization of the metabolically active material could be controlled by receptor sites, but that these sites regulate the reincorporation and breakdown of molecules that originated in any nearby cell (10). In other words, this raises the possibility of control of the matrix over multicellular zones and regions.

There is one additional observation about these cell-surface materials that should be considered when postulating functional roles. As we have seen from the DEAE profiles of trypsin-removable material, the mucopolysaccharides in general and heparan sulfate in particular can contribute a significant portion of the total radioactivity from ^{3}H-glucosamine. However, we have been impressed with the fact that they do not contribute much to the total mass (Table IV). These data are from growing monolayer CHO cells where a fair amount of the total cell-associated hyaluronate and chondroitin sulfate is also in the trypsin-removable fraction. Not counting the sialic acid residues that were not assayed, the mucopolysaccharides, as a whole, contributed only about 7.5% of the total sugar mass. Cell-surface heparan sulfate contributed 27% of the ^{3}H radioactivity but only a little over 2% of the mass.

The types of functions that we can envision for this type of situation are those relating to the enormous impact that small amounts of mucopolysaccharides can have on the properties of solutions and gels (11). Such 2% concentrations of heparan sulfate in the diffusion boundary of the cell surface could have a major impact on the movements of anions to and from the cell, as well as an important and versatile reservoir of cations such as calcium (12). I believe that we should look to these areas for the function of heparan sulfate (2).

TABLE IV Sugar Mass and Radioactivity of Trypsin-Removable Complex Carbohydrates from CHO Cells Labeled for One Generation of Monolayer Culture with ^{3}H-Glucosamine

		Specific Activity (cpm/μg)
Glycopeptides		
^{3}H cpm	232,200	
Fucose	3.2 μg	
Mannose	45.9	
Galactose	40.6	
Glucosamine	46.2	
Galactosamine	5.6	4,483
Hyaluronic acid		
^{3}H cpm	137,100	
Glucosamine	2.6 μg	52,731
Heparan sulfate		
^{3}H cpm	105,200	
Glucosamine	1.7 μg	61,882
Chondroitin sulfates		
^{3}H cpm	34,700	
Galactosamine	1.4 μg	24,786

ACKNOWLEDGMENT

This work was performed under the auspices of the United States Energy Research and Development Administration.

REFERENCES

1. Dietrich, C.P., Sampaio, L.O., and Toledo, O.M.S., Biochem. Biophys. Res. Commun. *71*, 1 (1976).
2. Kraemer, P.M., *in* "Surfaces of Normal and Malignant Cells" (R. Hynes, ed.), Wiley Interscience, New York (in press), 1977.
3. Kraemer, P.M., Biochemistry *10*, 1437 (1971).
4. DeLuca, C., Exp. Cell Res. *40*, 186 (1965).
5. Kraemer, P.M., J. Cell. Physiol. *71*, 109 (1968).
6. Silva, M.E., Dietrich, C.P., and Nader, H.B., Biochim. Biophys. Acta *487*, 129 (1976).
7. Kraemer, P.M., and Tobey, R.A., J. Cell Biol. *55*, 713 (1972).
8. Kraemer, P.M., and Smith, D.A., Biochem. Biophys. Res. Commun. *56*, 423 (1974).
9. Kjellen, L., Oldberg, A., Rubin, K., and Höök, M., Biochem. Biophys. Res. Commun. *74*, 126 (1977).
10. Neufeld, E.F., Lim, T.W., and Shapiro, L.J., Ann. Rev. Biochem. *44*, 357 (1975).
11. Laurent, T.C., *in* "Chemistry and Molecular Biology of the Intercellular Matrix" (E.A. Balazs, ed.), p. 703. Academic Press, New York-London, 1970.
12. Langer, G.A., and Frank, J.S., J. Cell Biol. *54*, 441 (1972).

HEPARAN SULFATE AND RELATED COMPLEX CARBOHYDRATES OF NERVOUS TISSUE

Richard U. Margolis and Renée K. Margolis

New York University School of Medicine and
State University of New York, Downstate Medical Center

Heparan sulfate and other glycosaminoglycans are discussed in relation to their structure, distribution, metabolism, and possible functional roles in brain and nervous tissue storage organelles.

In the past, nervous tissue has not been a popular choice of material for investigators interested in glycosaminoglycans and glycoproteins. However, neurochemists have recently devoted more attention to these complex carbohydrates, and this paper will summarize certain studies from our laboratories concerning their structure, distribution, metabolism, and possible functionl roles in brain and nervous tissue storage organelles (for reviews see (1) and (2)). Although the emphasis here will be on heparan sulfate, we have not been interested exclusively in this glycosaminoglycan. Therefore, comparisons will also be made with chondroitin sulfate, hyaluronic acid, and the glycoproteins of nervous tissue, in the hope that such comparative data may provide clues to the interrelationships and functions of these complex carbohydrates.

I. STRUCTURE

There is no convincing evidence that heparin occurs outside of mast cells in nervous tissue, but it has been established that significant amounts of heparan sulfate are present in brain parenchyma. Its concentration in adult rat brain is approximately 46 μg/g fresh weight, where it comprises 12-14% of the total glycosaminoglycans. Heparan sulfate has also been demonstrated to occur in comparable amounts in bovine, sheep, and human brain.

ISBN 0-12-484850-8

The heparan sulfate of rat brain can be fractionated into two components (HS-I and HS-II) by ion exchange chromatography on Dowex-1 (3). HS-I is eluted with 1.0 *M* NaCl and accounts for approximately one third of the total heparan sulfate, while HS-II, accounting for the remaining two thirds of the material, is eluted between 1.1 and 1.5 *M* NaCl. Both heparan sulfate fractions are of similar molecular size and contain the same proportion of N- and O-sulfate, although the content of total sulfate is 50% greater in HS-II as compared to HS-I. The finding that heparan sulfate fractions of slightly different composition may be obtained from brain indicates that in this respect brain heparan sulfate resembles that from lung and gastric mucosa, while only single fractions have been isolated from other tissues such as skin, aorta, and umbilical cord.

Nitrous acid degradation studies indicated that in contrast to the molecular structure proposed for heparan sulfate from bovine lung, the heparan sulfate of brain contains a relatively smaller proportion of uronosyl-N-sulfohexosamine disaccharide repeating units, and that much of the heparan sulfate of brain consists of large, completely N-acetylated segments containing a relatively high content of ester sulfate (3).

Alkaline-borohydride treatment of chondroitin sulfate and heparan sulfate isolated from rat or bovine brain following Pronase digestion of the lipid-free protein residue demonstrated that the polysaccharide chains in both of these sulfated glycosaminoglycans are covalently linked to a protein moiety by the usual type of O-glycosidic xylosyl-serine linkages (4). Thus, in brain as in other tissues, heparan sulfate occurs as a proteoglycan.

We have recently obtained evidence that heparan sulfate is closely associated with brain proteoglycans in which chondroitin sulfate is the major component. This material comprises 2-3% of the soluble protein of brain, from which it can be isolated by ion exchange chromatography and gel filtration (5,6). It accounts for essentially all of the soluble chondroitin sulfate of brain, and its presence in neuronal cell bodies and astrocytes leads us to believe that the proteoglycan is a cytoplasmic constituent of neurons and glia. It is composed of 75% protein, 13% glycoprotein carbohydrate, and 12% glycosaminoglycans (consisting of 83% chondroitin 4-sulfate, 5% chondroitin 6-sulfate, 6% heparan sulfate, and 6% hyaluronic acid), and differs in several respects from the better characterized material isolated from cartilage. These differences include its higher protein content, smaller molecular size (6.1 S), and the presence of heparan sulfate, hyaluronic acid, and glycoprotein oligosaccharides that remain with the proteoglycan even under dissociative conditions (4 *M* guanidine). Although the heparan sulfate may be derived from a contaminating proteoglycan, it is possible that it is covalently linked to a common protein core together with chondroitin sulfate, in a role analogous to that of keratan sulfate (which is not found in nervous tissue) in the cartilage proteoglycan subunits. Other investigators have also reported the presence of small amounts of heparan sulfate together with chondroitin sulfate proteoglycans in early stages of chondrogenesis (7).

II. DISTRIBUTION

After differential centrifugation of a brain homogenate (Table I), approximately 60% of the heparan sulfate is found in the microsomal fraction, which consists largely of fragments of endoplasmic reticulum and plasma membranes. Only 17% is soluble, in distinction to chondroitin sulfate, over half of which occurs in the form of a soluble proteoglycan (8).

The crude mitochondrial fraction contains 1-3% of the chondroitin sulfate and heparan sulfate and 5% of the brain hyaluronic acid. This fraction is composed of myelin and synaptosomes (pinched off nerve endings) in addition to mitochondria. Purification of these subfractions demonstrated that glycosaminoglycans are not present in myelin (9), and that synaptosomes and purified synaptic membranes contain only traces of sulfated glycosaminoglycans, which could be due to a small amount of microsomal contamination. Although we and others also found low concentrations of glycosaminoglycans, including heparan sulfate, in purified mitochondria from brain (8, 10), we are again inclined to attribute these results to a slight contamination of the mitochondria.

A low speed pellet containing nuclei, cell debris, unbroken cells, and blood vessels accounted for 21% of the total heparan sulfate and 12-19% of the chondroitin sulfate and hyaluronic acid (8). When highly purified rat brain nuclei were prepared and analyzed for their glycosaminoglycan and glycoprotein levels and composition (11), it could be calculated (from the yield of purified nuclei and their concentrations of glycosaminoglycans) that the nuclei themselves contain a maximum of 11-12% of the hyaluronic acid and chondroitin sulfate present in the crude "nuclei and cell debris," whereas less than 4% of the heparan sulfate found in this fraction is actually associated with nuclei. Much of the remaining heparan sulfate is probably present in cell membranes and unbroken cells, although a portion may occur as

TABLE I Distribution of Glycosaminoglycans in Subcellular Fractions Obtained by Differential Centrifugation of Rat Brain

	Hyaluronic acid		Heparan sulfate		Chondroitin sulfate	
Nuclei and cell debris	0.142[a]	19[b]	0.074	21	0.209	12
Crude Mitochrondrial Fraction	0.112	5	0.035	3	0.064	1
"Heavy" microsomes	0.126	28	0.071	34	0.190	19
"Light" microsomes	0.223	26	0.102	25	0.344	17
Soluble fraction	0.169	22	0.057	17	0.860	51

[a] Concentration expressed as μmoles of constituent hexosamine per 100 mg of lipid-free dry weight.

[b] Represents the percent of the total in whole brain which is found in each fraction; (sum of figures in each column = 100%).

a constituent of capillaries and smaller blood vessels.

It is notable that 60% of the heparan sulfate (and 36-54% of the chondroitin sulfate and hyaluronic acid) are found in the microsomal fraction obtained by differential centrifugation (8). When brain microsomes are subfractionated on a discontinuous sucrose density gradient, half or more of the hyaluronic acid and chondroitin sulfate is associated with membranes of low density that sediment on 0.5 *M* sucrose. In contrast, the heparan sulfate is present in membranes of considerably greater density (8). We have recently found that the glycosaminoglycans associated with low density microsomal membrane subfractions can be removed by various types of mild washing procedures and are closely related metabolically to the strictly soluble glycosaminoglycans (12). These glycosaminoglycans are components of large vesicles (with a high water content and therefore a low buoyant density) formed of smooth membranes which, on the basis of chemical and enzyme composition and morphology, appear to be derived from both plasma membranes and from smooth endoplasmic reticulum.

The concentration of chondroitin sulfate and hyaluronic acid in rat liver microsomes is only 5 to 10% of that in brain microsomes, although the concentration of heparan sulfate is half as great in liver as compared to brain. However, in certain higher density membrane subfractions from liver (sedimenting on 1.0 and 1.3 *M* sucrose) the concentration of heparan sulfate was found to be somewhat greater than in comparable subfractions obtained from brain, whereas the concentration of hyaluronic acid and chondroitin sulfate was lower in all of the liver membrane subfractions (Table II). These data suggest that heparan sulfate may share some common function in both brain and liver (e.g., as a component of cell surface or internal membranes), while hyaluronic acid and chondroitin sulfate may be associated with cellular structures and functions more peculiar to nervous tissue. This difference between brain and liver is especially marked in the case of chondroitin sulfate, which is the major glycosaminoglycan of nervous tissue, whereas even the small amounts present in liver appear to be of extrahepatic origin (13).

Although there are only very low concentrations of sulfated glycosaminoglycans at nerve endings (see above), heparan sulfate is present in neuronal cell bodies and axons isolated in bulk from rat and bovine brain, as well as in astrocytes and oligodendroglia (14). Since it has been demonstrated in several experimental systems that there is a rapid axonal transport of heparan sulfate and other complex carbohydrates from the nerve cell body down the axon (15, 16), it is possible that the transported heparan sulfate is a component of some synaptic structure or is involved in

TABLE II Distribution of Glycosaminoglycans in Rat Brain and Liver Microsomal Subfractions

	Hyaluronic acid			Chondroitin sulfate			Heparan sulfate		
	Percent of total		Conc. ratio (L/B)	Percent of total		Conc. ratio (L/B)	Percent of total		Conc. ratio (L/B)
	Brain	Liver		Brain	Liver		Brain	Liver	
0.8 M sucrose	76	6	0.02	70	14	0.02	45	14	0.38
1.0 M sucrose	9	24	0.51	13	19	0.12	22	27	1.17
1.3 M sucrose	9	44	0.56	9	37	0.20	20	40	1.17
2.0 M sucrose	6	26	0.20	8	30	0.09	13	19	0.36
Unfractionated	100	100	0.09	100	100	0.05	100	100	0.50

Data are expressed as percent distribution of glycosaminoglycans among the four subfractions from brain and liver microsomes, and the concentration ratio was obtained by dividing the concentration of glycosaminoglycan in liver microsomes by the concentration in the corresponding subfraction from brain (Conc. ratio L/B).

neurotransmission. It is of interest in this connection that low concentrations of heparin produce a three-fold stimulation of brain tyrosine hydroxylase activity and a seven-fold decrease in the K_m of tyrosine hydroxylase for its tetrahydropteridine cofactor, while much higher concentrations of hyaluronic acid or chondroitin sulfate showed only a very slight or no activation of the enzyme (17). Since the effects of heparan sulfate isolated from brain have been found to be similar to those of heparin (unpublished results), it is possible that this glycosaminoglycan may be important in the regulation of catecholamine biosynthesis through its ability to activate the rate-limiting enzyme, tyrosine hydroxylase.

The highest concentration of total glycosaminoglycans as well as of heparan sulfate is found in neuronal perikarya, where heparan sulfate comprises 17% of the glycosaminoglycans (Table III). This proportion is very similar to that found in axons and astrocytes (16-18%), whereas oligodendroglia have both a higher relative amount of heparan sulfate (27% of the total glycosaminoglycans) and a concentration of glycoprotein carbohydrate that is over twice that present in neurons. Since oligodendroglia are small cells with a high surface-to-volume ratio, it is possible that their relatively greater concentrations of heparan sulfate and glycoproteins reflect the localization of these complex carbohydrates in plasma membranes.

III. METABOLISM

The turnover half-times (determined in adult rat brain *in vivo*) for the polysaccharide backbone and for sulfate in the glycosaminoglycans, and for hexosamine, fucose, sialic acid, sulfate, and the protein moiety of brain glycoproteins, are summarized in Table IV (for references see (1) and (2)). It can be concluded from these data that two major metabolic pools are present. One has rapid turnover, with half-times in the range of one day to a week, while a pool of lower metabolic activity turns over with a half-time of two to six weeks. However, chondroitin sulfate is distinguished by having only a single metabolic pool. These data also indicate that the sulfate groups on the glycosaminoglycans turn over independently of and more rapidly than the polysaccharide chain. This independent turnover of sulfate on an intact carbon backbone may have functional significance by providing a mechanism for the addition and removal of anionic groups on cell membranes.

TABLE III Distribution of Glycoproteins and Glycosaminoglycans in Bovine Neurons and Glia

	Neuronal perikarya	Axons	Astrocytes	Oligodendroglia
Glycoprotein carbohydrate (% of lipid-free dry wt.)	1.1	1.1	1.9	2.4
Total glycosaminoglycans (μmoles hexosamine/100 mg lipid-free dry weight)	0.830	0.508	0.565	0.144
Percent of total GAG				
Hyaluronic acid	19	43	34	48
Chondroitin sulfate	64	41	48	24
Heparan sulfate	17	16	18	27

TABLE IV Turnover Half-Times (in Days) of Rat Brain Glycosaminoglycans and Glycoproteins

Glycosaminoglycans		
	Sulfate	*Hexosamine*
Hyaluronic acid	-	*9, 45*
Chondroitin sulfate	*7*	*21*
Heparan sulfate	*3*	*3.7, 10*
Glycoproteins		
Hexosamine	*4.6, 15*	
Sialic acid	*6, 30*	
Fucose	*1, 30*	
Sulfate	*2.5, 14*	
Threonine	*13, 38*	

There are no significant differences between neurons and astrocytes in the turnover of either the polysaccharide backbone or of sulfate in heparan sulfate and chondroitin sulfate, although the turnover of hyaluronic acid is more than twice as rapid in the neuronal cell bodies when compared to glial cells (14).

Labeling studies revealed that maximum specific activities of heparan sulfate, hyaluronic acid, and glycoprotein hexosamine are attained in the rough endoplasmic reticulum of brain by 2 hr after the administration of [^{3}H] glucosamine. At this time maximally labeled chondroitin sulfate has already moved to a lower density fraction (1.1 *M* sucrose) where high specific activity heparan sulfate, hyaluronic acid, and glycoproteins are also found by 18 hrs. There is then a progressive movement of these labeled complex carbohydrates to fractions (sedimenting between 0.7 and 0.9 *M* sucrose) consisting predominantly of smooth membranes and Golgi apparatus. Our studies did not indicate major differences in the time course of biosynthesis or intracellular transport of the sulfated glycosaminoglycans in brain. However, after a long interval (eight days) following pulse labeling with [^{3}H] glucosamine hyaluronic acid attains a relatively high specific

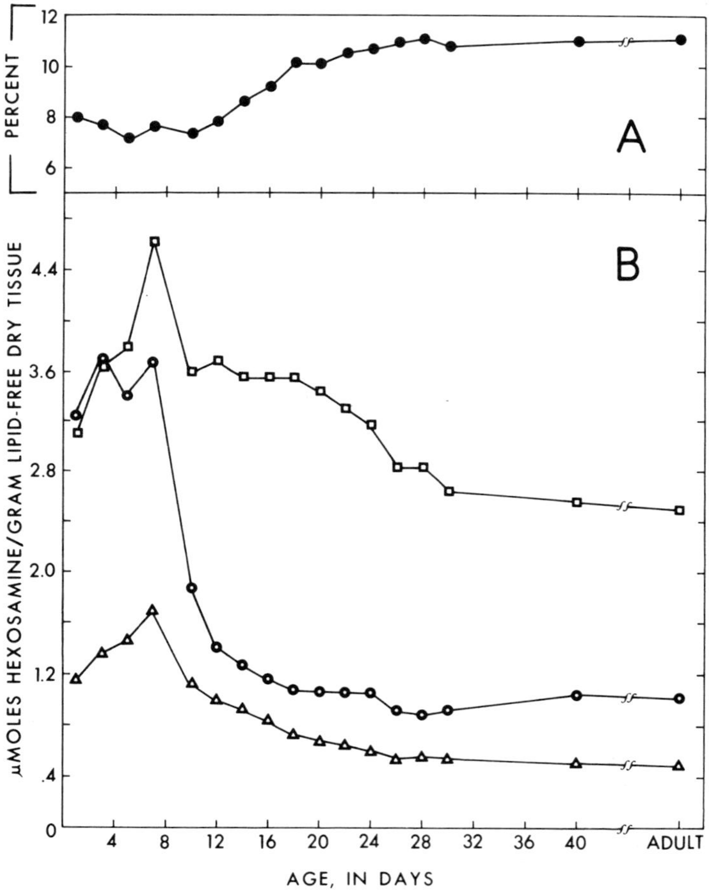

Fig. 1. (A) Lipid-free dry weight as percent of fresh weight of rat brain during postnatal development. (B) Concentration of glycosaminoglycans, expressed as micromoles of the constituent hexosamine per gram of lipid-free dry weight, as a function of increasing postnatal age. (□) Chondroitin sulfate; (○) hyaluronic acid; (△) heparan sulfate.

activity in membranes sedimenting on 0.9 *M* sucrose, suggesting that this fraction may contain the hyaluronate pool that we previously demonstrated to have a slow turnover ($t_{1/2}$ = 45 days).

IV DEVELOPMENTAL CHANGES

The levels of all three brain glycosaminoglycans increase after birth to reach a peak at seven days, after which they decline steadily, attaining by 30 days concentrations within 10% of those present in adult brain (Fig. 1). The greatest change occurs in hyaluronic acid, which appears to be present in a soluble form where it is relatively inactive metabolically (18).

TABLE V Incorporation of [^{3}H] Glucosamine into the Glycosaminoglycans and Glycoproteins of Rat Brain as a Function of Age

	Relative specific activity			
	1-day	7-day	16-day	Adult
Hyaluronic acid	1.0	1.0	1.0	1.0
Chondroitin sulfate	1.4	1.4	0.9	1.0
Heparan sulfate	2.2	2.8	4.6	9.0
Glycoprotein sialic acid	1.0	2.3	2.1	2.0
Glycoprotein hexosamine	2.8	3.9	4.5	4.7

The high concentration of soluble hyaluronic acid in very young brain may function in the retention of water and thereby form an easily penetrable matrix through which neuronal migration and differentiation may take place during brain development. The significance of the higher concentration of heparan sulfate and chondroitin sulfate in one-week-old as compared to adult brain is not clear, but it is interesting that only heparan sulfate showed a marked change in metabolic activity during development (Table V), as reflected in a fourfold increase in relative specific activity after labeling with [^{3}H] glucosamine (18). The increase in heparan sulfate turnover occurred mostly after one week of age, suggesting that it may be related to the involvement of this glycosaminoglycan in specific neural processes that do not develop fully until that time.

V. NERVOUS TISSUE STORAGE ORGANELLES

Fillion *et al.* (19) first reported indirect evidence for the presence of sulfated glycosaminoglycans in chromaffin granules of adrenal medulla, based on their finding that catecholamines, sulfate radioactivity, and hexosamine all had similar sedimentation patterns when a homogenate of adrenal medulla (labeled with [^{35}S] sulfate *in vivo*) was centrifuged through a sucrose density gradient. Although it was suggested by these investigators that glycosaminoglycans might play an important role in the binding and storage of catecholamines in chromaffin granules, similar to that proposed for protein-polysaccharide complexes studied in mast cells and platelets, our analysis of the concentration and chemical composition of glycosaminoglycans in purified chromaffin granules (20) indicated that the amounts present are much less than sufficient to account for the simple *ionic* binding of the high concentrations of catecholamines in these organelles.

In a more detailed study of the composition and biogenesis of complex carbohydrates in bovine chromaffin granules (21), we have recently found that heparan sulfate is present in a considerably higher concentration in the granule membranes (11% of the total glycosaminoglycans) than in the soluble contents, which contain 77% of the protein and 80% of the glycosaminoglycans (Table VI). These data are consistent with other studies described above, which indicate that heparan sulfate is more closely associated with membrane functions in nervous tissue than as a component of cytoplasmic or soluble proteoglycans.

Although the role of glycosaminoglycans in chromaffin granules is still unclear, we also found that acetylcholine stimulation of the perfused adrenal gland results in a 12- to 20-fold increase in the release of chondroitin sulfate and heparan sulfate, together with the expected stimulation of catecholamine secretion (22). Since we know that catecholamines are present in chromaffin granules in a nondiffusible form, it is possible that some type of structural interaction between the catecholamines and glycosaminoglycans, glycoproteins, or other proteins or low molecular weight constituents of the granules may be responsible for the high amine-binding capacity known to occur *in vivo*.

TABLE VI Distribution of Complex Carbohydrates in Bovine Chromaffin Granules

	Soluble	*Membrane*	*Total*[a]
Glycosaminoglycans (hexosamine)	*80%*	*20%*	*3.4*
Ratio of chondroitin sulfate/ heparan sulfate	*20:1*	*8:1*	*(16:1)*
Glycoproteins			
Hexosamine	*67%*	*33%*	*5.8*
Ratio of glucosamine/ galactosamine	*1:2*	*9:1*	*(1:1)*
Sialic acid	*82%*	*18%*	*5.4*
Neutral sugars	*61%*	*39%*	*9.3*
Gangliosides (sialic acid)	*4%*	*96%*	*1.6*
Protein	*77%*	*23%*	-

[a]*Whole granule concentration as μmoles/100 mg protein.*

Other studies have demonstrated the presence of small amounts of glycosaminoglycans, of which 50% is heparan sulfate, in "membraneless" prolactin secretory granules isolated from rat and bovine pituitary glands ((23) and Margolis *et al.*, unpublished results). The possible functional significance of these glycosaminoglycans and accompanying glycoproteins in the granule matrix remains to be determined.

In conclusion, we can say that heparan sulfate is both a soluble component of brain as well as a constituent of membranes in nervous tissue. In the latter case its role may be similar to that of heparan sulfate in membranes elsewhere, possibly in relation to intercellular adhesion and various types of cell-cell interactions. For example, in chromaffin granules heparan sulfate may be involved in the fusion of the granule membrane with the adrenal medullary cell prior to the release by exocytosis of the stored catecholamines. However, we can also expect that the role of heparan sulfate will be better understood as more definitive data become available concerning this glycosaminoglycan in other locations, and as we learn more about the function of glycosaminoglycans and glycoproteins in nervous tissue generally.

REFERENCES

1. Margolis, R.U., and Margolis, R.K., Int. J. Biochem. *8*, 85 (1977).
2. Margolis, R.K., and Margolis, R.U., *in* "Biochemistry of Brain" (S. Kumar, ed.), Pergamon Press, New York, in press.
3. Margolis, R.U., and Atherton, D.M., Biochim. Biophys. Acta. *273*, 368 (1972).
4. Margolis, R.U., Margolis, R.K., and Atherton, D.M. J. Neurochem. *19*, 2317 (1972).
5. Margolis, R.U., Lally, K., Kiang, W.-L., Crockett, C., and Margolis, R.K., Biochem. Biophys, Res. Commun. *73*, 1018 (1976).
6. Margolis, R.U., Lally, K., Kiang, W.-L., Crockett, C., and Margolis, R.K., Abstracts, Sixth International Meeting of the International Society for Neurochemistry, Copenhagen, 1977.
7. De Luca, S., Heinegård, D., Hascall, V.C., Kimura, J.H., and Caplan, A.I., J. Biol. Chem., in press.
8. Margolis, R.K., Margolis, R.U., Preti, C., and Lai, D., Biochemistry *14*, 4797 (1975).
9. Margolis, R.U., Biochim. Biophys. Acta *141*, 91 (1967).
10. Dietrich, C.P., Sampaio, L.O., and Toledo, O.M.S., Biochem. Biophys. Res. Commun. *71*, 1 (1976).
11. Margolis, R.K., Crockett, C.P., Kiang, W.-L., and Margolis, R.U., Biochim. Biophys. Acta *451*, 465 (1976).
12. Margolis, R.U., Margolis, R.K., Kiang, W.-L., Lally, K., and Crockett, C.P., Trans. Am. Soc. Neurochem. *8*, 236 (1977).
13. Oldberg, Å., Höök, M., Öbrink, B., Pertoft, H., and Rubin, K., Biochem. J. *164*, 75 (1977).
14. Margolis, R.U., and Margolis, R.K., Biochemistry *13*, 2849 (1974).
15. Elam, J.S., and Peterson, N.W., J. Neurochem. *26*, 845 (1976).
16. Karlsson, J.-O., and Linde, A., J. Neurochem. *28*, 293 (1977).
17. Kuczenski, R.T., and Mandell, A.J., J. Biol. Chem. *247* 3114 (1972).
18. Margolis, R.U., Margolis, R.K., Chang, L., and Preti, C., Biochemistry *14*, 85 (1975).

19. Fillion, G., Nosal, R., and Uvnäs, B., Acta Physiol. Scand. *83*, 286 (1971).
20. Margolis, R.U., and Margolis, R.K., Biochem. Pharmacol. *22*, 2195 (1973).
21. Geissler, D., Martinek, A., Margolis, R.U., Margolis, R.K., Skrivanek, J.A., Ledeen, R., König, P., and Winkler, H., Neuroscience, in press.
22. Margolis, R.K., Jaanus, S.D., and Margolis, R.U., Molecular Pharmacol. *9*, 590 (1973).
23. Giannattasio, G., and Zanini, A., Biochim. Biophys. Acta *439*, 349 (1976).

THE ROLE OF THE HEPARIN PROTEIN COMPLEX IN THE STORAGE OF HISTAMINE IN MAST CELLS

Börje Uvnäs

Karolinska institutet

When, about forty years ago, the metachromatic staining of mast cell granules was found to be due to their content of heparin, it was natural to ascribe to the mast cell and its heparin a functional role in the regulation of the coagulability of blood and tissue fluids. Years later histamine was observed to be stored in mast cells of various animals species and the interest then largely shifted towards the possible role of the mast cell and its histamine in regulation of the microcirculation and vascular permeability. The release of histamine from mast cells during anaphylactic reactions was taken to support such an idea. Today the list of active components stored in the mast cell granules has considerably increased to include enzymes like chymotrypsin and glucuronidase, as well as polypeptides like eosinophilic and neutrophilic chemotactic factors. The modes of storage and release of these various granule components are largely unknown, but they are probably all released to a greater or lesser extent during exocytosis and degranulation when the granules become exposed to the extracellular fluid. The battery of active factors then released will elicit complex reaction patterns in the surrounding tissue. The functional significance of the mast cell response to various releasing factors is still speculated upon, but it has been suggested as serving as an element in the local defense mechanisms by facilitating the accumulation of humoral and cellular defensive factors.

A role for heparin in such a defense mechanism is perhaps easy to imagine in animal species such as the dog and the guinea pig that have mast cells with granules that rapidly dissolve when exposed to the extracellular fluid, on exocytosis and degranulation of the cells. However, in other species, such as the rat, the mast cell granules do not dissolve. They can be seen retained in challenged mast cells or as phagocytosed particles in tissue macrophages for days or even longer. Which extracellular function - if any - heparin has in such species remains to be clarified.

The concomitant occurrence of heparin and histamine in the mast cell granules earlier led to the suggestions that these two biologically active compounds may be stored together as an inactive salt complex. The formation of such a complex

ISBN 0-12-484850-8

in vitro was taken to support the hypothesis. The *in vitro* complex arises from ionic binding between the ester sulphate groups of the heparin and the amino groups of the histamine. Desulphated heparin does not bind histamine. The complex has its maximum stability at pH 2-3, when histamine is divalent, and consequently both amino groups are able to take part in the complex formation (1).

From data on the composition of rat mast cell heparin (2) and the content of heparin and histamine in rat peritoneal mast cells (3), the maximal histamine binding capacity of the granule heparin can be calculated to be 920 neq of histamine/mg dried granule material. The amount of histamine actually found in the granules was 910 neq/mg. Theoretically, therefore, the heparin present in rat mast cell granules should suffice to bind all the granule histamine. However, a closer analysis of the *in vivo* situation makes such a storage mechanism less likely. In the first place the *in vitro* heparin-histamine complex has its maximum stability at pH 2-3, a strongly acid milieu rather unlikely to exist in the granules. Since at a neutral pH the granule heparin suffices to bind only a minor part of the normal histamine content - about 10% at pH 7.4 - the question arises: How is the rest of the histamine stored? Or, perhaps there is no heparin-histamine complex at all *in vivo* As mentioned above, the ester sulphate groups of the heparin are essential for its histamine binding ability. Are there such groups available for binding in the granules? Surprisingly little attention has been paid to the fact that one major component of the granule matrix is protein. This might be bound to heparin thereby making the acid groups required for the binding of histamine.

Mast cell granules can easily be obtained from disrupted rat peritoneal mast cells by differential centrifugation (4). Granules isolated from such cells destroyed by water lysis are devoid of surrounding membranes (Fig. 1), which means that the granule matrix is directly exposed to ions and other constituents of the suspension medium. As long as such granules are kept in deionized water they are still able to retain histamine. The histamine is however immediately released on suspending the granules in isotonic saline or other salt solutions (5,6). But no appreciable release of heparin occurs. In other words, the granule matrix, consisting almost exclusively of protein and heparin (Table I), remains undissolved. As will be illustrated below, the histamine depleted granules are able to reaccumulate and store histamine if resuspended in a histamine containing medium. However, titration of the granules does not indicate the presence of

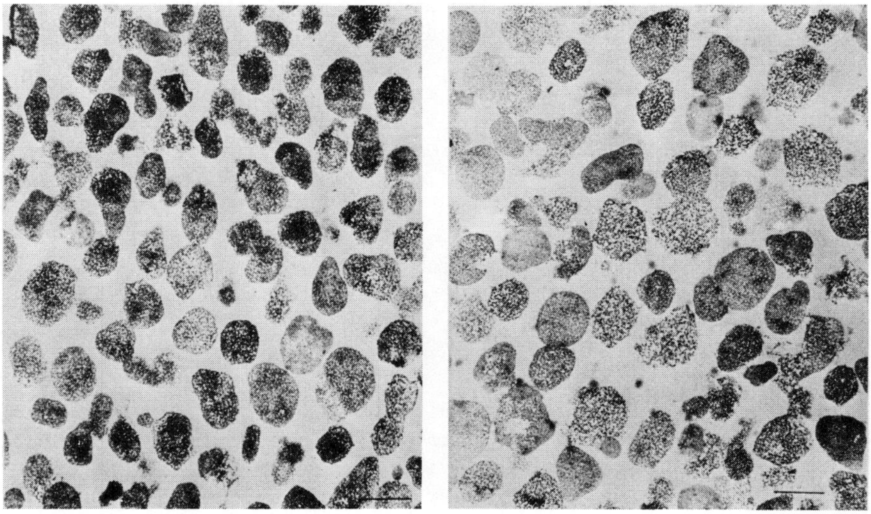

Fig. 1. Electron micrographs of granules isolated from cells: (a) degranulated by incubation with compound 48/80. x 8,600; (b) lysed by distilled water. x 8,600.

TABLE I Calculated Composition of Mast Cell Granules (from Uvnäs (3)).

Protein	*∿ 60%*
Heparin	*∿ 30%*
Histamine	*∿ 10%*
5-HT	*< 0.3%*
Phospholipids	*1-2%*
ATP	*< 0.2%*

any free strongly acid groups, i.e., ester sulphate groups. Only weakly acid groups, presumably carboxylic groups, are found. In other words, the ester sulphate groups of heparin are masked, presumably by protein in the granule matrix (7).

As already stated the granule matrix does not dissolve in isotonic sodium chloride solution but does so in 1-2 *M* NaCl. On column chromatography two main components - heparin and protein - can be separated from the dissolved granules. The major part of the protein is a basic polypeptide with a probable molecular weight of around 5600 (ultracentrifugation). The strongly basic character of the protein - isoelectric point around 9 - explains its tendency to form a complex with heparin and thereby to mask the latter's ester sulphate groups (8).

As mentioned above, histamine-containing granules release their histamine when sodium chloride is present in the suspension medium. However, the storage mechanism is also very pH-dependent. On acidification of the suspension medium (deionized water) the storage capacity is rapidly reduced to be practically abolished at pH 4-5 suggesting that ionized carboxyl groups are essential for the histamine binding ability of the granule. When the granules were also found to take up sodium, and the uptake curve for sodium was shown to be identical with the reversed carboxyl titration curve, the principle prerequisites existed for a granule storage mechanism based on a cation exchange principle (7). Further studies confirmed this idea. Isolated granules showed an unselective *in vitro* uptake of inorganic cations (Na+, Ca++, Zn++) and amines (PhEA,[a] TA, DA, NA, A, Hi, TrA, 5-Ht, etc.) (9). As illustrated (Fig. 2) for histamine and sodium, they were all taken up by the granules to about the same maximal level - 1000 neq/mg dried granule material. They competed for the same ionic sites on the granules, and when, for instance, histamine was released by sodium, there was an equivalent exchange between histamine and sodium in the granules. Titration of granule material for COO^-- groups indicated the presence of about 1000 neq/mg (7), a figure in good agreement with the maximal uptake of sodium, histamine, and other biogenic amines.

The observations cited above all agree with the idea of a heparin-protein complex in the granule matrix operating as a weak cation exchange material, the COO^-- groups of the protein acting as the ionic binding sites. This suggestion was further corroborated by the fact that the uptake values

[a] *PHEA - Phenylethylamine, TA - Tyramine, DA - Dopamine, NA - Noradrenaline, A - Adrenaline, Hi - Histamine, TrA - Tryptamine, 5-HT - 5 hydroxytryptamine*

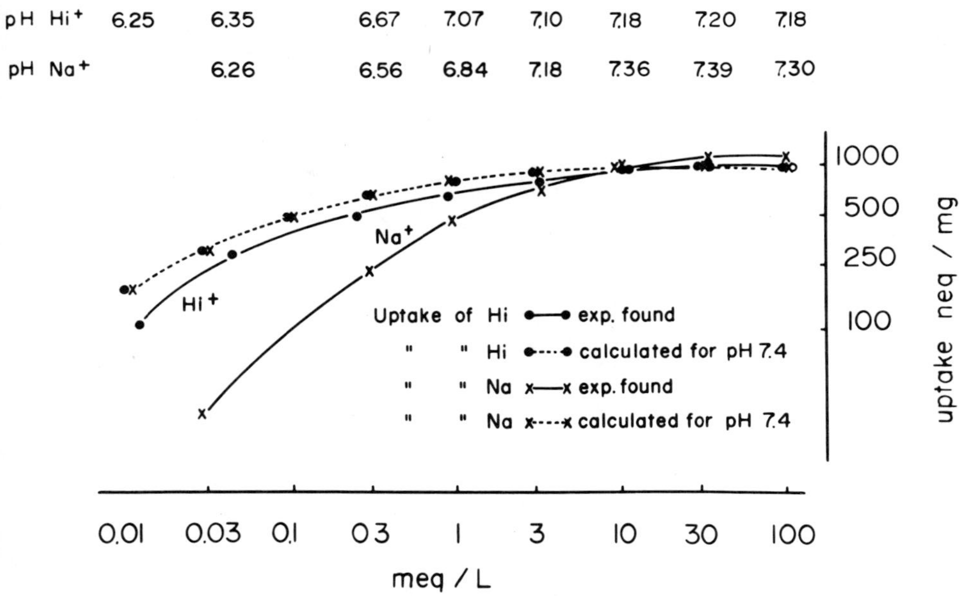

Fig. 2. Uptake by mast cell granules of Hi+ and Na+ (Uvnäs and Åborg (10)).

for histamine and sodium fitted the Rothmund-Kornfeld equation for weak cation exchangers (10). The equation implies that when two cations compete for the ionic sites of an ion exchanger, plotting the log of the ratios between the concentration of the two cations in the exchanger versus the log of the corresponding concentration of the cations in the suspension medium will give a straight line. In the granules the two cations competing for the binding sites will be hydrogen ions and the cation under investigation, i.e., sodium or histamine. Since the maximal uptakes for the two ions in the same batch of granule material are identical, and the pH and the cation uptake known, the validity of the exchange equation for the cation binding properties of the granule material can be tested. As shown in Fig. 3, the uptake values fit the cation exchange equation. It is noteworthy that above pH 7 the two lines for sodium and histamine not only run parallel but also very close to each other, indicating almost identical affinities for the granule binding sites of these two cations. Below pH 7 the histamine curve deviates. This is due to the increasing divalency of the histamine with falling pH.

Let us for a moment go back to Fig. 1, showing the concentration dependence of the uptakes of sodium and histamine by the mast cell granules. We experimentally found uptake values indicating a slightly higher affinity of the

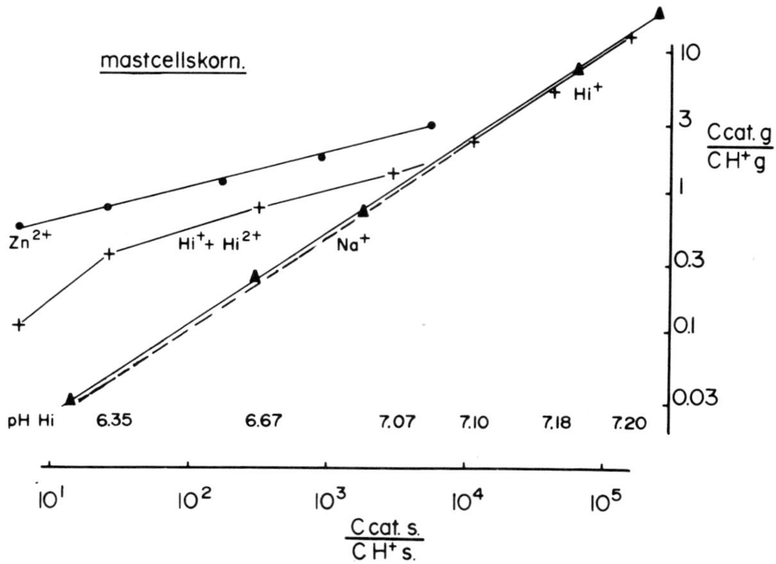

Fig. 3. Plot of the logs of the ratios between the concentrations of Na+, Hi+, and Zn++ ions over the concentrations of ions in mast cell granules versus the logs of the corresponding concentration ratios in the suspension medium. For symbols see the figure. Note the straight lines obtained (from Uvnäs, Åborg (10)).

granule storage sites for histamine than for sodium. As also seen from the figure, at lower concentrations the buffer capacity of the medium is insufficient to prevent a slight shift of pH towards acidity. Due to the consequent suppressing of the dissociation of carboxyl groups even such small shifts should result in reduced uptakes of the two cations. At the same time the reduced uptake of histamine should be counteracted by its higher affinity for the storage sites due to increased divalency at acid pH. Hence, the apparent higher affinity for histamine than for sodium. However, if the experimentally found values were recalculated for pH 7.4 according to the Rothmund-Kornfeld equation, the uptake curves for sodium and histamine became identical (Fig. 1).

To summarize, our observations indicate that the mast cell granules operate like a weak cation exchange resin with carboxyl groups of the protein serving as ionic binding sites.

Since the affinities of histamine and sodium for the granule sites are equal and the concentration of sodium present in the extracellular fluid (150 mM) is between 100-200 times higher than required to saturate the granule binding sites (1-3 mM), histamine will immediately be released by cation exchange when mast cell granules devoid of surrounding membrane are exposed to the extracellular fluid during exocytosis and degranulation (Fig. 4).

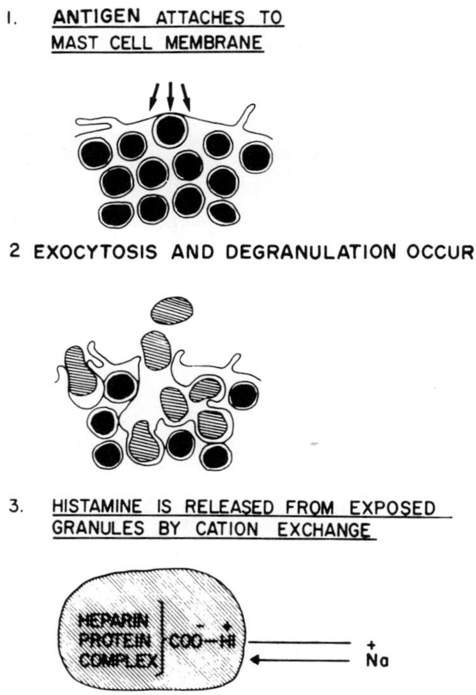

Fig. 4. Suggested mechanism of action of compound 48/80 (Uvnäs (4)).

So far the amine storage and release mechanism has only been studied in rat peritoneal mast cells. As far as I know, the basophil granules in mast cells of other animal species also contain heparin or closely related sulphomucopolysaccharides. Therefore, it seems plausible that these cells also store and release amines in an analogous way. However, a storage and release mechanism based on cationic exchange is so attractive in its simplicity and possible applications that a search for such mechanisms in connection with the storage and release of other amines, hormones, etc., might be rewarding. We have in fact observed that granules isolated from ox adrenal medullary cells (10) and from ox splenic nerves (Uvnäs *et al.*, to be published) contain binding material. In their cation binding properties these materials behave like mast cell granules, i.e., like weak cation exchange resins. The functional significance of these observations for the understanding of the storage and release of transmitter amines is still obscure, as is the chemical composition of the cation binding material. It is true that we (11,12) like others (13) have identified mucopolysaccharides in granule material from ox adrenal medulla and also in adrenergic vesicle preparations from various tissues and nerves. However, it is doubtful whether the amounts of sulphomucopolysaccharides present in these granule materials would suffice to account for the binding of appreciable amounts of the transmitter amines present. However, these amines are supposed to be separated into various compartments, releasable and storage pools, etc., and whether sulphomucopolysaccharides or related substance are involved in the storage of any such pools remains to be investigated. However, be that as it may, there are many other situations in the body, where storage and release mechanisms based on cation exchange principles might be found.

REFERENCES

1. Uvnäs, B., Life Sci *14*, 2355-2366 (1974).
2. Schiller, S., and Dorfman, A., Biochem. Biophys. Acta. *31*, 278-280 (1959).
3. Uvnäs, B., 2nd Int. Symp. Blackwell Scientific Publ. (1971).
4. Uvnäs, B., Biomembranes, Cells, Organelles and Membrane Components. *in* "Methods in Enzymology" (1972).
5. Uvnäs, B., Ann. New York Acad. Sci. *116*, 880-890 (1964).
6. Uvnäs, B., and Thon, I.L., Proc. Int. Wenner-Gren Symp. *in* "Mechanisms of Release of Biogenic Amines." Pergamon Press. Oxford, 361-370 (1966).
7. Uvnäs, B., Åborg, C.-H., and Bergendorff, A., Acta Physiol. Scand. Suppl. *336* (1970).
8. Bergqvist, U., Samuelsson, B., and Uvnäs, B., Acta Physiol. Scand. *83*, 362-372 (1971).
9. Bergendorff, A., and Uvnäs, B., Acta Physiol. Scand. *87*, 213-222 (1973).
10. Uvnäs, B., and Åborg, C.-H., Acta Physiol. Scand. *99*, 476-483 (1977).
11. Blaschke, E., Bergqvist, U., and Uvnäs, B., Acta Physiol. Scand. *97*, 110-120 (1976).
12. Åborg, C.-H., Fillion, G., Nosál, R., and Uvnäs, B., Acta Physiol. Scand. *86*, 427-429 (1972).
13. Margolis, R.K., and Margolis, R.U., Biochemistry *9*, 4389-4396 (1970).

DO MAST CELLS SECRETE THEIR GRANULES?[a]

Jacques Padawer

Albert Einstein College of Medicine

I. INTRODUCTION

The words *secrete* and *secretion* get short shrift in our textbooks: they do not even appear in the indexes of several well known college and medical school physiology or biochemistry treatises. Dictionaries, at least, all have appropriate entries, but the range of variations represented is startling. Officially, secretion is almost whatever one wishes; it's a matter of choosing the desired authority.

It therefore seems imperative that we define our terms at the outset. I have settled on a definition that is a composite of several given in standard or medical dictionaries. For this essay, the following will be meant:

Secrete (se-kret) (Fr. L. *Secretus*, separated). To elaborate some physiologically useful substance (e.g., by a cell) and to release it directly, in response to physiological control mechanisms (e.g., hormonal or neural) into blood, tissue, or body cavity.

Among the views held today, are the beliefs that mast cells normally secrete histamine and heparin, two substances they synthesize and store in surprisingly large quantities. Some of the evidence mustered in support of these views is questionable, while other data clearly argue against them. My purpose here is to challenge current wisdom regarding mast cells and their putative function(s), and to focus on intracellular events rather than on degranulation, for I believe these to be more germane to the normal physiology of mast cells. Heparin, the focus of this conference, and other components of mast cell granules, could play as critical a role intracellularly as has been proposed for them if they were secreted into the tissue spaces.

---

[a] *The following abbreviations are used in the manuscript: AB - antibody; Ag - antigen; ATP - adenosine triphosphate; CH - commercial heparin; ECF-A - eosinophyl chemotactic factor of anaphylaxis; Ig - immunoglobulin; MMH - macromolecular heparin; PAPS - phosphoadenosylphosphosulfate; RES - reticuloendothelial system.*

ISBN 0-12-484850-8

II. DEGRANULATION: THE JOKER IN THE MAST CELL DECK?

If a crab is seized by a claw, or a lizard by the tail, the animal will sever that body part and escape to live another day. Autotomy unquestionably has survival value, but the normal function of a claw or tail is not merely to await autotomy as a means of escape from predators. Of itself, the process of autotomy is fascinating, but were we to understand it in its minutest biochemical detail it would still tell us precious little about the function of claws. And thereby hangs a tale...which I hope to develop in this essay.

Mast cells, under a variety of conditions, can, if you will, *autotomize* their granules, i.e., degranulate, though I must emphasize that much as autotomy is a response to stimuli outside the organism, degranulation is not similarly initiated by the cell, but rather it is impressed upon the cell by extracellular agents. I do not care to carry the analogy to its extreme, for the animal no doubt autotomizes by an active process, whereas mast cells, in my view, are degranulated passively. Degranulating agents perhaps subvert some mast cell reactions normally engaged in some unrelated activity, and if so, the fact that cyclic AMP, altered calcium flux, oxygen uptake, or glucose utilization, for instance, participate in the degranulation process may not in fact be proof that degranulation is a physiological event, for these reactions may be equally pertinent to whatever function(s) mast cells normally perform on an ongoing basis. More pointedly, these and other biochemical processes shown to come into play during degranulation are essentially basic reactions in the armamentarium of cellular mechanisms: they are universal, can lead to any number of effects depending on the cell involved, and thus cannot be taken as evidence for any one particular process or response.

Degranulation of mast cells, like autotomy for the crab, can be a matter of life and death for the host organism. As one allergic to animal hair and other allergens, I follow with interest the findings of my degranulation-centered colleagues. I wish them well, for the pathology of allergy hangs over me like the sword of Damocles. Were the thread to break, semantic arguments pitting secretion versus degranulation would be academic.

Thus, lest there be confusion regarding the thrust of this paper, it must be stressed at the outset that the fact mast cells can be degranulated under some circumstances is not questioned. Nor is the fact that, when degranulation occurs, it evidences biochemical reactions that also are found to be associated with secretion. Rather, the message I hope to convey is, quite simply, that mast cells *do not* secrete their granules in order to carry out their normal function(s).

But first one must ask whether any function is served by mast cell granules *in situ*, i.e., when *no* degranulation is involved.

III. DO MAST CELL GRANULES FUNCTION *IN SITU*?

Several observations strongly suggest that mast cell granules must have a function *in situ*, and that neither the granule as a unit nor any known granular component leaves the cell in the process. That being the case, one ought to look for functions that do not depend on degranulation.

The basis for these statements derive from observations of very disparate and independent nature, including: *1* Mast cells are small in young animals (e.g., rat, mouse, hamster, gerbil). They grow larger and larger as the animal ages (1,2). One would not expect this if granules were continuously secreted from the cell. On the other hand, this would happen, of necessity, if granules were *not* secreted and if more were elaborated as their substance became slowly committed as they function, or if physiological demand for their activity increased with aging of the animal. *2* Mast cell granules *mature* over a long time period, possibly weeks to months, in that their tinctorial properties with some dyes change with time and in parallel with cell size (3,4). One would not expect this if the granules were secreted apace on an ongoing basis. *3* Mast cells display the cytological features of endocytic rather than absorptive or secretory cells (5,3). They can endocytize various substances, under conducive conditions, and they then deposit the ingested material onto some of their specific metachromatic cytoplasmic granules (6,7,8,9). *This is unexpected for secretion granules*. *4* Deposition of ingested material on granules is not indiscriminate. Only a few granules are involved in any one cell, and these often are clustered in close proximity to each other (8). *5* If the endocytized material is an indigestible metal oxide marker (e.g., colloidal thorium dioxide), labeled granules can be seen in the cells for a substantial portion of the animal's life span -- at least 10 months in the rat (10). If granule secretion were a physiological process, such markers should be lost in the course of secretion. *6* When mast cells are degranulated by histamine liberators, mitochondrial and cytosol enzymes do not leak out into the medium (11); the cells remain viable and will regenerate new sets of granules (12). Regeneration is very slow -- several weeks are needed for complete recovery. This does not support the view that granule secretion is a continuous event. *7* If mast cell granules are damaged experimentally or inactivated *in situ*, feedback mechanisms become operative, the cell undergoes a form of blastogenesis, and active synthesis of new granules occurs (13). If granule secretion were a continuous process, granule synthesis would be more evident in the normal cell. *8* Granular components, namely histamine, heparin, or serine protease(s), appear to *not* turn over with time (10,3). Their release from the cells can be demonstrated only in conjunction with overt degranulation, or at least marginal damage. This is not compatible with ongoing secretion of granules. *9* The granular proteases, chymotrypsin or trypsin-like in nature exist within the granules in enzymatically active forms (14) rather than as inactive zymogen precursors. This contrasts with granule enzymes of secretory cells in which proteases are present as inactive zymogens. *10* Mast cells deformed by centrifugation under high hydrostatic pressure relax to their original spheroidal shape rapidly in young rats but slowly in older ones. Small cells relax faster and differently than large ones (15,16). One would not expect this if the cells were short-lived or turned over rapidly. It may reflect the granule load that must be moved during the relaxation process. *11* Mast cells are deformed by exposure to colchicine (17,18), but sensitivity to the drug decreases from birth to advanced age of the animal (19). This suggests a long-term evolution of the mast cell response, and thus implies the cells have a very long lifespan. It may reflect the granule load that must be moved during the deformation period.

In contrast to these observations, is the fact that mast cells nuclei are of essentially constant size regardless of overall cell size (Padawer, unpublished). Since cells generally possess a characteristic nuclear-cytoplasmic ratio, this suggests that mast cell granules do not enter into the *cytoplasm* factor of the equation.

What can we infer from these findings?

First, it is clear that mast cells are active participants in the economy or ecology of the body, an inference that flows directly from the existence of feedback mechanisms. It is startling to think that only two decades ago one could still propose that mast cells were the mummified corpses of once polysaccharide-laden cells (20). The ingenious proposal that mast cell granules are released into the ground substrate so as to trap and neutralize toxic substances as a prelude to disposal by tissue phagocytes (21,22,23) must also be reinterpreted; although such an effect is indeed demonstrable under certain pathological or experimental conditions, it does not follow that this is the way mast cells function.

Second, we can infer that the physiological role that

mast cells play is not only an ongoing one, since the changes they undergo as the animal ages are progressive, but one that involves a very low level of synthetic activity. Indeed, their ultrastructure in mature animals suggests a minimal, almost resting level of biosynthetic involvement (3); when mature they have only a few, small mitochondria, a small Golgi apparatus, a barely noticeable nucleolus, little rough endoplasmic reticulum, etc. Their plasmalemma, on the other hand, is characteristically thrown into numerous folds, especially in solid tissues where these features can reach a remarkable development. These surface features have often been described, erroneously, as microvilli. Microvilli are generally associated with absorptive (e.g., intestinal epithelium) or secretory (e.g., gastric parietal cells) processes. Hyaloplasmic veils, on the other hand, are indicative of endocytosis (both pinocytosis and phagocytosis), including the interiorization of soluble materials that adsorb onto the cell surface. Thus the ultrastructural features of mast cells suggest one ought to look for functions with qualitative impact, perhaps an involvement with trace substances, and in which endocytosis may have special significance.

Abundant synthesis of cytoplasmic granules for secretory purposes appears most unlikely at this time. The above detailed ultrastructure would argue against mass synthesis of proteins or high molecular weight proteoglycans. These arguments are not meant to deny secretion of some trace substance(s). Indeed, synthesis of trace substances could not readily be gauged from ultrastructural observations, especially if the secretory products were discharged as fast as produced. Yet, such trace substances might be of great import were they lymphokine-like materials, superantigens, or informational molecules for instance. This possibility is well worth considerable thought, but we currently lack data to even speculate on that point.

IV. PHAGOCYTOSIS BY MAST CELLS: A CLUE TO THEIR FUNCTION?

A. Endocytosis of Particular Matter

Mast cells are unquestionably phagocytic (24,25,26,27, 6,7,13,8,9,28,29). This has been established only recently. Phagocytosis by mast cells was incontrovertibly demonstrated only when the peritoneal cavity was used as an experimental reaction site and the *right* particulates selected (26,6,8,9). As a matter of record, Michels, in his definitive review of the literature to 1938 (30), concluded that mast cells were not phagocytic. This, in a period that covered the enunciation of the reticuloendothelial system (RES) as a concept. In an even more ambitious summing up of our knowledge to 1965, Selye (31) reiterated that very conclusion. Yet, early workers should not be faulted: colloidal carbon and Trypan Blue, the two traditional substances used to delineate the RES are not taken up by mast cells (32,8). Furthermore, peritoneal fluid does not restrict access of particles to the mast cells the way the gelatinous connective tissue ground substance does, and this favors uptake which must depend on chance collisions between cells and particles because mast cells are not effectively ameboid. Still, mast cells are apparently phagocytic even in solid tissue sites, so long as the particles abound in their immediate vicinity and can drift into contact with the mast cell membrane (25, 28,29,33,34). Even in peritoneal fluid, where their phagocytic ability is most readily demonstrated, rat mast cells run very poor seconds to other cell types, especially macrophages, as far as uptake of most foreign particulates is concerned (7). But that is not an absolute situation, as there are particles which when introduced intraperitoneally are phagocytized by mast cells but *not* by eosinophils or diapedesing neutrophils, cells greatly predisposed to phagocytosis. It must also be noted that phagocytosis by mast cells is even less impressive in other species, such as the mouse, hamster, or gerbil (26).

There is much misunderstanding and confusion regarding these observations. Are mast cells part of the RES? What would they normally phagocytize, especially in solid tissues of untreated animals? All cells take up particulates under some circumstances, even cells highly specialized for mechanical function (35), but phago- and pinocytosis are primitive mechanisms referable to cellular nutrition, and thus may be of no special significance, except for RES cells which specialize in phagocytosis for bactericidal and tissue scavenging purposes.

Such arguments miss the mark.

Phagocytosis by mast cells is primarily an experimental curiosity. Its importance derives from the several implications it carries, namely, that mast cells bind extracellular materials to their plasmalemmal folds, and subsequently endocytize these materials. That, of itself, would hardly be arresting. What *is* remarkable is that the ingested material is deposited onto the specific cytoplasmic granules and that this occurs in a directionally-polarized way that indicates the granules are interconnected in a specific manner. The particulate substances I chose for my several studies were selected not because of any physiological significance, but rather because they could be recognized readily and with certainty in electron micrographs, i.e., they were operationally significant. The manner in which the cell disposes of these, it can be expected to similarly dispose of macromolecules such as IgE-Ag complexes (5), for instance, but further studies with radioactive or fluorescence-tagged macromolecules are needed to demonstrate uncontrovertibly the truth of that assumption.

The variety and disparity in size, electric charge, and chemical nature of the particles that mast cells will ingest is remarkable (8), and admittedly baffling. Most likely, however, foreign particulates quickly become coated upon injection with adsorbed tissue fluid proteins (or proteoglycans?), and the unifying concept might be that the adsorbed material rather than the particles themselves is what determines whether uptake by mast cells will occur. It has been shown that fresh serum greatly enhances the uptake of zymosan by rat mast cells *in vitro* (36,37), but that heated serum does not have such an effect. Thus, perhaps, adsorption of complement might be a prerequisite for phagocytosis of zymosan by mast cells since zymosan is known to adsorb complement (heat-labile) most effectively (particularly the properdin components). On the other hand, IgE is also denatured when serum is heated to destroy complement activity. Thus it might be that particles which adsorb IgE are thereby rendered *palatable* to mast cells also. There would seem to be promising research opportunities in this area.

B. Endocytosis of Immune Globulins

Mast cells are clearly involved in immune reactions, one of the most intriguing being their affinity for IgE, and their subsequent degranulation upon presentation of the IgE-specific antigen. A variety of other findings also link mast cells to immune mechanisms; I have briefly reviewed some of them elsewhere (3).

A question of particular interest is how mast cells might relate to B or T lymphocytes. Differentiation of lymphocytic cells into mast cells in tissue culture has been reported; thymic epithelioid elements are not needed for this transformation. Pure populations of either B or T lymphocytes have not been tested in this way and thus it is not known which line, or whether both lines, might be the precursor(s). Studies with congenitally athymic (nude) mice, however, are most revealing in that such animals may have more rather than fewer mast cells than nonnude animals (nu/+, +/+) of the same strain. Nude mice are not prone to increased incidence of spontaneous tumors, and thus their surveillance system

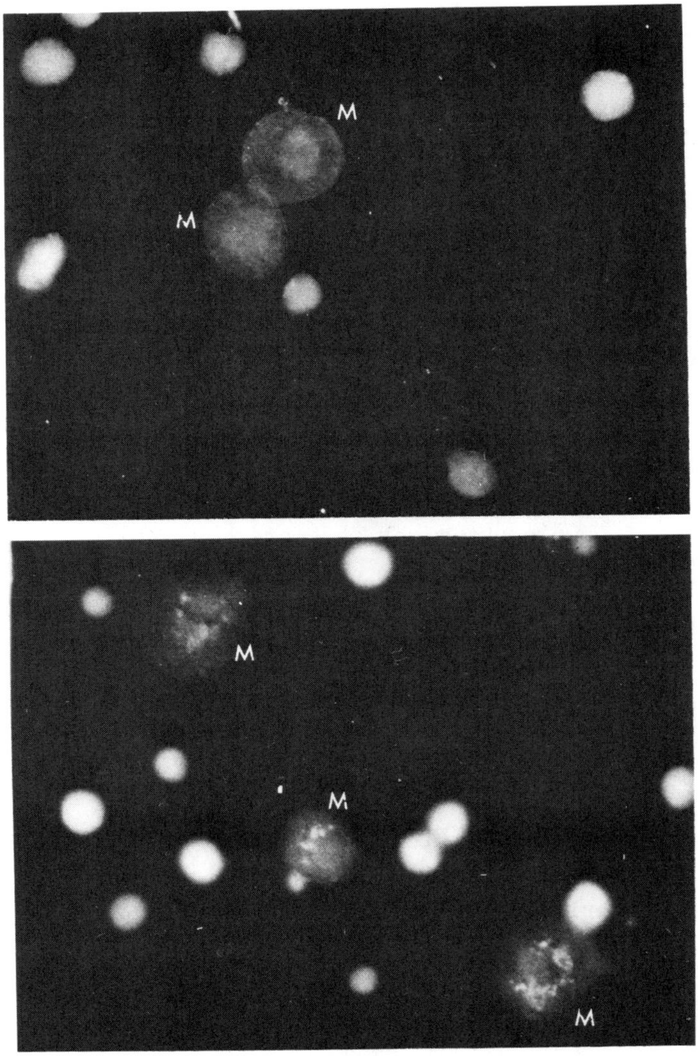

Fig. 1. A) Binding of fluorescein-tagged rat IgE[b] *myeloma protein to air-dried, aldehyde-fixed rat peritoneal mast cells. Perinuclear foci of irregular size and shape are seen in all three mast cells (M). Virtually all the mast cells in the IgE-treated area responded in this way. Nonmast cells are strongly fluorescent, but comparison with B) indicates this is nonspecific (probably due to fixation). B) Untreated cells from a portion of same slide not exposed to IgE reagent. The mast cells (M) lack foci of fluorescence.*

appears to be operative, even though they lack plasmocytes and circulating immunoglobulins. Precursor T cells are present, however, and these can be induced to differentiate in the presence of thymic epithelioid elements. Furthermore, a small proportion of nude mice lymphocytes are killed by antitheta serum, although nude mice are though to be devoid of T cells. IgG and IgE, but not IgM, are thymus-dependent immunoglobulins, and so one might assume little or no IgE is synthesized in nude mice. On the other hand, suppressor T cells can also inhibit IgE production (38). Whether or how this relates to mast cells remains to be explored.

These observations support the suggestion of Viklicky *et al.* (39) that mast cells do not originate from thymus cells, and that they are not to T cells what mature plasmocytes are to B cells, as proposed by Burnet (40,41). Mature fully granulated mast cells can undergo mitosis, but this would not necessarily preclude concurrent continued differentiation from lymphocytic or mesenchymal precursors that could then enter the pool of mitosing mast cells. Mitosis of mast cells appears to be far more common in young animals. It remains to be seen whether it occurs throughout life.

The fact that mast cells become degranulated upon complexing of Ag to the IgE they bind need not signify that degranulation is an essential component of the normal Ab-Ag response. Indeed, degranulation might occur only when much antibody has been fixed and antigen then presented too rapidly. These are the very conditions selected for in many experiments, and it may give us a fortuitously biased view. Though storm drains may overflow during an excessively severe downpour, it does not signify their purpose is to flood the surrounding land. The analogy may well be applicable to mast cells if their role is to process IgE, i.e., drain it away from extracellular fluids. The vanishingly small amounts of IgE normally extant suggest that mast cells normally are not faced with the need to cope with mich Ag-Ab complexing on their surface. And the suggestion that IgE is endocytized by mast cells (5) has now received some support from experiments by Orr (42) who noted the intracellular IgE (40) showed there is an affinity between gamma globulin and

---

[b] *The preliminary nature of these observations must be emphasized. Only a single IgE preparation was used to date, and its binding capacity was only 20%. Control studies, with heat-deactivated IgE, with anti IgE, or with unlabeled IgE blocking have not yet been done. Other immunoglobulins have not been examined in this model system; neither have trace amounts of free fluorescein.*

mast cell granules in sectioned material, though their experiments with heat-treated serum would seem to have ruled out IgE. In analogous, preliminary experiments, I have examined the affinity of air-dried, aldehyde-fixed rat peritoneal mast cells for fluorescein-tagged IgE (ex rats bearing monoclonal IgE-secreting tumors, courtesy Dr. H. Metzger, NIH). Whereas Simson *et al.* (43) found that all the mast cell granules bound immunoglobulin indiscriminately, I find binding of IgE to be confined to a number of perinuclear sites of varying size and shape (Fig. 1). Inasmuch as only light microscopy was involved in my experiments to date, it is not clear whether specific mast cell granules or some other organelles are involved, but on the basis of their size, shape and distribution pattern, it may well be that these sites are identified with the younger, developing granules to which endocytized materials are normally first brought. Experiments of Mayrhofer (44) are of particular interest in this respect. He showed IgE localized to the granules of intestinal mast cells in rats infected with a worm parasite, but in lymph nodes of these same animals the fluorescence was limited to the cell surface. It seems most probable that this dichotomy arises from differences in availability of antigen. In the gut, worm antigens abound, and their complexes with specific IgEs bound to mast cell surfaces are apparently endocytized and deposited on the mast cell granules. By contrast, antigen may not reach the lymph nodes in appreciable amounts and mast cell surface-bound IgE remains localized at the cell-environment boundary. A careful examination of Mayrhofer's illustrations (his figures 3,3a,5, 6,7) suggest that IgE is unevenly bound within the cells and preferentially so to paranuclear sites -- the cells have a scalloped boundary that suggests peripheral granules are unstained. His illustrations differ somewhat from my own preliminary ones (Fig. 1) in that in his figures many have granules that are reactive. This may just be a matter of technique - either more binding or greater sensitivity due to enhancement by the goat antirabbit-FITC sandwich procedure. Mayrhofer wouldn't assert whether the IgE was "... in the granules or in the soluble cytoplasm" (p. 181), and he indicated he was "... not convinced that (peritoneal mast cells) are the same as the mucosal mast cells" (p. 180).

It seems likely that cross-linking of receptors on the cell surface is required to induce capping and endocytosis. In a sense, large particles -- and all particulates are *large* in comparison with macromolecules -- probably bind to many receptors simultaneously and thus effect *cross-linking* when they bind to the mast cell surface and are phagocytized. This suggests that the physical interlocking of receptors at the cell surface may be more critical than any change in the receptor molecule itself.

C. Fate of Endocytized Matter

Studies with digestible particulate markers (zymosan, sperm nuclei) reveal that mast cells cannot readily digest the materials they take up (5,9); they are poorly endowed with lysosomes and their specific granules which contain only 2 enzymes -- a peptide and a glycosidase, are therefore lysosomoid at best. This, too, sets mast cells apart from *professional* phagocytes whose abundant lysosomes are replete with many kinds of enzymes which, in concert, can rapidly degrade almost anything. Macrophages, upon phagocytosis, redistribute their lysosomes around the ingested particles and these pour their contents into the phagosome to yield secondary lysosomes. Additionally, macrophage acid phosphatase activity increases markedly upon phagocytosis. Mast cells do not respond similarly. They posses only a few punctate sites of cytochemically demonstrable acid phosphatase activity (7,45), and these neither become redistributed around ingested zymosan particles nor do they proliferate upon particle ingestion. That may not be the case for other particulates, however (27).

This limited digestive capability of mast cells may have immunological import, for phagocytosis is needed as an early step in the chain of events that lead to immunity, whether humoral or cell-mediated, and whereas partial digestion of the antigen may be acceptable or even necessary, complete digestion down to amino acids and/or low molecular weight saccharide components might not be conducive to a good immunological response. Conventional macrophages may eat to forget; mast cells may eat to remember. If so, mast cell endocytosis may have special significance.

D. Inferences Derived from Mast Cell Endocytosis

The phagocytosis experiments clearly demonstrate that mast cell granules cannot fairly be compared cytologically to granules in other cell types. In the latter, each granule is individually enclosed within a membrane, much as the meat of an orange is completely enwrapped by the peel. For secretion of granules by a variety of cells, fusion of peri-granular membranes, first with the plasmalemma and subsequently with nearby granules located deeper within the cytoplasm, apparently occurs and leads to the formation of labyrinthine channels to which contiguous granules are consecutively joined and given access to the extracellular space. This process has been demonstrated clearly for exocrine (46) and for endocrine cells (47,48) of the pancreas and for salivary gland cells (49,50). This membrane fusion process allows the extracellular compartment to flood the granular material which then is dissolved by it. It has been termed *noncytotoxic secretion* in a review by Morrison (personal communication). Uvnäs (51) and Lagunoff (52) have argued that the very same events occur during mast cell degranulation. On the basis of available data, I do not believe these views can be defended. Indeed, there is much evidence that mast cells differ from the secretory cells mentioned above in that their granules are more readily compared to a chain of sausage links than they are to oranges (7). Nevertheless, the membrane-limited domains within which sets of granules are sequestered can also be merged with the extracellular compartment if some external agent acting on the cell surface induces potential plasmalemmal pores to open at the termini of the granule-laden channels, in which case all of the granules held within the particular set are affected simultaneously. That is what I believe occurs when polycations (this includes well-known liberators such as Compound 48/80 or Polymyxin B sulfate) are applied to mast cells. These agents somehow interact with receptors at the mast cell surface (53) and induce a wave of granule swelling and/or degranulation which is propagated centripetally. If extracellular tracers are applied concurrently, these flood the elicited labyrinthine channels, as demonstrated conclusively by Uvnäs and collaborators (54) and by Lagunoff (55) with various tracers such as hemoglobin, lanthanum nitrate, ferritin, or ruthenium red. Under these conditions, it is the mature peripheral granules that are contacted first (52,56; see also Fig. 6 of 51). This is also the case when another polycation, namely polylysine, is used alone (13) or as a coating on plastic microspheres (8). With polylysine, the extreme swelling of the granules that usually accompanies degranulation does not occur, and both the cytoplasmic channels and the induced surface pores become clearly delineated (13). Though clumping of mature granules occurs with polylysine, very immature ones are not drawn into the aggregates, probably because they lack the heparin component. If the polylysine is adsorbed onto plastic microspheres, the ingested particles are seen to attach to mature granules rather than to immature ones (8), indicating these are the ones contacted first.

These degranulation-associated developments are the *opposite* of what happens when nondegranulation particulate tracers are phagocytized or when mast cell damage occurs spontaneously *in vitro* in absence of polycations. Indeed spontaneous aggregation of granules (a sign of cell damage) after a sojourn *in vitro* arises within the deeper areas of the cell (57). When spontaneous degranulation occurs *in vitro* (also a sign of cell damage), granules deep within the cell are affected first, and the wave of swelling granules proceeds centrifugally. When particulate tracers are phagocytized by undamaged mast cells, they first make contact with immature granules (7,8).

Clearly, the granules are held within channels that have polarity -- immature granules at one end (the proximal one, near the outer face of the Golgi apparatus) and mature ones at the other end (the distal one, near the cell periphery) and it is possible, under different circumstances, for extracellular substances to enter the granule channels from either direction. If uptake into the cell is under cellular control via endocytic vacuoles, access into the granular channels occurs at their proximal end, and there is no degranulation. If entry (forced?) is effected from the distal end, degranulation occurs. The difference may be that extracellular fluid can be modified (*cleaned up* by removal of offensive cations) by the cell in the course of transferring endocytic vacuoles to their fusion sites at the proximal segment of granule channels, whereas no such opportunity exists when direct access is gained through the distal plasmalemmal pore termini of the channels. Mast cell granules isolated from cells disrupted in nonionic saccharide media do not swell, and they retain their histamine (58). Addition of trace amounts of inorganic cations (Na^{+}, K^{+}, Ca^{++}, Mg^{++}, it does not seem to matter) to the isolated granules causes their immediate disruption (swelling) and an explosive concomitant release of histamine (52,59). Ionophores can induce degranulation (60,61) but it is not clear whether that is in response to influx of cations into the cytosol or to the transfer of cations across the membrane that delimits the granular channels. In view of their mechanism of activity, it is more likely that ionophores carry ions across all the cellular membranes including those that delimit organelles. Direct microinjection of calcium *into the cell* achieved the same results (62), but the method did not differentiate between delivery of the ion into the intergranular cytosol in contrast to intraluminal deposition within the granular channels. K^{+} and Mg^{++} did not lead to degranulation, which suggests that granular channels were not penetrated. It would be of great interest to know whether Zn^{++} might act similarly to Ca^{++} when microinjected as per Kanno *et al.* (62). Their results suggest that the stimulus for degranulation is not at the cell surface but rather within the cytosol, perhaps the microtubule-microfilament system I have suggested orchestrates the endocytosis- peristalsis-pore discharge events associated with granule channel activity (3). Evidently, common ions of either the intra or extracellular *milieux* are incompatible with granule integrity; they *must* be eliminated if degranulation is to be eschewed. I have speculated elsewhere (3,5,8) on how this may be achieved, but it is worth re-emphasizing that normal mast cell function is probably unrelated to and independent of degranulation by polycationic substances or by IgE.

By contrast with mast cells, when other cells having specific granules (e.g., neutrophilic or eosinophilic leucocytes, Paneth cells) phagocytize particulate substances, the ingested material remains sequestered within endocytic vacuoles to which lysosomes are transported individually and into which they discharge their contents thereby losing their integrity; there is apparently no transfer of endocytized material to the specific secretory granules (63,64).

But polyanionic macromolecules, e.g., polyglutamic or polyaspartic acids, do not elicit fusion of mast cell granules *in vivo* though much basic protein is present within the granules to cross-link with the polyanion (13). Even the heparin present in the granules fails to act analogously to polylysine and to fuse neighboring granules to each other by virtue of their basic protein contents. Perhaps the heparin precludes binding of granule cationic proteins with the perigranular membrane which is anionic. Eosinophil granules are not linked to each other; they flow freely and independently during leukopedesis. This may be why they do not fuse when exposed to polyelectrolytes. This suggests that the connections between the mast cell granules within each set may be putative, i.e., not necessarily patent at all times, and that they may open in response to polycations. I have theorized on the role of endocellular polycations elsewhere (3,5).

Thus the postulated pores on the mast cell surface evidently endow mast cells with special reactivity toward polycations, and the manner in which the granules are disposed in sets within the cells leads to an explosive chain reaction of swelling and histamine release once pore integrity has been violated.

E. Protective Mechanisms

It seems probable that the same mechanism underlies the response to all polycations. At first blush, this is not consonant with the phenomenon of tachyphylaxis in which partial degranulation and amine release in response to one dose of releaser precludes further release by a second dose of that same releaser or of a closely related one (65,66). Furthermore, the pK of the releaser does not invariably parallel releasing ability. Thus the cationic complement components *C3a* (pK > 9.5) and *C5a* (pK ∼8.5) both cause mast cell degranulation, but the latter is more effective despite its lower pK (67).

Tachyphylaxis, or desensitization, of mast cells would appear to be a protective mechanism that can prevent the degranulation of mast cells. Indeed, Morrison has found (personal communication) that exposure to doses of drug that do not yield detectable amine release in a very sensitive assay are nevertheless effective in blocking the response to a subsequent substantial dose of that same activator. It seems most probably that conditions that engender tachyphylaxis *in vitro* normally predominate for many substances *in vivo*. In fact, tachyphylaxis has been demonstrated for IgE as well as for degranulating complement factors, and thus it must be viewed as having *in vivo* significance.

This raises an interesting question of clinical import. Many substances cause histamine shock either by allergic or other mechanisms. Antibiotics, sulfa drugs, and x-ray visualization media are notorious examples. Could an injection of a minute amount of the drug a few minutes prior to the bulk of the dose preclude morbidity or mortality? This practice deserves examination.

A second protective mechanism may also operate *in vivo*. It has been shown by Morrison *et al.* (66) that small concentrations of albumin ($\sim$ 0.5%) inhibit amine release elicited by some activators, an inhibition the authors ascribe to interaction with the cell surface rather than with the activator. This effect was demonstrated with *C3* but not with exogenous releasers (Cpd 48/80, Polymyxin B). Inasmuch as tissue fluids contain about 0.5-1% albumin, it seems likely that it prevents degranulation of mast cells *in vivo* when the stimulus is applied at a slow rate. Interestingly, albumin does not interfere with tachyphylaxis (Morrison, personal communication).

Thus the spectacular massive amine release that commands attention may only be induced when there is an overwhelmingly rapid rise in the concentration of a new factor sufficiently unrelated to those the organism is exposed to on an ongoing basis.

These two protective mechanisms might be expected to synergize in protecting mast cells from endogenous cations and possibly noncationic degranulation as well. The presence of such antidegranulation mechanisms supports the idea that mast cell function and degranulation are mutually exclusive.

V. THE MAST CELL

A. Chemical Considerations

Mast cell granules are remarkable. They contain enormous quantities of heparin, protease(s), amine(s), and zinc. An

N-acetyl-β-glucosaminidase, chemotactic peptides, and at least two undefined basic proteins are also present. Experimental data indicate that these substances exhibit no significant turnover in the absence of cellular damage or degranulation.

The function of these various components has yet to be defined, as do their interaction(s). Does the heparin, which in its native state may contain a peptide core, serve as a substrate for the chymotrypsin? That seems unlikely if that core contains only serine and glycine. Why does the chymotrypsin not digest the glucoaminidase? Or itself, for that matter? There are beta linkages in heparin; does the glycosidase act on any of them? Are there endoglycosidases in normal mast cells, as there are (68) in neoplastic ones?

The chemical organization of mast cell granules remains unresolved, particularly as pertains to the role of heparin. It is generally assumed that, because of its strongly acidic groups, it is the heparin that binds the granular amine(s). Yet, Uvnäs and his group (69, see also this volume) have convincingly argued that the amines are bound to protein. Kerp (70) has examined the role of zinc in altering the stoichiometry of heparin-histamine complexing. Would zinc similarly affect the stoichiometry of protein-histamine or heparin-protein complexing?

These studies obviously suffer from oversimplification and ought to be complemented by others that approximate more closely the many possible interactions *in situ*. Specifically *reconstituted granule* models ought to be examined, in which all the various known granular components or their analogs are present at concentrations reflecting the *in vivo* conditions, i.e., in extremely concentrated solutions (or near-solid state?). Data on the complexing of amine or metal ion in relation to the conformation of macromolecules in such reconstituted systems would be of greater interest.

B. Biophysical Consideration

In vitro biophysical studies re conformation of heparin-protein complexes, even in the most simplified systems, must have direct pertinence to the morphological appearance of mast cell granules in cytological preparations. For instance, histamine release is generally accompanied by granular swelling - some 30-fold by volume (about 3-fold increase in diameter of granules). Even air-dried, methanol-fixed granules can swell upon exposure to water, and then precipitously shrink back to their original volume if cations are added (71). Could this involve conformational changes in the heparin-protein complex from random coil to helix?

Could optical rotatory dispersion, laser scattering, and other sophisticated biophysical methods be adapted to single cells viewed through the microscope? Such studies might yield interesting data re macromolecular conformation of native components in swollen versus nonswollen or recondensed granules.

From the standpoint of this Symposium, it would therefore appear that heparin chemists and biophysicists might profitably redirect some of their investigations to include conditions more analogous to those that exist within the mast cell granule. For instance, in studies of ionic interactions with heparin, zinc is conspicuously absent despite its very large concentration in mast cells. Also, the concentrations of constituents within the granules are so great as to suggest solid-state interactions; such have not been studied in model system, save perhaps for x-ray diffraction studies. Furthermore, the conformation of the heparin complex within the granule appears critical from a morphological point of view; this should be amenable to study *in vitro*. And in view of the data reported by Yurt (72), and Silbert (this symposium), a greater emphasis on native macromolecular heparin is indicated.

C. Functional Considerations

I have hypothesized elsewhere (3,5) that mast cell granules interact with components of the modified extracellular fluid that the cell takes up and percolates over them. The chymotrypsin, and possibly the N-acetyl-β-D-glucosaminidase, are present not only in surprisingly high concentrations, but in active form. Is there so much percolate, and is transit time so short, that only high concentrations of enzyme can adequately perform whatever enzymatic modification(s) of it are required?

The granules, in any one mast cell, are evenly spaced from each other, and all are of virtually the same size, though that size can vary from cell to cell (5). Studies on ingestion of colloidal thorium dioxide revealed that the tracer could be restricted to the granule surface, could be embedded within the granule substance, or could be disposed in narrow veins meandering across the granular matrix (7,10). These observations are readily explained if one entertains that granular substance is plastic, that the granules are indeed held in sets within membrane-limited channels, sausage link-fashion, and that a peristaltic process sweeps back and forth over these channels, driving fluid over them and occasionally kneading the granules in the process. In presumably analogous systems, i.e., the rabbit uterus and colon, perstaltic waves distribute the luminal contents (several ova, or fecal pellets, respectively) equidistantly from each other.

Additionally, the kneading action of the rabbit gut molds the fecal material into pellets of remarkably uniform size and shape. The forces involved, and the physics of peristalsis, are no doubt responsible for the spacing and, where applicable, the sizing and shaping of the material within the lumen. It seems likely that the same mechanisms operate to size, shape, and space mast cell granules by microperistalsis at the intracellular level.

I have discussed elsewhere in some detail both the hypothetical function(s) of mast cells and the roles the various granular constituents might play in the process (3,5). Briefly, two lines of reasoning appear most attractive, and may even be interrelated. One proposal is that mast cells take up extracellular components, such as IgE, other immune globulins, or perhaps other substances, that they percolate these over their granules which effect some enzymic modification, and that they then return the altered material to the extracellular compartment. For instance, mast cells might function to destroy IgE or to liberate some fragment of Ag-Ab complexes that might have *informational* value to other cells of the immune system. The second proposal is that the granules act as binding sites for some component(s) of the percolate (antigens or antibody-antigen complexes?), and that they retain those *on file* on a long-term basis for some as yet undefined purpose.

These two hypotheses are not mutually exclusive. Indeed, whereas chymotrypsin is a peptide it can also function in transpeptidation, and similarly whereas N-acetyl-β-D-glucosaminidase is a saccharide-splitting enzyme it can also function in transglycosylation. Generally, transglycosylases will effect the transfer of only one monosaccharide at a time but some, particularly endoglycosidases, can transfer blocks of 10-12 monosaccharides at one time, as a rule to a protein. For the most part, the glycosyl transferases are extremely specific, and it seems unlikely that heparin would itself be a substrate for the granular glycosidase -- sulfatase and sulfamidase action would first be required. It therefore seems more likely that the granular enzyme might act on some exogenous substrate. Could IgE be covalently bound via its carbohydrate component?

In very broad terms, one might wonder whether mast cell granules might transfer to their matrix some fragment(s) of IgE for long-term retention, fragments that might even retain the ability to bind their specific antigens, as IgE does when bound to the plasmalemma via its Fc moiety. Such a scheme would endow the granules with the properties of an affinity chromatography resin. Alternatively, internalization and binding of the Ag-Ab complex, performed at the cell surface, may occur; current evidence favors this latter possibility.

Or, mast cells could transfer some hapten fragment to antigens before releasing them again, and so enhance their antigenicity. Could mast cells transfer ECF-A to antigens and thereby render them chemotactic for eosinophils?

Cytophilic antibodies are normally widely distributed on the surface of lymphocytes but, upon complexing with antigen, capping occurs and the complex is then interiorized (73). Capping has been shown to occur in mast cells also (74). This does not seem in harmony with proposals that view localized degranulation as a response to IgE-antigen complexing. If Ag complexing is a prerequisite to endocytosis, then binding of the Ag-Ab complex (or part of it) to the granules would occur in preference to uncomplexed IgE, but this would not materially affect my hypotheses. As already suggested, capping and endocytosis would occur as antigen *slowly* attached to the mast cell surface, whereas degranulation would occur when Ag-Ab complexing outpaces the rate of capping and interiorization. Experimental conditions in this field of research are intentionally set with degranulation and amine release as conveniently operational end points, and this may be very misleading.

The hypothetical concepts advanced above may admittedly turn out to have no basis in fact. Should that be the case, I would not view it as a set-back, because my purpose here is not so much to come up with definitive answers as it is to open us to more imaginative approaches. There must be more to mast cells than currently accepted dogma.

VI. HEPARIN AND MAST CELL GRANULES

This being an international symposium on heparin, it is appropriate to focus on the role that heparin might play as a granular constituent.

Pertinent to that question are several others, namely: *1*-how is heparin distributed within the mast cell? *2*-what are the characteristics of mast cell heparin? *3*-how does heparin arise in mast cells? *4*-do mast cells secrete heparin? and *5*-why do mast cells elaborate heparin?

A. Distribution of Heparin in Mast Cells

Inasmuch as heparin is the substance that imparts metachromasia to mast cell granules, it is evident that it is located within the granular matrix. There have been recurrent reports in the literature that some metachromasia could also be seen in the intergranular ground cytoplasm. This could represent either artifactitious diffusion or heparin as a result of, for instance, inadequate fixation, subsequent treatment including type of stain formulation, or species involved.

The granules, in some species, are water soluble, by which is meant that the metachromatic substance diffuses readily away upon death of the cell. Some fixatives, e.g., formaldehyde, are very ineffective for retaining granular substance when used in aqueous solution, and must be incorporated in formulations that contain some organic solvent (about 30% by volume) such as ethanol or a glycol. Glutaraldehyde is far more satisfactory for aqueous solutions, but it tends to reduce subsequent stainability. Even if alcoholic formaldehyde is used, *fixation* can be incomplete and subsequent transfer to aqueous solutions, e.g., during rinsing or dehydration will allow partial to complete dissolution of the granules (depending on species involved). Water solubility is not all or none: fixation may be adequate when preparations are stained after only 30 minutes, and yet after 2-3 days' fixing time mast cells may be undemonstrable altogether. Alkaline reagents are particularly effective in solubilizing granular matrix, and will do so even with mast cells of the rat which are water insoluble (at least as far as metachromatic substances is concerned). So do moderate concentrations of inorganic salts.

These statements refer to normal mast cells rather than to mastocytoma cells. In the latter (P-815 mouse mastocytoma, Dunn-Potter-derived lines), granule size varies enormously, from 1-2 micra down to a size well below the resolving power of the light microscope. As a result, many mastocytoma cells show *intergranular* metachromasia, and some display a metachromatic hue throughout their cytoplasm in which no granules are apparent at the light microscopic level (17). Mastocytomas, even when descended from a particular source, have become increasingly heterogeneous as they have evolved along different paths in various laboratories. Comparison of data published at different times and/or in different places can be risky. It is of interest, however, that mastocytomas secrete chondroitin sulfate rather than heparin, and that some do not display granules even at the electron microscope level (75).

B. Mast Cell Heparin(s)

1. *Nature of Mast Cell Heparin(s)*

This symposium seems hardly the place where I, a morphologist cell biologist, should expound on the properties of mast cell heparin. One does not carry coals to Newcastle! However, it may still be worthwhile to present a morphologist's viewpoint, as it complements those of the chemists and pharmacologists who are enlightening me so here. Enormous pains are being taken to purify heparins to their utmost, as must obviously be done for the purposes at hand. From where I stand, however, this can at best result in pristine artifacts that do not exist as such in mast cells! Extrapolation back to live, functioning mast cells thus presents many risks, which acts as leveler for us all; if I jump to false conclusions, I am likely to be in good company! The question, *What is heparin?* is no less pertinent to the cytologist-cell biologist than it is to the biochemist and physiologist. It seems equally pertinent to ask the converse, namely what heparin is not. Both questions have meaning primarily in terms of how they relate to the material(s) as it (they) occur(s) *in situ* within mast cells, i.e., *native* heparin.

L.B. Jaques, to whom this symposium is dedicated, has raised such questions himself (76) with respect to the chemist's or physiologist's heparin; he focused on four meanings of *heparin*. He did not furnish any answer, but merely warned us to watch our language! Good advice, that: We ought to heed it for *native heparin* as well, especially since the metachromatic substance of mast cell granules may differ significantly from species to species.

I need not emphasize to this audience that the chemist's heparin is not a single substance, but rather a family of compounds showing overlapping spectra of structural features and properties not yet fully characterized. The heterogeneity involved is dizzying, as shown for a small area of the problem by our Conference organizer (77, McDuffie, this Symposium), among others (78).

There are macromolecular heparins (79, and this monograph, 80), which are apparently polyheparins held together by a polypeptide core structure (68,72, Silbert, this monograph), from which cleavage can be effected nonenzymatically by ascorbate, or enzymatically by heparin depolymerase (81). Heparins occur in various molecular weights and differ widely in anticlotting potency or other properties, and this cannot be ascribed solely to methods of purification. Commercial (low molecular weight) heparins release lipoprotein lipase efficiently from tissues, but macromolecular heparins inhibit this activity (81,82, see also this monograph). The chemical constituents of heparins vary quantitatively from species to species; even in a given species, different heparins are found in different tissues (81). Lindahl *et al.* (68) have recently stated that the structural properties of heparin "... are now *reasonably* well established" (emphasis added). They underscore that "...heparin is not a homogeneous compound but rather a group of polymers within an extremely heterogeneous family of polysaccharides," part of a spectrum that includes the heparan sulfates. In light of such findings,

I find it baffling that one could infer that the heparin detectable in blood (83) is derived from mast cells when in fact the identity between blood and mast cell heparins has not been established. It seems to me that the presence of extracellular heparin *can not* at this time be taken to mean that it originates from mast cells or, conversely, that mast cells secrete the heparin they synthesize.

On the other hand, Yurt and co-workers (72) have extracted heparin from isolated rat mast cells by procedures much milder than those used for commercial preparations. They report that a single molecular species is present, although in varying degrees of polymerization. The commercial process is extremely crude. Tissues such as intestinal mucosa shipped in large unrefrigerated tank cars, often cross country under nonsterile conditions, are then extracted and digested extensively before isolation of the *pure* product. It is clear that the starting material contains a host of polysaccharides, many closely related, and that tissue and bacterial enzymes have ample opportunity to alter whatever native heparin is present. From a clinical standpoint, this presents problems in standardization of the product, but these have been manageable as evident from the wide and safe use of heparin *in vivo*. From a biological viewpoint, however, the shortcomings are far more telling. It is becoming increasingly difficult to extrapolate with confidence from the commercial *Gemisch* to material that must be present in the cell.

Mast cells take up radiosulfate avidly upon intravenous injection (84,85,86), a fact that might suggest a rapid turnover. The mature granules seem to become heavily labeled within a matter of hours. They retain that radioactivity for very long periods (86), which paradoxically argues for a slow turnover. These findings are difficult to interpret, however, because the sulfate pools in bone, cartilage, and ground substance so dwarf the one in mast cells, that they could easily replenish any losses incurred by the mast cells and thus mask any turnover *in vivo*. That swamping of the mast cells by exogenous sulfate pools is not the entire story is evident from the fact their SO_4 half-life is not the same for all body sites (87); this is countered, however, by the fact that uptake of $^{35}SO_4$ is avid and rapid in sites that have the long half-life. Also, ^{35}S heparin is an unstable variant that might turn over much faster than normal heparin (88).

In the face of these paradoxical findings, Lagunoff (89) proposed that mast cell heparin is a structural component of the granules rather than a secretory product. Barring new evidence, this still seems as good a proposal as any, particularly since the presence of serine and glycine in heparin suggests it may normally be bound covalently to protein(s). This is rarely emphasized by mast cell researchers, who commonly assume that polyanionic heparin simply binds electrostatically to cationic granular protein(s) the way it binds, for instance, to protamine. Both types of linkage are apparently present.

The heparin of rat mast cells has been found to be of the macromolecular type (81,72, Silbert, this symposium). Heparin depolymerases that cleave macromolecular heparins into low molecular weight fragments are present in gut and other tissues (81), but such an enzyme has yet to be reported as present within rat mast cells. Horner has suggested that whether or not a species is prone to thrombotic disorders or atherosclerosis may depend on whether its mast cells contain heparin depolymerase; he suggests that macromolecular heparin is synthesized first, and that it is cleaved into smaller heparin fragments as a prelude to secretion (81), the secreted low molecular weight heparin then affecting lipid metabolism by activating lipoprotein lipase. If so, rat mast cells should certainly possess such depolymerase activity, as this species is notoriously refractory to experimental atherosclerosis. In parallel with my suggestion (3,5), re: mast cell chymotrypsin and N-acetyl-α-D-glucosaminidase, it may be worthwhile to examine whether heparin depolymerases might also function as transheparinases or as endoglycosidases.

It is of interest that highly purified heparin still retains glycine and serine after extensive proteolytic treatment. Serine is commonly a site of attachment of carbohydrate to proteins, and it has been suggested that a polypeptide of serine and glycine is the core structure of macromolecular heparin (68). This would be of special interest in terms of the possibility I have raised, viz., that the chymotrypsin of mast cell granules might perform in transpeptidation, as these peptides might furnish the necessary substrate. This could be a mechanism for transferring portions of IgE (the antigen specific variable region?), for instance, to granular heparin.

One may also speculate regarding ECF-A, the eosinophil chemotactic factor that is present in mast cell granules (90). That *factor* is an equimolar mixture of two tetrapeptides, namely *Ala*. *Gly*. *Ser*. *Glu*. and *Val*. *Gly*. *Ser*. *Glu*. The glycine and serine in heparin apparently alternate in the core peptide and one wonders whether *Gly*. *Ser*. dipeptides might somehow be contributed toward the formation of ECF-A in the course of the transpeptidation mechanisms I have speculated about. Or could ECF-A contribute to formation of the core peptide instead? Chymotrypsin, as a peptidase, has special affinity for valyl, and to some extent also alanyl peptides. Is there any significance to the fact that these very two amono acids are components of the ECF-A peptide? Could this also pertain to transpeptidase activity?

Caution is advised when extrapolating from mastocytoma to normal mast cells. Indeed, P-815 mastocytoma cells in tissue culture secrete their amines and heparin into the medium directly, the cellular heparin having a half-life of 2-3 days, whereas for the same cells *in vivo* it is appreciably longer. In normal mast cells, on the other hand, the half-life appears to be measured in weeks. Similarly, mastocytoma cells release histamine apace in tissue culture; sporadic episodes of flushing can occur in mastocytosis (urticaria pigmentosa) patients, but there is no evidence for histamine turnover in mast cells of intact rats (10).

Intuitively, principles of conservation would lead one to expect normal cells to be very similar to their tumor counterparts. This may be fallacious for mast cells: some mastocytoma lines have lost one synthetic ability or another, some produce a mixture of very disparate mucopolysaccharides, and some have even lost the ability to elaborate storage granules altogether (75). If an intestinal epithelium cell nucleus can be made to initiate embryogenesis when introduced into an enucleated frog's egg it seems clear that all cells have enormous potentialities, but it seems equally clear that what they could do and what they actually do may be very different things. Mastocytoma cells and normal mast cells may exhibit more differences than similarities.

Thus mastocytoma cells can tell us what might be biochemically or physiologically feasible, not necessarily what is probable for normal mast cells.

2. *Heparin(s) and Mast Cell Staining*

Mast cells stain metachromatically with basic (cationic) dyes such as Toluidine Blue or Safranin. It is important to stress that this type of staining reaction involves a *single* dye. All too often, reports in which blood stains have been used (e.g., Wright-Giemsa) mention metachromasia as evidence that mast cells are identified. Whereas indeed mast cell metachromasia is certainly present in those instances, the fact these stains are mixtures of basic and acid (anionic) dyes so complicates the matter as to render references to metachromasia meaningless, because, for instance, a mixture of red and blue dye cannot be distinguished from the metachromatic shift in a blue dye alone, especially to the naked eye.

Metachromasia, in its true sense, derives from extensive binding of dye cations to the closely spaced anions of heparin, and the resultant ability of correspondingly closely spaced bound dye molecules to interact with each other through the intermediary of intercalated water molecules. Depending on pH, carboxyl, phosphate, and sulfate groups all can bind the dye, and thus the amount of dye bound -- and the consequent metachromasia -- can be elicited with many if not most tissue components merely by raising the pH of the dye solution. Other factors, namely electrolytes and nonpolar solvents also affect metachromasia. It follows that details of staining procedures used to stain mast cells must be given in appropriate detail when reported in the literature. All too often, the matter is simply dismissed by the cursory statement ...*mast cells were stained with toluidine blue*.

Other basic dyes also deserve special mention, including Alcian Blue, Astra Blue, Safranin, and Astraphloxine.

Mast cells also stain well with Alcian Blue, a cationic copper phthalocyanine dye, down to pH 1.0. This dye can stain polysaccharides in general, including some nonsulfated ones (91), and thus it is able to bind to carboxyl groups. Alcian Blue does not stain metachromatically.

Astra Blue is another excellent dye for staining mast cells (92). It has not gained the popularity it deserves. This basic dye (erroneously reported in many published reports to be a copper phthalocyanine) binds very selectively to mast cell granules at pH 0.5 to 1.0, and at that pH binds to sulfate (and sulfamate?) groups. It does not stain metachromatically.

Astraphloxine is yet another basic dye (red) that stains mast cells readily at low pH (8). It does not appear to yield metachromasia. It has not gained general use.

These various dyes can bind to carboxyl, sulfate, or sulfamate radicals as a function of pH. This is tricky business, though, for artifacts can occur rapidly as slides are processed through subsequent rinsing and dehydration steps, unless the appropriate pH is maintained by addition of acetic or hydrochloric acid to all the reagents that follow the staining step or other precautions taken (91).

Basic dyes can be used singly to stain mast cells, and those that yield a metachromatic shift at low pH and defined conditions lend additional aid in identifying mast cells. They can also be used in combination to yield additional data. Several sequential procedures have been proposed in the literature, one developed by Spicer *et al*. (93) currently being the most popular. I have used a mixture of two dyes as a single dye bath with much advantage (3). Both approaches reveal that mast cells are heterogeneous.

The Spicer procedure is a useful two-dyes sequence of Alcian Blue followed by Safranin. In this method, Alcian Blue staining reveals the more highly sulfated heparins (94).

I have been working with a method that allows two dyes to compete for heparin binding sites simultaneously in a single dye mixture rather than sequentially as in the Spicer method. The two dyes, already mentioned above, are Astra Blue and Astraphloxine, and they are dissolved in a complex mixture of salts, organic solvents, and other reagents that can simultaneously act as fixative. By that method, individual mast cells in a population stain variously blue, purple, or red, this spectrum resulting from varying ratios of blue to red-staining granules (3); nonmast cells are virtually unstained.

Both the Spicer method and the single-step Astra Blue-Astraphloxine method make it clear that normal mast cells may indeed contain more than a single species of heparin, and that what can be extracted from them might be a heterogeneous mixture of closely related substances. The heterogeneity in staining could derive from differences in binding constants between the two dyes and various anionic groups of heparin (carboxyl, O-sulfate, N-sulfate). On the other hand, it might depend on differential extraction by the dye solution, or on the molecular weight of the polysaccharide being stained. There are precedents for the latter thought. For instance, the Methyl Green-Pyronin method similarly consists of two basic dyes in a mixture, the one dye binding to high molecular weight DNA, the other to lower molecular weight RNA. Also, starch-iodine complexes can appear blue or red depending on the molecular weight of the polysaccharide. Could there be two (families of) heparins in mast cells, one of low molecular weight, the other macromolecular, each binding a different dye from the mixture? Curiously, if mice are killed and peritoneal fluid samples secured after a delay of 30-45 minutes at room temperature for staining by the Astra Blue-Astraphloxine procedure, all of the mast cells take on a red coloration. Do *post mortem* changes occur in mast cell heparin? Horner (81) has reported that macromolecular heparin might be depolymerized rapidly *post mortem*.

These thoughts prompted me to examine the staining of *artificial granules*, in a model system consisting of substances deposited on filter paper (Whatman #50). The substances, all dissolved in distilled water, were commercial heparin (CH), macromolecular heparin (MMH, from rat skin, courtesy, Dr. A.A. Horner), α-chymotrypsin (bovine pancreas, Worthington Biochemicals), and zinc acetate. Various combinations of these substances were also examined. The paper strips were stained, as if they were histological slides, with Toluidine Blue, Astra Blue or Astra Blue-Astraphloxine.

In these experiments zinc did not stain in any instance. Chymotrypsin yielded a very faint spot after staining with Astra Blue, but not after toluidine Blue. All spots containing either CH or MMH stained metachromatically with

Toluidine Blue, sky blue with Astra Blue, or purplish with the Astra Blue-Astraphloxine combination. The addition of zinc and then chymotrypsin to spots of either CH or MMH tended to shift the staining with Toluidine Blue toward a somewhat less metachromatic hue (from purplish red to bluish). There was no noticeable effect with the other two stains. Presumably, zinc and chymotrypsin bind to heparin and might be expected to interfere with dye binding. Whatever the explanation, there was very little interference in the model system. Thus a first attempt to see if the molecular weight of the heparin affects staining properties failed to support my postulate, but one must emphasize that negative data are generally meaningless in cytochemistry. It should also be noted that in the model system, the test substances could at best bind electrostatically rather than covalently, and thus that they may have been dissociated and/or dissolved by the dye solutions all of which contained salts, acids, and water.

Against that background, the data of Yurt *et al*. (72, see also Silbert, this volume) are of particular interest in that these authors report finding a single species of heparin in rat peritoneal mast cells subjected to very mild extraction procedures. Further experiments will be needed to determine the reason for this apparent discrepancy - whether their methodology lacks sufficient sensitivity (unlikely), whether the molecular weight of the proteoglycan is indeed determining, whether bound material that compete with the dye(s) is present, or conceivably whether some other factor is involved. On the other hand, measurements of fluorescence decay of rat mast cells stained with Acridine Orange led West *et al*. (95) to conclude that two different polysaccharides are present in the granules, as also suggested by the Alcian Blue-Safranin and the Astra Blue-Astraphloxine methods. This strongly suggests that the biochemical analytical data may represent an average of the two components. Could Silbert's speculations (this volume) be somewhat premature?

Incidentally, staining procedures, of themselves, can sometimes lead to the degranulation of mast cells even when the cells are dead. Indeed, when air-dried, methanol-fixed preparations of rat peritoneal fluid are exposed to water, mast cell granules swell considerably and displace each other in the process. Subsequent exposure to cations, including basic dyes, causes a rapid shrinkage of the granules, and they are retracted back toward the center of the cell mass rather than shrink in place where they have become dislocated during swelling; as this occurs, many granules can be left stranded at the periphery of the once swollen mass (71). It is most unlikely that this phenomenon involves any of the biochemical reactions, viz., oxygen consumption, cyclic AMP, calcium flux across membranes, etc..., that have been noted during *secretion*/degranulation of live cells, denoting that there are biophysical factors at play. These perhaps include conformational changes (in heparin?) as the granular matrix imbibes water, and again as the cation effects recondensation of that matrix. Of itself, this could not explain the pulling in of peripheral granules back into their original position. One must therefore postulate that some contractile fibrillar system must remain anchored to or associated with the granules; it might be entwined about the membranous channels in which the granules reside (3). Macrophages and eosinophils in the same fixed preparations do not swell and shrink in parallel to the mast cells.

It is clear that the possibility of technique artifacts must be kept in mind when evaluating degranulation. This may be especially true for methods that involve air drying of tissue spreads or of cell suspension.

C. Origin of Mast Cell Heparin(s)

Mature mast cells possess all the organelles needed to synthesize cellular constituents, albeit most of these organelles are poorly developed. Mast cells are not post-mitotic cells, as they incorporate thymidine into their DNA (96,97,17,3) and undergo mitosis (98,99,96,100,1) even when well differentiated. As already mentioned above, more granules accumulate slowly but steadily in mast cells as the animals, and their mast cells, age. This, incidentally, contrasts sharply with the basophilic leukocyte which can neither mitose nor replace its granule.

The presence of amino acids in macromolecular heparin suggests that the cells may synthesize the core peptide first, and that the carbohydrate portion is subsequently added to it in the Golgi apparatus, as has been demonstrated for various glyco and mucoproteins of other cell types. This was already suggested from cytochemical considerations (94). It needs to be reconciled with the biochemical concepts advanced by Silbert elsewhere in this monograph.

Electron microscopic autoradiography after radiosulfate administration suggests that the Golgi apparatus is also where sulfation of the polysaccharide takes place (101). However, the demonstration that mast cell granules not overtly associated with the Golgi continue to mature tinctorially for an extended period of time suggests that the polysaccharide is only partially sulfated in the Golgi (via PAPS), and that some low molecular weight sulfate donor, also made in the Golgi, might then transfer additional sulfate groups to the maturing granules' polysaccharide matrix via transsulfation and/or transsulfamidation. This suggests the possibility of sulfate turnover within the heparin. Such a turnover may occur in heparan sulfate of the nervous system (Margolis, this Symposium), though it would seem at variance with Silbert's conceptions (this monograph). Mast cells evidently differ from cells that secrete their sulfated acid mucopolysaccharide products (e.g., goblet cells) in that in those there is neither sulfate exchange with nor continued sulfation of mature secretory granules (102).

D. Do Mast Cells Secrete Heparin(s)

There is no direct proof at this time either for or against the suggestion that mast cells secrete their heparin. However, indirect evidence supports the view that they do not do so.

Mastocytomas of varying degrees of differentiation occur in man, rodents, cattle, cats, and dogs. Blood coagulability is not generally affected, even when large tumors are present. Neither is clotting time affected in *urticaria pigmentosa* (103).

The data discussed in previous section re the extended lifespan of both mast cells and of their granules, as well as the continuing maturation of these granules, all argue against turnover of granular matrix.

Granular components studied directly, namely histamine and chymotrypsin, do not turn over measurably (3) in the rat. The persistence or radiosulfate labeling also argues against rapid turnover, within the provisos already discussed in a previous section.

Lastly, the amounts of heparin involved in sites other than mast cells (assuming the same heparin is involved!) may be pertinent to the present considerations. It is not fully resolved whether there is any heparin in plasma (83); at best (assuming the same heparin is involved), concentrations are relatively low. So must be the amounts associated with lipoprotein lipase. Were these the total body needs for heparin, the total body mast cell population would most likely excede needs by many orders of magnitude, especially since some of that nonmast cell heparin may be recycled. Engelberg, however, has alluded to some theories of Heilbrun's according to which heparin might play a role in the cytoplasmic sol-gel transformations of all body cells. If this is indeed so, a much larger supply of heparin might be needed. Heilbrun's concepts would need to be re-examined by modern experimental techniques, however; they lack credibility at this time.

E. Why Do Mast Cells Need Heparin(s)?

If heparin is not synthesized *for export*, there ought to be a *raison d'etre* for its presence *in situ*.

Several possible roles for granular heparin have already been mentioned, namely, *1*-to insolubilize the enzymes and other basic proteins of the granules, *2*-to extract (bind) substances from the interstitial fluid mixture percolated over the granules, and *3*-to act as a matrix for covalent attachment of peptide or carbohydrate fragments cleaved from some substance(s) in that percolate.

Other possibilities deserve consideration, among them a possible role of heparin to stimulate, stabilize, and/or inhibit the activity of granular enzymes. Stimulation of enzyme activity has been described for antithrombin. In lipoprotein lipase systems, there may also be a stabilizing (protective) effect on the enzymes, or at least protection against inhibition (104). Inhibition might involve especially the granular chymotrypsin, and might operate to prevent proteolysis of the undefined basic proteins, or self-digestion of the chymotrypsin which, it will be recalled is present in surprisingly high concentration and in enzymatically active form. The *inhibition* I have in mind could derive from trapping the enzyme(s) in a heparin gel, i.e., keeping their molecules physically separated from each other. The gel could allow permeation by smaller molecular weight substrates -- a sort of natural exclusion chromatography perhaps.

Another possible role for heparin might be to bind intracellular cations that play a role in the contractile system(s) involved in milking fluid over the granules (3). Calcium binding by heparin has been studied, and tentatively ascribed to carboxyl rather than sulfate groups (105). Interaction with zinc, which abounds in mast cell granules, does not appear to have been studied by heparin chemists, despite the expected pertinence of this ion to mast cell function.

Heparin has a special affinity for the serine proteases of the coagulation and fibrinolytic systems (106). This suggests that it might be the granular chymotrypsin to which the heparin may be bound in contradistinction to other basic proteins of the granule, and that ECF-A may similarly be bound by virtue of its serine content. Acid polysaccharides are commonly found in association with basic proteins in the secretory granules of many cell types (107). Thus there may be a general principle at work in all storage granules. Complexing of high molecular weight anions (MMH?) with multiple cations of lower molecular weight (the basic proteins and metals) would reduce osmotic pressure, and charge neutralization and would minimize Donnan effects. In that way, heparin could be a most useful constituent to increase the specific activity of the granule per unit volume.

The affinity for serine proteases also suggests the possibility that it is one or more enzyme(s) of the coagulation or fibrinolysis systems that the cell takes up from the extracellular fluid for deactivation by the granules. ECF-A could also be implicated, if it originates from some other cell type, such as macrophages (3).

VII WHEREFORE MAST CELLS?

A. Getting it All Together

This dicussion which complements one published elsewhere (3), has deliberately focused on aspects of mast cell behavior that do *not* involve degranulation. My thesis has been that degranulation is a response to unusual conditions, probably best viewed as pathological. I have argued that normal physiological mast cell function requires the granules to perform *in situ*. Degranulation, in fact, would interrupt mast cell function. Furthermore, I have argued that the ultrastructural organization of mast cells differs significantly from other granule-laden cells, and that this is intimately related to their function(s).

Briefly, and the reader is referred to a complementary discussion (3) for material not covered in this paper, I am proposing that mast cells adsorb material(s) from the intercellular fluid. Likely candidates are complement or derived products, IgE, some component(s) of the clotting cascade, or some self-nonself recognition factor, e.g., tumor antigen, proteoheparans, antitumor antibody, but many other possibilities must obviously be entertained. Currently, I would favor IgE or some undefined gamma globulin involved in self-nonself mechanisms that may be similar to IgE and cross-reactive with it.

As I see it, whatever is preferentially bound to the mast cell surface (by multiple receptors?) is eventually endocytized, and any extracellular fluid simultaneously endocytized in the process is *cleaned up* prior to deposition of the endocytic vacuolar contents onto morphologically and chemically immature granules.

The granules of mast cells, contrary to those in other cell types, do not occur individually as independent entities but rather occur in sets held collectively within extended membranous channels which order the granular matrix material in a polarized manner and impose a unidirectional percolation of the endocytized material(s) over the length of the granules' channels via a subcellular peristaltic mechanism drive and orchestrated by a microtubular-microfilamentous system (3). Interaction between the granules and the percolate are postulated. Altered percolate is thought to then be returned to the extracellular *milieu* through transient pores at the mast cell surface.

The possibility must be entertained that the granule channels conceived for the mast cells represent a persistent and unusually extensive form of the Golgi-Endoplasmic Reticulum-Lysosome (GERL) complex, described by Holtzman *et al.* (108) and further by Novikoff *et al.* (109), in which the final step of severing the individual granules away from the organelle complex does not occur. Some variations in the nature of GERL in various cell types have been entertained recently by Hand and Oliver (110) and would allow for the lack of acid phosphatase activity in mast cell granules.

Likely interactions between granules and percolate are *1*-enzymatic degradation by the granular peptidase(s) and or glycosidase(s), *2*-translocation of some molecular fragment(s) from the percolate to the granular matrix; heparin and/or protein-components could act as acceptors, and *3*-transfer of some molecular fragments to percolate components.

The first possibility might furnish the means to destroy IgE, the function of which is still unknown. If this be the case, it is an inefficient mechanism, as tissue PCA reactivity lasts for some 6 weeks (111,112), and tissue IgE turnover is slow (113). But one might have to differentiate between the ways the cell deals with IgE in its uncomplexed as compared to its complexed state.

The second possibility would transform mast cells into antigen storage units, or specialized memory cells. Were this the case, how to *read the file,* and to what end, would be major questions. Large polymeric anions, e.g., poly AU, can function as adjuvants for immune reactions; it is of particular interest that dextran sulfate, but not dextran itself, is counted among such adjuvants (112). Although administered heparin is not antigenic and normally depresses immune reactivity, the possibility that it might have an adjuvant function *in situ* might be entertained, as might the possibility that *information* might be exchanged between macrophages and mast cells (33) and/or between mast cells and lymphocytes. Further conjectures on these points must await experimental evidence for such an antigen storage function.

B. Epilogue

Mais revenons a nos moutons. Do mast cells secrete their granules? If my arguments have any force, we must answer that query with a resounding *No!*

That being the case, we must begin to explore in earnest what function(s) mast cells might perform in the absence of degranulation. In this essay and elsewhere (3), I have purposefully gone out on a limb in order to force us into broader perspectives. I hope others will join me in sorting out the many hypotheses, conjectures, postulates, and wild guesses I have unabashedly advanced. The challenges are greater and more exciting than ever, as are the potential rewards, both intellectual and practical. Though the frustrations of mast cell research by many -- we have yet to define their function(s) after a full century of at times intensive effort; -- fortunately so are the hopes and promises. I myself have studied the mast cell for some 25 years so far, and I'm hooked on her; she has become my paramour, which may be why I see her as interesting, captivating, useful. I trust these are not merely the self-delusions of a lover, but be they that, I plead with Tennyson that

"T's better to have loved and lost
Than never to have loved at all."

Paramours being what they are, it is tempting to wax lyrical, and I would like to share with the reader a summary I feel does justice to the thrill of our quest:

ODE TO THE MAST CELL

Oh pretty mast cell with granules so bright
You've held your secrets both long and tight.
You've fooled us often, drove us to the wall,
As we searched and researched for your special role.
Your granules, we thought, are secreted apace,
But maybe they aren't and you made us lose face!
You even confuse us as to what lies within,
Whether enzymes, amines, metals, or heparin.
Your role in allergy, so mean and portentous,
May yet be secondary in terms of what you give us.
For if self from nonself is what you tell apart,
You protect us from cancer, bless your little black heart!
And we must grant, Oh Mast Cell, with no further ado,
That you know more about us than we know about you!

REFERENCES

1. Padawer, J., J. Reticuloendoth. Soc. *14*, 462 (1973).
2. Padawer, J., and Gordon, A.S., J. Gerontol. *11*, 268 (1956).
3. Padawer, J., in "Modern Concepts and Developments in Immediate Hypersensitivity" (M.K. Bach, ed.), p. 301. Marcel Dekker, New York, 1978.

4. Yong, L.C., Watkins, S., and Wilhelm, D.L., Pathol. *7*, 307 (1975).
5. Padawer, J., Am. J. Anat. *141*, 299 (1974).
6. Padawer, J., Proc. Soc. Exp. Biol. Med. *129*, 905 (1968).
7. Padawer, J., J. Cell Biol. *40*, 747 (1969).
8. Padawer, J., Lab Invest. *25*, 320 (1971).
9. Padawer, J., and Fruhman, G.J., Experientia *24*, 471 (1968).
10. Padawer, J., Exp. Molec. Path. *20*, 269 (1974).
11. Johnson, A.R., and Moran, N.C., Am. J. Physiol. *216*, 453 (1969).
12. Meyer, S.L., and Saunders, A.M., J. Histochem. Cytochem. *17*, 56 (1969).
13. Padawer, J., J. Cell Biol. *47*, 352 (1970).
14. Lagunoff, D., and Benditt, E.P., Nature *192*, 1198 (1961).
15. Padawer, J., Marsland, D., and Pankove, J.I., Exp. Cell Res. *21*, 316 (1960).
16. Padawer, J., Marsland, D., and Pankove, J.I., Exp. Cell Res. *25*, 65 (1961).
17. Padawer, J., Ann. N.Y. Acad. Sci. *103*, 87 (1963).
18. Padawer, J., and Gordon, A.S., Proc. Soc. Exp. Biol. Med. *88*, 522 (1955).
19. Padawer, J., J. Gerontol. *20*, 515 (1965).
20. Policard, A., Collet, A., and Prégermain, S., Rev. Hématol. *5*, 374 (1960).
21. Higginbotham, R.D., Ann. N.Y. Acad. Sci. *73*, 186 (1958).
22. Higginbotham, R.D., and Dougherty, T.F., R.E.S. Bull. *2*, 72 (1956).
23. Higginbotham, R.D., and Karnella, S., J. Immunol. *106*, 233 (1971).
24. Archer, G.T., Robson, J.E., and Thompson, A.R., Pathol. *9*, 137 (1977).
25. Clark, J.M., J. Reticuloendoth. Soc. *11*, 437 (1975).
26. Fruhman, G.J., Proc. Soc. Exp. Biol. Med. *141*, 101 (1972).
27. Kamiyama, A., and Spicer, S.S., Lab. Invest. *32*, 485 (1975).
28. Sato, S., and Kukita, A., Acta Dermatovener *54*, 113 (1974).
29. Sato, S., Kukita, A., and Sato, S.I., J. Invest. Dermatol. *53*, 183 (1969).
30. Michels, N.A., in "Handbook of Hematology" (H. Downey, ed.) Vol. *1*, p. 232, 1938. Reprinted in Ann. N.Y. Acad. Sci. *103*(1), 1963.
31. Selye, H., "The Mast Cells". Butterworths, Washington, 1965.
32. Fruhman, G.J., J. Reticuloendoth. Soc. *14*, 371 (1973).
33. Simson, J.A.V., and Spicer, S.S., J. Cell Biol. *52*, 536 (1972).
34. Spicer, S.S., Simson, J.A.V., and Farrington, J.E., Am J. Path. *80*, 481 (1975).
35. Garfield, R.E., Chacko, S., and Blose, S., Lab. Invest. *33*, 418 (1975).

36. Fruhman, G.J., J. Reticuloendoth. Soc. *13*, 424 (1973).
37. Fruhman, G.J., and Padawer, J., J. Cell Biol. *43*, 41 (1969).
38. Gallapudi, S.V.S., and Kind, L.S., Int. Arch. Allergy Appl. Immunol. *53*, 395 (1977).
39. Viklický, V., Síma, P., and Pritchard, H., Folia Biol. Praha. *19*, 247 (1973).
40. Burnet, F.M., Persp. Biol. Med. *16*, 1 (1972).
41. Burnet, F.J., "Immunology, Aging and Cancer". Freeman, San Francisco, 1976.
42. Orr, T.S.C., Acta Allergol. Suppl. IX *30*, 13 (1975).
43. Simson, J.A.V., Hintz, D.S., Munster, A.M., and Spicer, S.S., Exp. Molec. Path. *26*, 85 (1977).
44. Mayrhofer, G., in "Ciba Symposium, Immunology of the gut", #46 p. 155. North Holland, New York, 1977.
45. Fruhman, G.J., Anat. Rec. *175*, 502 (1973).
46. Ichikawa, A., J. Cell Biol. *24*, 369 (1965).
47. Esterhuizen, A.C., and Howell, S.L., J. Cell Biol. *46*, 593 (1970).
48. Gabbay, K.H., Korff, J., and Schneeberger, E.E., Science *187*, 177 (1970).
49. Amsterdam, A., Ohad, I., and Schramm, M., J. Cell Biol. *41*, 753 (1969).
50. Hand, A.R., J. Cell Biol. *44*, 340 (1970).
51. Uvnäs, B., in "Mechanisms in Allergy; Reagin- Mediated Hypersensitivity" (L. Goodfriend, A.H. Sehon, and R.P. Orange, eds.), p. 369. Marcel Dekker, New York, 1973.
52. Lagunoff, D., J. Cell Biol. *57*, 252 (1973).
53. Morrison, D.C., Roser, J.F., Cochrane, C.G., and Henson, P.M., J. Immunol. *114*, 966 (1975).
54. Rölich, P., Anderson, P., and Uvnäs, B., J. Cell Biol.. *51*, 465 (1971).
55. Lagunoff, D., Biochem. Pharmacol. *21*, 1889 (1972).
56. Bloom, G.D., Fredholm, B., and Haegermark, Ö., Acta Physiol. Scand. *71*, 270 (1967).
57. Padawer, J., Am. J. Anat. *127*, 159 (1970).
58. Uvnäs, B., Ann. N.Y. Acad. Sci. *103*, 278 (1963).
59. Thon, I.L., and Uvnäs, B., Acta. Physiol. Scand. *71*, 303 (1967).
60. Cochrane, D.E., and Douglas, W., Proc. Natl. Acad. Sci. U.S. *71*, 408 (1974).
61. Kagayama, M., and Douglas, W.W., J. Cell Biol. *62*, 519 (1974).
62. Kanno, T., Cochrane, D.E., and Douglas, W.W., Can. J. Physiol. Pharmacol. *51*, 1001 (1973).
63. Erlandsen, S.L., and Chase, D.G., J. Ultrastruct. Res. *41*, 296 (1972).

64. Erlandsen, S.L., and Chase, D.G., J. Ultrastruct. Res. *41*, 319 (1972).
65. Morrison, D.C., Roser, J.F., Cochrane, C.G., and Henson, P.M., Int. Arch. Allergy Appl. Immunol. *49*, 172 (1974).
66. Morrison, D.C., Henson, P.M., Roser, J.F., and Cochrane, C.G., in "Leukocyte Membrane Determinants Regulating Immune Reactivity" (V.P. Eijsvogel, D. Roos, and W.P. Zeijlemaker, eds.), p. 551. Academic Press, New York, 1976.
67. Johnson, A.R., Hugh, T.E., and Müller-Eberhard, H.J., Immunol. *28*, 1067 (1975).
68. Lindahl, U., Höök, M., Bäckström, G., Jacobsson, I., Riesenfeld, J., Malmström, A., Rodén, L., and Feingold, D.S., Fed. Proc. *36*, 19 (1977).
69. Uvnäs, B., Åborg, C.-H., and Bergendorff, A., Acta. Physiol. Scand. *78*, *Suppl. 336*, 3 (1970).
70. Kerp, L., Int. Arch. Allergy *22*, 112 (1963).
71. Padawer, J., Proc. Soc. Exp. Biol. Med. *120*, 318 (1965).
72. Yurt, R.W., Leid, R.W., Austen, K.F., and Silbert, J.E., J. Biol. Chem. *252*, 518 (1977).
73. Unanue, E.R., Perkins, W.D., and Karnovsky, M.J., J. Exp. Med. *136*, 885 (1972).
74. Pontefract, R., and Perelmutter, L., Acta Allergol. *31*, 184 (1976).
75. Freilich, L.S., Lewis, R.G., Reppucci, Jr., A.C., and Silbert, J.E., J. Cell Biol. *72*, 655 (1977).
76. Jaques, L.B., Adv. Exp. Med. Biol. *52*, 139 (1975).
77. Nader, H.B., McDuffie, N.M., and Dietrich, C.P., Biochem. Biophys. Res. Commun. *57*, 488 (1974).
78. Lasker, S.E., Fed. Proc. *36*, 92 (1977).
79. Horner, A.A., J. Biol. Chem. *246*, 231 (1971).
80. Ögren, S., and Lindahl, U., J. Biol. Chem. *250*, 2690 (1975).
81. Horner, A.A., Fed. Proc. *36*, 35 (1977).
82. Horner, A.A., Proc. Nat. Acad. Sci. *68*, 3469 (1972).
83. Engelberg, H., Fed. Proc. *36*, 70 (1977).
84. Bélanger, L.F., Anat. Rec. *118*, 755 (1954).
85. Curran, R.C., and Kennedy, J.S., J. Path. Bact. *70*, 449 (1955).
86. Jorpes, E., Ödeblad, E., and Boström, H., Acta Haemat. *9*, 273 (1953).
87. Jennings, M.A., Florey, H.W., Robinson, D.S., and Salaman, M.R., Ann. N.Y. Acad. Sci. *103*, 313 (1963).
88. Lloyd, A.G., Balazs, E.A., Emberg, G., and Wusteman, F.S., Biochem. J. *98*, 34 (1966).
89. Lagunoff, D., in "Conference on Mast Cells and Basophils" (J. Padawer, ed.), Ann. N.Y. Acad. Sci., *103(1)*, 446 (1963).
90. Goetzl, E.J., and Austen, K.F., Proc. Natl. Acad. Sci. U.S. *72*, 4123 (1975).

91. Lev, R., and Spicer, S.S., J. Histochem. Cytochem. *12*, 309 (1964).
92. Bloom, G.D., and Kelly, J.W., Histochemie *2*, 48 (1960).
93. Spicer, S.S., Horn, R.G., and Leffi, T.J., in "The Connective Tissue", Internat. Acad. Path. Monogr. #17, p. 251. Williams and Wilkins, Baltimore, 1967.
94. Combs, J.W., Lagunoff, D., and Benditt, E.P., J. Cell Biol. *25*, 577 (1965).
95. West, S.S., Golden, J.F., Menter, J.M., and Love, L.D., J. Histochem. Cytochem. *24*, 59 (1976).
96. Allen, A., Lab. Invest. *11*, 188 (1962).
97. Padawer, J., Angiology *12*, 538 (1961).
98. Allen, A., Anat. Rec. *139*, 13 (1961).
99. Allen, A., J. Nat. Cancer Inst. *28*, 1125 (1962).
100. Bloom, G.D., in "The Inflammatory Process" (B.W. Zweifach, L. Grant, and R.I. McCluskey, eds.), 2nd Ed., *Vol. 1*, p. 545. Academic Press, New York, 1974.
101. Young, R.W., J. Cell Biol. *57*, 175 (1973).
102. Lane, N., Caro, L., Otero-Vilardebo, L.R., and Goodman, G.C., J. Cell Biol. *21*, 339 (1964).
103. Sagher, F., and Even-Paz, Z. (ed.), "Mastocytosis and the Mast Cell", p. 282 (Karger) Phiebig, 1967.
104. Iverius, P.H., Lindahl, U., Egelrud, T., and Olivecrona, T., J. Biol. Chem. *247*, 6610 (1972).
105. Perlin, A.S., Fed. Proc. *36*, 106 (1977).
106. Rosenberg, R.D., Fed. Proc. *36*, 10 (1977).
107. Spicer, S.S., Staley, M.W., Wetzel, M.G., and Wetzel, B.K., J. Histochem. Cytochem. *15*, 225 (1967).
108. Holtzman, E., Novikoff, A.B., and Villaverde, H., J. Cell Biol. *33*, 419 (1967).
109. Novikoff, P.M., Novikoff, A.B., Quintana, N., and Hauw, J.J., J. Cell Biol. *50*, 859 (1971).
110. Hand, A.R., and Oliver, C., J. Cell Biol. *74*, 399 (1977).
111. Humphrey, J.H., and White, R.G. (eds.), "Immunology for Students of Medicine", 2nd Ed. Davis, Phila., 1964.
112. Eisen, H.H. (ed.), "Immunology", Harper and Row, New York, 1974.
113. Tada, T., Okumura, K., Platteau, B., Beckers, A., and Bazin, H., Internat. Arch. Allergy Appl. Immunol. *48*, 116 (1975).

HEPARIN AND ENDOTHELIUM

L.M. Hiebert

Department of Physiology
University of Saskatchewan

The best known pharmacological action of heparin after injection has been its action as an inhibitor of the coagulation system. The interest in this anticoagulant action has masked the other effects that heparin may have in the blood vessel environment, namely on the blood vessel wall. Some of these effects were observed by Dr. Jaques and co-workers in 1934-1935 (1) who noticed that heparin prevented venous thromboembolism after endothelial damage in dogs. Heparin is also known to release the enzyme lipoprotein lipase from endothelium. In addition many medical devices in contact with blood require a heparinized surface for use (2). Srinivasan *et al.* have observed that heparin increases the negative charge across the blood vessel wall (3). Thus there is much concurrent evidence that heparin affects the endothelium after injection.

We have attempted to observe more directly the relationship of exogenous heparin to the endothelium. Aortic endothelium was removed by applying cellulose acetate paper. The cellulose acetate paper was then removed with the endothelial cells sticking to it. The endothelium was extracted from cellulose acetate paper with acetone according to the method of Hiebert and Jaques (4). The endothelial powders were then applied to microelectrophoresis slides according to the methods of Jaques and Wollin (5), and the amount of heparin present was determined.

Figure 1 shows the quantity of heparin on endothelium after *in vitro* application of heparin with variation in several parameters including: minutes of application; concentration of heparin; source of heparin; and source of endothelium. Basal conditions for all experiments, unless otherwise specified, dog aortic and vena caval endothelium, with bovine mucosal heparin applied at 40 units/ml for 15 min. The aorta and/or vena cava was removed and heparin was applied for the given time in Locke's solution to the exposed endothelial surface. The endothelium was rinsed and removed. Heparin was determined as above and is expressed here in units/cm^2 of endothelium. Heparin found with endothelium averaged 140 times that in the bathing solution.

ISBN 0-12-484850-8

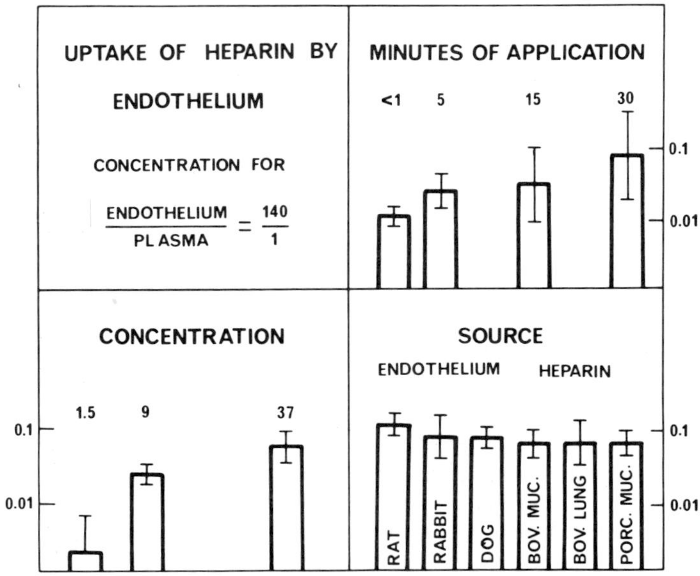

Fig. 1. The quantity of heparin found with endothelium in units/cm^2 after in vitro application when time of application, concentration applied, source of endothelium, and source of heparins are varied.

When time of application was varied (panel A) at <1,5,15 and 30 min the amount of heparin removed from endothelium increased with the minutes of application, although significance was reached only when < 1 min of application was compared with 30 min. When concentration was varied, (panel B) at 1.5, 9,37 units/ml the amount of heparin found on endothelium increased significantly with concentration. When source of endothelium (panel C) was varied between rat, rabbit or dog endothelium, the amount of heparin found with the different endothelium was relatively the same. When heparins from three sources, (panel C) including bovine mucosal (Abbott Labs. Ltd.), bovine lung (Upjohn Co.), and porcine mucosal (Upjohn Co.), were applied, the amount of heparin found with endothelium was similar for all heparins applied. It was also observed that when the endothelial surface previously exposed to heparin was bathed in Locke's solution for 10 min there was no loss of heparin from the endothelium into the bathing solution, and the quantity of heparin found was the same as compared to not bathing in Locke's solution.

Heparin has been observed on endothelium after injection. Figure 2 shows the comparison of heparin concentration in blood and endothelium after intravenous, subcutaneous, and intraperitoneal injection of 1000 units per rat. The limit of detection for heparin on endothelium by the method of Hiebert and Jaques is 50 units/ml. This is due to the quantity (1 to 2 mg) of endothelium that can be obtained from one rat aorta. After intravenous injection of 1000 units (panel A), the amount of heparin found in blood decreases rapidly with time, possibly at 2 different rates. The amount of heparin found with endothelium is expressed as a regression line with standard error of the estimate. Heparin was found on aortic endothelium of all 17 rats. The concentration of heparin found

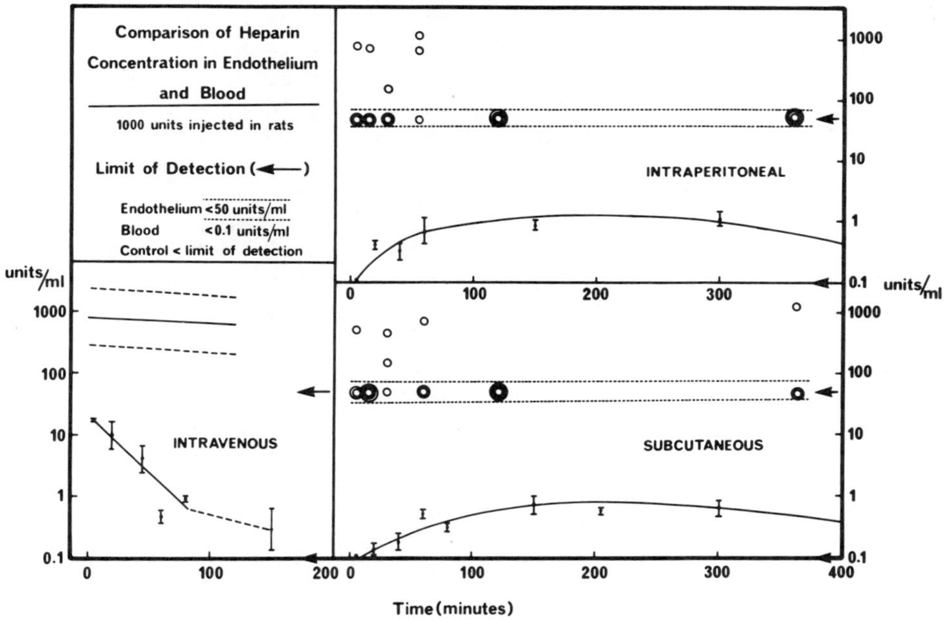

Fig. 2. The quantity of heparin found with endothelium and blood in units/ml at various times after intravenous, intraperioneal, and subcutaneous injection. Heparin in endothelium was determined by the method of Hiebert and Jaques (4). Heparin in blood was determined by the method of Jaques et al. (7).

with endothelium is 100 to 1000 times the concentration in the blood. The amount of endothelial heparin decreases slowly with time in comparison to the decrease in blood concentration. This suggests that the amount of heparin with endothelium is not in equilibrium with that in the blood.

After intraperitoneal injection (panel b), the concentration of heparin in the blood rises slowly and ranges from 0.1 to 1 units/ml when measured up to 400 min after injection. The concentration of heparin on endothelium in some rats is between 100 and 1000 units/ml at 5, 15, 30, and 60 min after injection. Heparin could not be observed on endothelium of other rats at these times and on rats at 2 and 6 hr after injection. It is possible that heparin *is* present on the endothelium but the concentration is below the limit of detection (50 units/ml).

After subcutaneous administration, (panel c) results were similar to those after intraperitoneal injection. The amount of heparin found at 5, 15, 30 and 60 min was variable. Heparin was found on endothelium of one rat at 6 hr after injection and could not be found on many other rats.

It is interesting to observe that heparin can be found on endothelium at 5 and 15 min after intraperitoneal and subcutaneous injection when blood concentrations are very low. It is likely that some heparin immediately leaks into the circulation after injection and becomes attached to endothelium. The wide variation in response, after intraperitoneal and subcutaneous injection, may reflect variation between animals due to variation in distribution from the injection site.

Heparin has been observed on endothelium after intrapulmonary administration. In Table I, is shown heparin detected on endothelium at 15 min after intrapulmonary administration. When 2000 units of cold heparin is administered, plasma levels are from 0.36 to 1.5 units/ml, as measured by the method of Yin and Wessler. Heparin was found on endothelium by the method of Hiebert and Jaques when concentrations were 1 to 15 units/ ml in plasma. When heparin in the plasma was at lower concentrations, heparin was not found and was considered below the limit of detection (50 units/ml). By measuring the radioisotope ^3H at 15 min after administration of 50 units, heparin can be detected on endothelium when heparin levels in the plasma were 0.25 units/ml.

TABLE I. Heparin in Blood and Endothelium 15 min after Intrapulmonary Instillation in Rats

Heparin administered total units	*Heparin in plasma μ/ml*	*Heparin in aortic endothelium μ/cm^3*
	Yin and Wessler	*Hiebert and Jacques*
2000	*0.72*	*50*
	1.5	*1750*
	0.36	*50*
	1	*50*
	Radioisotope ^3H	*Radioisotope ^3H*
50	*0.25*	*20*

Since chondroitin sulfate is similar to heparin in structure, it was attempted to determine if chondroitin C was taken

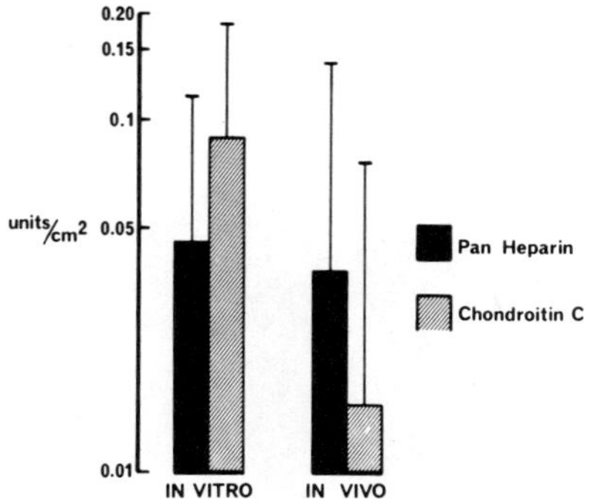

Fig. 3. The quantity of heparin or chondroitin C found with endothelium after in vivo or in vitro administration expressed in units/cm^2.

up on endothelium as well. In Fig. 3 is shown the quantity of heparin and chondroitin sulfate C (Chondroitin sulfate C, Sodium, P-L Biochemicals Inc., Milwaukee, Lot 330361) found with endothelium after *in vivo* and *in vitro* application expressed in units/cm^2. As can be seen the amount of chondroitin C found with endothelium is similar to the amount of heparin found with endothelium after *in vivo* and *in vitro* application. Thus one can conclude that uptake on endothelium is not specific but can occur with other substances.

The presence of heparin on endothelium after application has been observed histologically. We have observed in a previous publication (6) that there is metachromatic staining with toluidine blue around nuclei and on the endothelial cell membrane 10 min after *in vitro* application of 100 units/ml of heparin as compared to blue staining endothelial nuclei with application of Lockes solution alone. Preliminary studies in electron microscopy have shown an increase in the endo-endothlial layer on endothelial cells stained with Ruthenium Red, 5 min after intravenous injection of heparin as compared to controls (4).

These studies have been extended here. In Fig. 4 are shown endothelial cells from four different rats. In Fig. 4(a) is a cell from rat aorta stained with Ruthenium Red at 15 min after intravenous injection. Many dark staining particles can be seen in the abluminal vesicles and below the surface of the cell in the basal lamina. In Fig. 4(b) is a cell from rat aorta at 30 min after intravenous injection. Many dark staining particles are present in the basal lamina, and there is a thick endo-endothelial layer on the cell surface.

In Fig. 4(c) there is a control endothelial cell showing only very few dark staining particles in the basal lamina. It is possible then that these dark staining particles in experimental animals are heparin or are due to the affect of heparin on the endothelial cell.

a

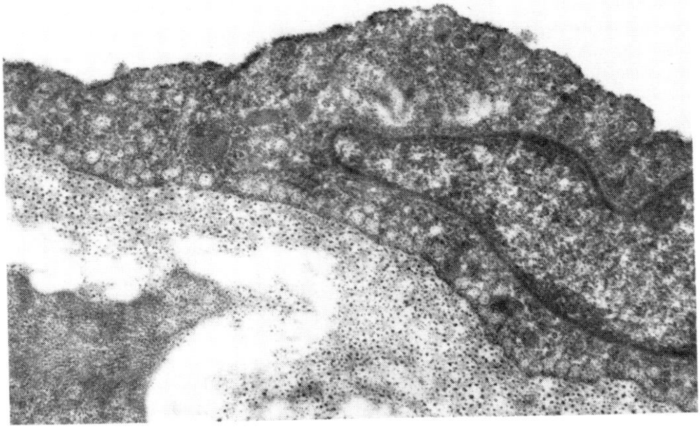

b

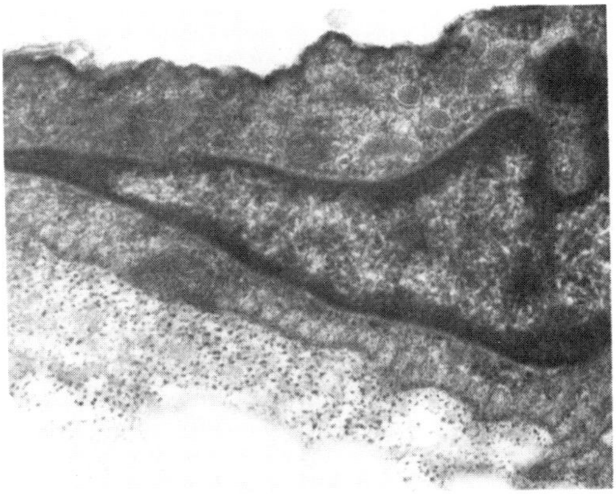

Fig. 4. Endothelial cells of rat aorta stained with Ruthenium Red during fixation, and further stained with uranylacetate and lead citrate. (a) Taken 5 min after intravenous injection of 1000 units of heparin indicating particles in vesicles and in the basal lamina 42,000x. (b) Taken at 30 min after intravenous injection of 1000 units of heparin showing a dense endo-endothelium layer with many particles in the basal lamina 42,000x.

c

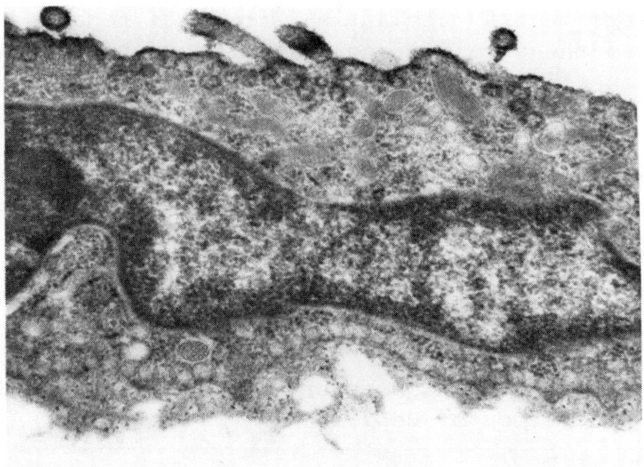

d

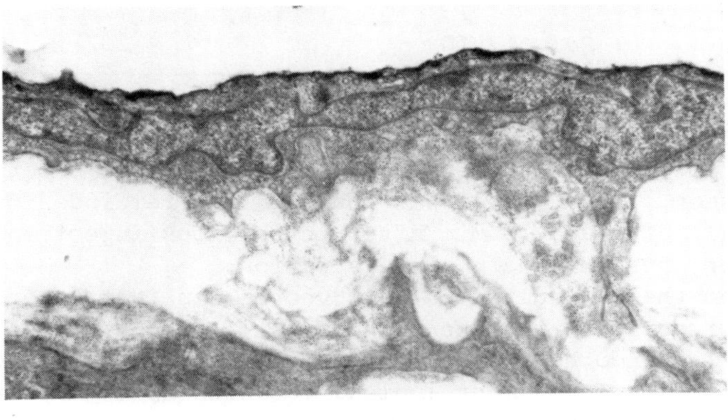

Figure 4 (continued) (c) Endothelium taken from an untreated rat showing few particles in the basal lamina 50,000x. (d) Endothelium 30 min after intraperitoneal injection of heparin showing a dense endo-endothelial layer with some particles in the basal lamina 25,000x.

In Fig. 4(d) are shown endothelial cells at lower magnification taken at 30 min after intraperitoneal injection. Here is shown a thick dark endo-endothelial layer with few dark staining particles below the endothelial surface. One may speculate that a substantial amount of heparin may just have entered the aortic circulation and much heparin is still on the endothelial cell surface.

The difficulty with the present electron microscopic study is the use of Ruthenium Red. Since it can stain many mucosubstances and is not specific for heparin we cannot be certain that all of these dark staining particles are heparin. This is a subject for further study. However we do have other evidence that heparin is passing through the endothelial cell. In Table II is shown the radioactive counts obtained from the aortic wall.

TABLE II. Radioactive Counts on Aorta Stripped of Endothelium after Administration of Heparin ^3H

Heparin Administration			*Cpm/cm^2*
Route	*Time (min)*	*Dose units*	*on aorta*
I.V.	*5*	*50*	*455*
I.V.	*15*	*50*	*174*
I Pul.	*15*	*50*	*207*

after intravenous, or intrapulmonary administration of heparin. After heparin administration, rat aorta was removed and stripped of endothelium by cellulose acetate paper. As can be seen, the ^3H label was found in the remainder of the aorta wall at 5 and 15 min after intravenous injection and 15 min after intrapulmonary administration.

From these results one can hypothesize that heparin when in the circulation is taken up against a concentration gradient on the endothelial surface and then into the vesicles. The vesicles are the most logical location of transport since they are considered the large pore system (8). The heparin then passes by vesicular transport through the endothelial cells to the basal lamina and into the vascular wall.

In summary, it can be concluded that heparin is definitely taken up on endothelium after *in vitro* application and intravenous, intraperitoneal, subcutaneous, and intrapulmonary administration. This uptake occurs at concentration as low as 0.25 units/ml of plasma. The uptake increase with concentration of heparin in blood and can be 100 to 1000 times that concentration observed in blood. This property is not confined to heparin, but has been observed with a similar negative polyelectrolyte Chondroitin C. Heparin may be passed through the endothelial cell via the vesicles into the vessel wall. The endothelium then represents part of the cellular pool, which may act as a site of distribution, metabolism or action of heparin.

ACKNOWLEDGEMENTS

This work was supported by grants from the Saskatchewan Heart Foundation. I am indebted to Robert Goodman and Mark Armanious who provided data for this paper.

REFERENCES

1. Jaques, L.B. "The Action of Heparin in Vivo", Thesis for the Degree of Master of Arts, University of Toronto, May (1935).
2. Gott, V.L. "Heparin Structure, Function and Clinical Implications" (R.A. Bradshaw and S. Wessler, eds.). Adv. Exp. Med. Biol. *52*, 351 (1974).
3. Srinivasan, S., Aaron, R., Chopra, P.S., Lucas, T., and Sawyer, P.M. Surgery *64*, 827 (1968).
4. Hiebert, L.M. and Jaques, L.B. Thromb. Res. *8*, 195 (1976).
5. Jaques, L.B. and Wollin, A. Anal. Biochem. *52*, 219 (1973).
6. Hiebert, L.M. and Jaques, L.B. Artery *2*, 26 (1976).
7. Jaques, L.B., Monkhous F.C. and Stewart, M. J. Physiol. *109*, 41 (1949).
8. Simionescu, N., Simionescu, M., and Palade, G.E., "Atherogensis" (R.A. Gamerini-Davalos, E.L. Dierman, W. Redisch, D.B. and Zilversmit, eds.). Ann. N.Y. Acad. Sci. *275*, 64 (1976).

HYPOTHESIS ON THE PHARMACOLOGICAL ACTION OF SUBCUTANEOUS "LOW-DOSE" OR "SMALL-DOSE" HEPARIN

C. Raby and H. Bertrand

Institut Choay

I. INTRODUCTION

The efficacy of subcutaneous heparin in the prevention of postoperative deep-vein thrombosis and pulmonary embolism has been proven, both for Kakkar's low-dose scheme (3) and for J.G. Sharnoff's small-dose scheme (7,8).

In atheromatous arterial disease (coronary and arteritic cases), long-term intermittent calcium heparinate treatment in small subcutaneous doses produces spectacular functional recovery and remarkable prevention of local and remote rethrombosis following reparative surgery (4).

In these two major indications for small-dose subcutaneous heparin administration, the prevention of thrombosis cannot be attributed only to the medication's anticoagulant effect. After a subcutaneous injection of 5000 to 7000 IU, the presence of heparin in the circulating blood is short-lived and is as brief as the coagulant potential is pathological. It is difficult to explain the observed preventive effect when in 24 hr the patient is far longer unprotected than protected.

An experimental study pointed our way towards a different pharmacological action.

We were drawn to the work of J.D. Whiffen *et al.* (9) who showed that heparin attached to vascular prostheses coated with graphite via benzalkonium chloride, endowed such surfaces with the property of resisting thrombus-formation. The same authors also showed that graphite-benzalkonium surfaces inserted in venae cavae of heparinized dogs associated with circulating heparin.

P.B. Samuel *et al.* (6) showed elsewhere, using toluidine blue as the usual heparin stain, the anticoagulant's affinity for the "cement lines" of vascular endothelium.

More recently, L.B. Jaques and his team (1), using an electrophoretic micro method on agarose and toluidine blue coloring, detected and evaluated heparin that remained associated with venous and arterial endothelium after soaking in various heparinized media followed by rinsing. They found that the amount of heparin taken up increased with the

ISBN 0-12-484850-8

time of contact and heparin concentration in the medium and was unaffected by the source of heparin used (cow, pig, lung, mucosa).

In a new study (2) these authors used the same method of measurement to determine heparin taken up by endothelium after single *in vivo* injections in rats by intravenous, subcutaneous and intraperitoneal routes. The capacity of endothelium to take up heparin regardless of the mode of administration was thus established. In addition, they localized heparin on the cell membrane and in the cytoplasm inside vesicles by electronmicroscopy with ruthenium red staining.

Using sulfur-labelled (^{35}S) heparin, we sought to find the uptake and release capacity of the vessel wall in relation to injected quantity, number, frequency, and type of injection.

II. METHODS AND MATERIALS

Animals

Animals used were Burgundy fawn rabbits weighing from 2500 to 3500 g. Heparin was injected intravenously or subcutaneously depending on the test. Animals were isolated in surveillance areas during experimentation. Aortae and venae cavae were removed after anesthesia by nembutal.

Heparin

Heparin used was supplied by Laboratoire Choay (Calciparine $^{(R)}$), strength 10,000 IU/ml. Amounts injected were expressed in units/kg of weight. Tagged ^{35}S heparin, (N-sulfonate ^{35}S heparin, sodium salt) was furnished by Amersham-Searle, specific activity 32.9 mCi/g. Radioactivity of one unit of heparin was measured before each test.

Preparation of vessels

When called for by the experiment, the aorta and vein were removed from the anesthetized animal and thoroughly rinsed with Locke's solution by syringe under pressure. Vessels were slit open lengthwise, washed in three Locke's baths, spread flat, and measured to estimate area. A venous blood sample was taken simultaneously for a circulating heparin search by specific coagulation test.

Measurement of Radioactivity

Elements were incubated for 3 hr at 60°C in the solvent medium (NCS 0.6 *M* - Amersham-Searle). After cooling to ambient temperature, the scintillant mixture (PPO/POPOP) was added and measuring was performed on a liquid scintillation spectrophotometer (Intertechnique, Type SL30). Noise was deducted after each measurement.

III. EXPERIMENTAL PROCEDURES

Trial Number 1

Three 2.5 kg rabbits were given 400 IU/kg, 1200 IU/kg, and 2000 IU/kg, respectively, in single 1 ml intravenous injections at time 0. Blood samples were taken 30 and 120 min after the injection; heparinemia assessed simultaneously by coagulation tests and radioactivity measurement. The animals were killed and vessels removed 6 hr after the injection.

Results (see Tables I and II) After a single intravenous strong dose of ^{35}S heparin, plasma heparin measured at 30 and 120 min by coagulation test (variable-concentration thrombin time) is very close to that reached in radioactivity measurement (the latter yielding a very slightly lower value). Six hours following injection, there is no more heparin in the circulating blood and the amount retained by arterial and venous walls is small (between 43 and 56 x 10^{-4} IU/cm^2 for the aorta) and independent of the dose injected.

Trial Number 2

Two 1000 IU/kg-injections were administered at 12-hr intervals for three days, *intravenously* in three rabbits and *subcutaneously* in three others. The animals were killed and vessels removed exactly 17 hr after the final injection following verification of the absence of circulating heparin.

Table I Heparinemia IU/ml of Plasma

I.V. heparin IU/kg	30 min		120 min	
	R	C	R	C
400	1.00	1.2	0.45	0.5
1,200	2.35	2.4	0.70	0.8
2,000	3.85	>3.0	1.15	1.3

R = radioactivity, C = coagulation

Table II Heparin in Vessel Walls (10^{-4} IU/cm^2) 6 hr after Single I.V. Injection

I.V. heparin IU/kg	Aorta	Vena Cava
400	56	19
1,200	43	23
2,000	45	28

Results Figure 1 shows mean quantities of heparin retained by arterial walls when injections were subcutaneous (391×10^{-4} IU/cm^2) and intravenous (128×10^{-4} IU/cm^2). Mean values of heparin uptake by veins were, respectively, 214×10^{-4} IU/cm^2 and 110×10^{-4} IU/cm^2. These findings demonstrate the part played by the mode of administration: the subcutaneous route is highly favorable to fixation of heparin to arterial and venous walls.

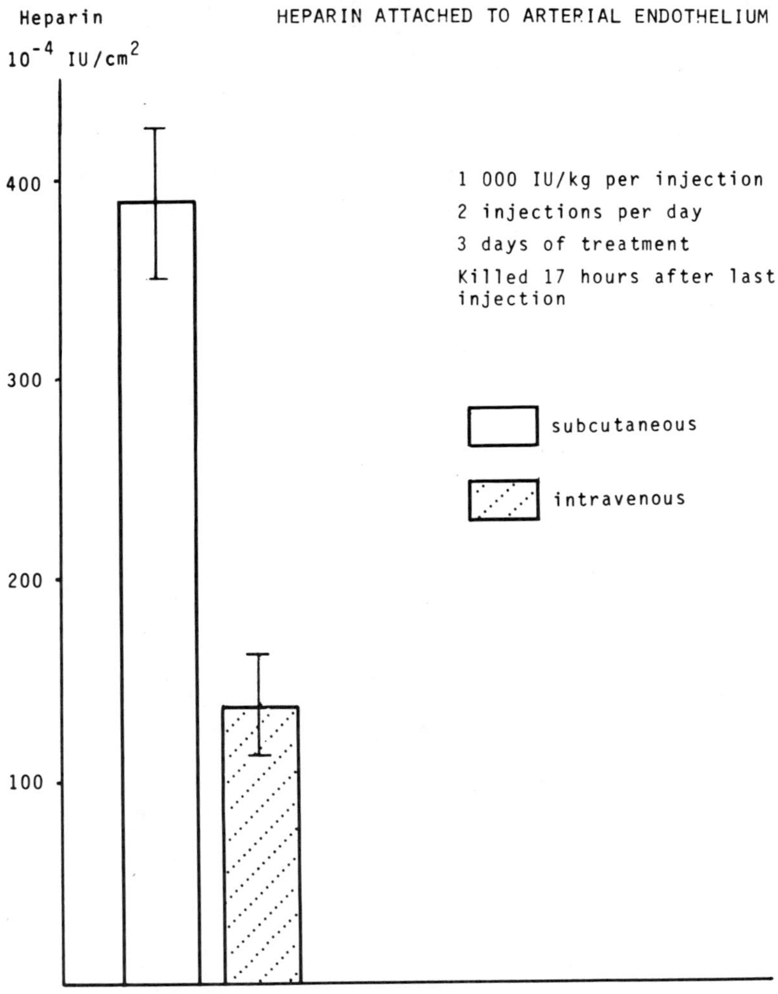

Fig. 1 Heparin attached to arterial endothelium.

Trial Number 3

Three rabbits were given totals of 1000, 2000, and 3000 IU/kg spread over unit injections (subcutaneous of 250 IU/kg (morning) and 500 IU/kg (evening) during 2, 4, and 6 days of treatment, respectively. All animals were killed and vessels removed exactly 6 hr after the last 250 IU/kg injection.

Results As shown in Fig. 2 for each total dose of heparin, the aortal walls retained, respectively, 68×10^{-4}, 80×10^{-4}, and 150×10^{-4} IU/cm^2. These findings demonstrate the cumulative effect brought about by repeating low doses, as was also found in venous wall values of 18×10^{-4}, 48×10^{-4}, and 62×10^{-4} IU/cm^2, respectively.

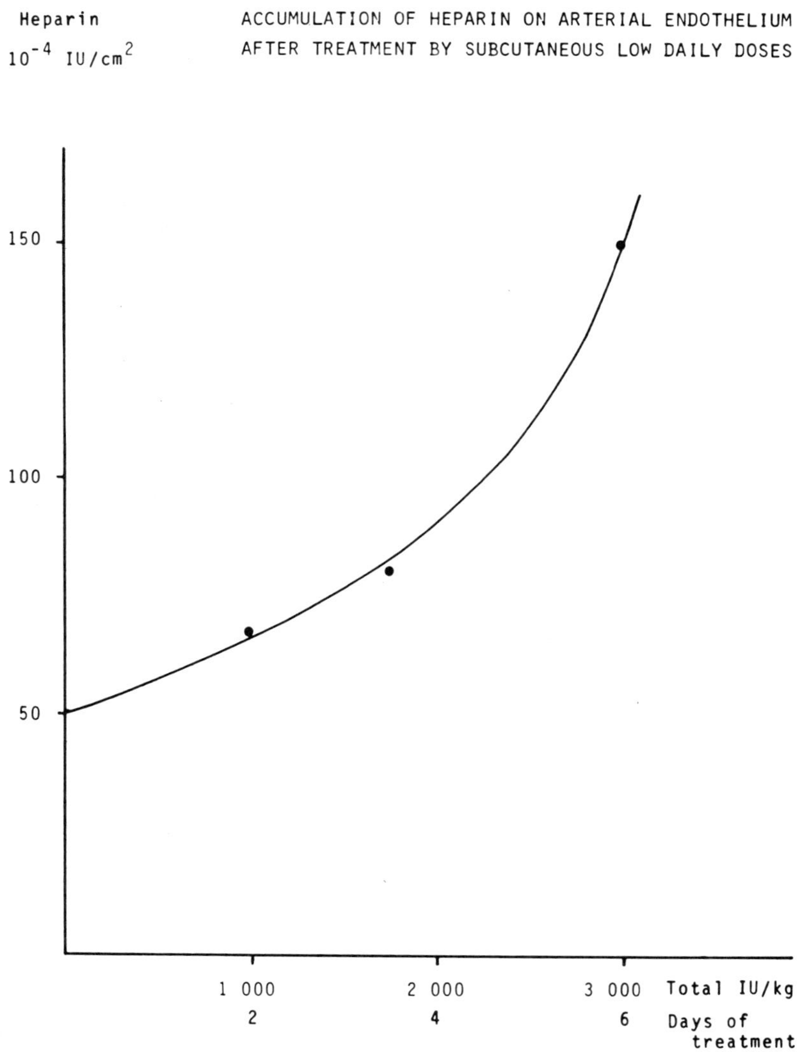

Fig. 2 Accumulation of heparin on arterial endothelium after treatment by subcutaneous low daily doses.

Trial Number 4

Six rabbits were given 12-hr-spaced morning and evening subcutaneous 1000 IU/kg injections of heparin for 3 days (total, 6000 IU/kg). Animals were killed and vessels removed, 17, 21, 24, 30, 38 and 48 hr after the final injection. Systemic blood was submitted to an hourly circulating-heparin check from the 12th to 17th hours.

Results Residual values of heparin associated with vessel walls are listed in Table III and Fig. 3. In systemic blood, circulating heparin found by thrombin time disappears between the 15th and the 17th hours. In the 48th hour, 85×10^{-4} IU of heparin were still found per cm^2 of arterial wall, i.e., 4½ times less than found after 17 hr (390×10^{-4} IU/cm^2), which represents an hourly loss of approximately 10×10^{-4} IU/cm^2.

Table III Heparin in Vessel Walls (10^{-4} IU/cm^2)

Hours after last injection	*Aorta*	*Vena cava*
17	*391*	*214*
21	*373*	*160*
24	*273*	*180*
30	*195*	*112*
38	*138*	*64*
48	*85*	*65*

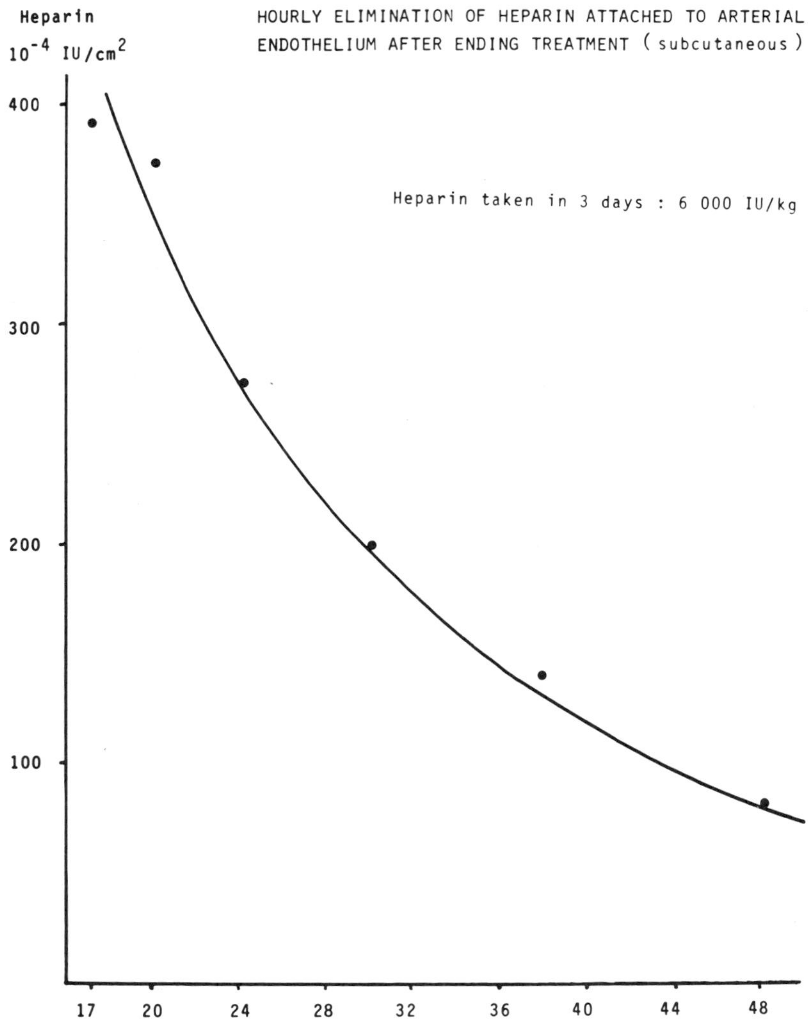

Fig. 3 Hourly elimination of heparin attached to arterial endothelium after ending treatment (subcutaneous).

Trial Number 5

Two rabbits received 2 daily subcutaneous injections at 12-hr intervals for 8 days, 250 IU/kg in one case (4000 IU/kg total) and 750 IU/kg in the other (12,000 IU/kg). They were killed and their vessels removed on the 9th day exactly 20 hr after the final injection.

Results Table IV sets forth values measured on the artery and vein of each animal that confirm the close proportionality between total heparin doses administered subcutaneously over a given time and the amounts retained by the arterial and venous walls, as well as the cumulative effect brought on by subcutaneous repetitive injection of medium doses. An idea of the attachment capacity of the vessel wall is also given.

Table IV Heparin Retention on Vessel Walls

	Total quantity of heparin taken	
	4,000 IU/kg	*12,000 IU/kg*
Aorta 10^{-4} *IU/cm*^{2}	*305*	*811*
Vena cava 10^{-4} *IU/cm*^{2}	*92*	*325*

IV. DISCUSSION

The very good correlation between assessment of heparin in systemic blood measured simultaneously by coagulation test and by radioactivity allows a real value to be attributed to subsequent trials, in localization and in quantitative assessments of heparin after ^{35}S labeling (trial number 1).

Treating anatomical elements prevents histological localization of the heparin found, but systematic verifying, by a specific coagulation test, of the absence of heparin in the circulating blood prior to each specimen-taking, points to a *parietal attachment* of the anticoagulant. Recent work by L.M. Hiebert and L.B. Jaques affirms beyond doubt that the association takes place on endothelium, that endothelial cells take an active part in rapid elimination of heparin from circulating blood and its integration in vessel walls.

This active role of endothelial cells seems to be confirmed by the fact that the amount of heparin retained by the wall is related more to the time of heparin presence in circulating blood than to the actual heparin value; after a single intravenous injection of 400 IU/kg and of doses three and five times as high (trial number 1), heparin level rises with the number of units injected but is short-lived (under 6 hr in all cases), and the amount of heparin retained by the wall, whatever dose is injected, remains small.

When injections of identical number, frequency, and unit dosage are repeated and only the route of administration differs, after a given time three times as much heparin remains on the artery and two times as much on the vein if administration is subcutaneous (trial number 2).

This difference most likely stems from high but short-lived heparinemia after intravenous administration resulting in rapid elimination of heparin from circulating blood, which "wastes" considerable amounts of anticoagulant.

The repetition of subcutaneous low-doses, on the other hand, results in accumulation of heparin on vessel walls (trial number 3), although the anticoagulant still vanishes from the circulating blood after each injection in about the same lapse of time for a given patient and dosage.

Trial number 4 shows that after only three days of subcutaneous treatment, heparin is still found in quite significant quantities on artery and vein 48 hr after termination of treatment; the hourly loss can be estimated at 10×10^{-4} IU/cm^2. As the attachment capacity of the vessel wall can be at least doubled (trial number 5) according to the dose injected or the length of treatment, it can only be concluded that heparin in sufficient quantities could stay in association with the wall four to five days after treatment is ended.

If, as several authors feel (1, 6), the faculty of heparin to attach to endothelial cells gives it antithrombotic properties connected to or independent of its anticoagulant effect, it is highly likely that the remarkable preventive effect of subcutaneously-administered small doses of heparin arises from this mechanism, rather than from possible selective action on a coagulation factor (activated factor X).

This kind of pharmacological action might also explain our excellent results with small dose intermittent ambulatory heparin therapy in long-term prevention of relapse and complications in arteritic and coronary patients.

Finally, the persistence of noteworthy quantities of heparin on vascular endothelium four to five days after subcutaneous treatment is ended would also explain the value, for high-risk patients and in thrombogenic interventions, of *preoperative preventive heparin treatment*, which we and others (5,7) have advocated for many years. Ambulatory subcutaneous administration of 7000 to 10,000 IU twice daily for 8 to 10 days before surgery makes it possible, when major immediate-postoperative hemorrhagic risk exists (thoracic surgery, urology, etc.), to postpone postoperative prevention a few days by considerably reducing the thromboembolic risk in the first 48 hr.

The remarkable effectiveness of minimal-dose subcutaneous heparin-therapy in short- and long-term prevention of arterial and venous thrombosis appears not to be attributable to the anticoagulant activity of the drug. It more probably results from the property of associating with and concentrating on vascular endothelium, which heparin insulates from cellular and plasmatic thrombogenic agents through a mechanism yet to be described.

REFERENCES

1. Hiebert, L.M., and Jaques, L.B., Artery *2*, 26 (1976).
2. Hiebert, L.M., and Jaques, L.B., Thromb. Research *8*, 195 (1976).
3. Kakkar, V.V., Field, E.S., Micolaides, A.N., Flute, P.T., Wessler, S., and Yin, E.T., Lancet *2*, 669 (1971).
4. Raby, C., Traitements anticoagulants et antiagrégants alternés. Colloque International d'Angéiologie, Paris, 26-29 April 1977.
5. Raby, C., Bertrand, H., and Servelle, M., *in* "Probl. Réan" (5ème série), J. Réan. Méd.-Chir., Nancy 1968, p. 1081.
6. Samuels, P.B., and Webster, D.R., Surgery *136*, 422 (1952).
7. Sharnoff, J.G., Rosen, R.L., Sadler, A.H., Ibarra-Isunda, G.C., J. of Bone and Joint Surgery *58-A*, 913 (1976).
8. Sharnoff, J.G., Modern Medicine March 15, 54 (1977).
9. Whiffen, J.D., and Gott, V.L., Surgery, Gynecology & Obstetrics *121*, 287 (1965).

Thursday, July 7, 1977 5:00 p.m.

LINKER, Salt Lake City I have a question for Dr. Kraemer. There have been reports showing cells in culture and suspension very readily pick up glucosaminoglycans and actually bind them fairly tightly. Now, in a sense I'm splitting hairs, because the cells you have shown obviously do make the polysaccharides, but they are an integral part of the membrane or is this material that they have made and picked up again?

KRAEMER, Los Alamos I'm sorry I didn't make that a little clearer in the talk. I tried to indicate that I had been of the opinion for many years, it was in fact an integral part of the membrane with the peotide moiety rooted in the plasma membrane as a transmembranous glycoprotein. I have been impressed by the work of Magnus Hook and his coworkers on this binding question. While various sorts of uptake have been in the literature for some time, that is conceptually different from binding sites that are specific, reversible, and saturable. So, as a consequence, I must say now that I am open on that issue.

WEST, Birmingham I just want to make a brief comment on the use of metachromasy which has been referred to a number of times and used perhaps to identify heparin. Metachromasy, a general phenomenon, can occur for a great many reasons and it can indeed be used specifically, however, it takes a great deal more than visual observation of a change in color to decide what the substrate has been. The mere presence of metachromasy does not guarantee that a particular biopolymer is present. Heparin or one of the other mucopolysaccharides, as well as other substances, can also serve to give a metachromatic effect, even the dye alone under proper conditions.

SILBERT, Boston I would like to comment on the question before, that Dr. Linker raised, and point out that Dr. Kraemer has shown that the material that comes off of cells with trypsin appears to be larger than a single chain substance. We have also seen, with fibroblast cultures, that treatment of the cells with trypsin results in a product that is larger than what is found if treated with alkali. This suggests very strongly to me that the substance is a component of cell surface. Unless we're taling about preparation or absorption of proteoglycan onto the cell surface, which then is not released from the cell surface except by proteolytic treatment. This is not absolute, but I think it would incline one to believe that it really is a portion of the cell surface. Perhaps it would be possible to solubilize cell surface

ISBN 0-12-484850-8

material as a proteoglycan, in other words get it off the cells without treatment with proteolytic enzymes, let's say with SDS or some sort of lipid solvent. It might be possible to establish that it truly was a portion of the cell surface as a proteoglycan, this remains to be done.

KRAEMER, Los Alamos I tried to get release of what we call cell surface heparan sulfate by all the usual ways that would not destroy the integrity of a membrane completely. It is clear that I will rush right home now and try to see whether I can bump off prelabeled surface heparan sulfate with heparin or heparan sulfate. In Hook's work they have yet to describe the binding as a function of all of the parameters of the N-sulfated glycosaminoglycans that they might like. In other words, what does the peptide moiety or other features of the specific molecules that bind, contribute. If there is some specificity at the microchemical level to this binding, it could be possible to use cells as an affinity column to perhaps isolate certain types of interesting subsets of molecules.

LINDAHL, Uppsala I'm not aware of the exact figures but I know that quite recently Magnus Höök carried out these actual experiments you described with cultured liver cells and could release a large fraction of prelabeled liver cell heparan sulfate by administering heparin.

LINKER, Salt Lake City I have a question to Dr. Margolis. He has isolated this brain proteoglycan that contains chondroitin 4 sulfate, chondroitin 6 sulfate, heparan sulfate, and hyaluronic acid, now indeed it would be extremely interesting to know if these compounds all sit on one peptide chain. I'm quite aware of the difficulties of this system, but have you tried any other fractionation method besides centrifugation?

MARGOLIS, New York We are somewhat skeptical about this result ourselves because it does seem like such a complex and unusual type of molecule, if indeed it is one molecule. We have tried several procedures not only density gradient centrifugation under dissociative conditions in cesium chloride. We also tried separation on the basis of molecular size on sepharose in 4 *M* quanidine. We find, for example, also that this proteoglycan is adsorbed by Concanavalin A sepharose-affinity columns and can be eluted by α-methyl-glucoside which is presumably due to the mannose containing oligosaccharides on the glycoprotein, another component, which you didn't mention. On the other hand, if we release chondroitin sulfate chains by beta elimination then these won't stick to the Concanavalan A columns as one would expect. They go to the bottom of the cesium chloride density gradient. If we take our sepharose column in 4 *M* quanidine and look at the composition of various cuts through the peak, although the material is polydisperse in terms of size, the composition is relatively the same through the four cuts. Incidently this material has been labeled with tritiated glucosamine so we could see other peaks of radioactivity in addition to just analysis of hexosamine and uronate. We don't have any evidence that we can separate this on the basis of the wide variety of conditions and we're still trying. On the other hadn, by trypsin digestion we can get smaller fragments that have pieces of the glycoprotein oligosaccharides together with the chondroitin sulfate and we are working on some of these more accessible things.

DIETRICH, São Paulo Dr. Margolis, have you found any difference in heparitin sulfate turnover between neonatal tissues and adult tissues?

MARGOLIS, New York No, we haven't actually done the turnover studies as such in neonates because one can't do this by the usual method of following decay since one doesn't have steady-state conditions because the concentrations are changing. We did look at changes in relative specific activities of five components, all of which were synthesized from a common precursor pool of UDP and acetylhexosamine. This would eliminate various differences in the actual content of the glycosaminoglycan as far as changes in penetration of precursor into brain, changes in pool size, etc. The only glycosaminoglycan that we found any appreciable change in was heparan sulfate between about two weeks in adult and a slight change in glycoprotein sialic acid specific activity.

DIETRICH, São Paulo I'm trying to relate the heparan sulfate turnover with the division and multiplication of cells, also correlating that with Dr. Kraemer's previous work on the desquamation of cell surfaces. Adult brain tissues do not show a very high multiplication of cells.

MARGOLIS, New York Well, the turnover is relatively low when one considers it in terms of days to weeks. Even though one is not getting cell division or anything of this sort these things are still not completely stable metabolically. In terms of what one considers to be very stable brain membrane such as myelin there is a quite significant turnover, actually more rapid than people originally thought, of myelin proteins and other things.

PADAWER, New York Did I understand correctly that the sulfate is turning over faster than the hexosamine and would I be correct in interpreting that to mean that perhaps there is desulfation and resulfation of polysaccharides and could this be something that could also occur with heparin in the mast cells? Does anybody have any information on that, because mast cells will pick up tremendous amounts of radioactive sulfate very fast and then they hold on to it for quite a while. Perhaps the basic heparin can stay in there but the sulfate part of that heparin might be exchanged in some way.

LINDAHL, Uppsala We have not found evidence for desulfation of heparin intracellularly in the mast cells after pulse labeling *in vivo* or *in vitro*.

SILBERT, Boston It is very difficult to explain away the findings of the Margolis's, it doesn't coincide with our preconceived notions of the mechanism of synthesis of the proteoglycan. In general the proteoglycans are synthesized or sulfated at the time that the polysaccharide chain is formed. The sulfation takes place probably in the same location in the membrane. Since we find no evidence of nonsulfated proteoglycans present in the tissues this implies that desulfation would have to take place in spottly places on the molecule and then resulfation would take place again with PAPS as a precursor on that molecule after it was formed. Now this creates all sorts of problems. The biosynthesis takes place in mast cells in the golgi apparatus and the material that the Margolis's are looking at is to a large extent in the cytosol, so we have to suggest a totally different form of exchange or of synthesis. It's entirely possible it's a different tissue, and it may very well be operating in a different way. I think that this finding of theirs, this difference in rate of turnover, is very interesting and really does present a lot of problems in terms of reconcilliation with other methods of biosynthesis.

CARR, Saskatoon Well, can I kick off by saying how delighted I was by Dr. Padawer's very scintillating combination of fact and imagination. I hope that several people are going to have a go at him. As an ignoramus in mast cells, I would just like to put one or two points. First of all, I think it would be a very convincing demonstration of the truth of the idea that the sausage-shaped granule of Padawer acts as an ion exchange column if you could actually follow ions into it by electron probe microanalysis. This is technically feasible and I think it would make a very pretty experiment.

Second, a recent demonstration suggests that during mast cell granule release there is an apparently purposive segregation of various proteins away from the point where the mast cell granule is bursting out. This implies purposeful mast cell granule release. The third point that I would like to make to Dr. Padawer is a philosophical one since he was being philosophical, I accept entirely his idea which is a splendid one. I don't think it necessarily or totally replaces the idea that mast cells may also release their granules and that's important because there is an important parallel that is the neutrophil polymorph which does, among many other things, two important things, it uses its granule within the cell in phagocytosis and most people would now agree that the granules are released outside the cell and form an important part in the perpetuation of chronic inflammation. These are one or two points from an ignoramus. I would hope the cogsnocenti would have some more.

PADAWER, New York The electron probe analysis experiment is an interesting one. I've done some of that, unfortunately on borrowed equipment. We are not equipped to continue. Would you expand your second point?

CARR, Saskatoon The second point is that in Raff's idea of mast cell granule release there is a segregation of various proteins on the membrane away from the point of release of the granule. (Raff, M.C., Sci. Amer. 234(5), 30, 1976.) There were several proteins involved and it was done by several techniques and this appears to imply that it is not just a sort of random bursting out of the granules happening in a non-purposive way but that there is really something happening here. I wonder what you think of this idea.

PADAWER, New York If I recall correctly he was using heterologous IgE antibody to cause an immune reverse anaphylactic reaction on the cell. I would expect that something would happen unevenly on the membrane because the pores that I'm postulating (either open pores, or closed pores), may be in a different area in the membrane. If you get a reaction that effects those areas, of course something is going to happen. I visualize the microtubule-microfilament system homing in on these areas and acting like either a chemical or physical sphincter of sorts, that would allow the material that is being percolated by microperistalsis over the granules to be pushed out so that there can't be any back flow. If there were back flow Uvnäs' release mechanism, e.g., exposure to small amounts of ions that come in from pores, would cause the cells to degranulate. Therefore, degranulation is something that one imposes on the cell that is not something that the cell does purposefully. Since the pores are not present in all places, and since we must have a mechanism that can voluntarily control these pores, it seems quite reasonable that if we can find something that will trick the cell and open it when the cell doesn't want to, when it is not prepared to keep the back flow out, then, of course we will get this kind of degranulation. With respect to your third question about the PMN's the situation is somewhat different there, although I don't know how different. You may have a point. Normally the lysosomes, which are the granules that you are taling about in the PMN's, are brought into contact with the phagocytic vacuoles and dump their material in them. This has been demonstrated with bacteria or with zymosan particles which are bigger than the cells themselves, in this case the lysosomes were beginning to discharge even before the vacuole membrane had completely closed around the ingested particules. In our example we are in effect bringing the substrate to lysosomes, if you want to call them that, they are at best lysosomoid, they are inactive in many ways and they are permanent. The neutrophil, once it loses a lysosome, it's gone, and it will never replace it, whereas here we have a very neat system which remains available for a long time. I think the point to emphasize is that it stays there for a long time, we don't digest anything and I want to emphasize the possibility that we have a cell which is, if you wish, is a little FBI with a very good file and it's putting things in there that it can keep reading on for a long time. Or, perhaps the fact that it's doing it so slowly, it means that it can take antigen antibody complexes and by hydrolyzing them slowly, can keep releasing the antigen in a slow way and provides better stimulation. I don't know. I purposely wanted to be challenging because that's how I think we're going to really find out whether these make any sense or not.

SUE, Saskatoon A comment from Dr. Raby, please. I think he showed beautifully the uptake of heparin by endothelial cells and he reminded us of the beneficial effect clinically. When heparin is taken up by the cells on the endothelial surface, will the heparin still produce an antithrombotic effect? In Dr. Hiebert's presentation she indicated that heparin was taken up intracellularly, this should block any beneficial effect clinically. Secondly, if I remember correctly, Dr. Raby showed heparin taken up in higher amount on the arterial rather than the venous side of the circulation, however, clinically, heparin is most effective in venous thrombosis.

HIEBERT, Saskatoon I wonder if I could comment. First of all, I have shown that the heparin goes inside the endothelial cells but that is not to say that there isn't planty of it left on the surface. In all of my slides I showed that, although the heparin was inside the cells, there was still a lot on the surface which could act on antithrombin.

RABY, Paris I have said heparin was on or in the vessel wall and Dr. Hiebert shows and proves, I think, it was on endothelium and in endothelial cells and I believe her.

HIEBERT, Saskatoon Raby has shown a difference in the arterial wall, the aorta, and vena cava, with the aorta having more radioactive counts representing more heparin. We should remember that the arterial wall is thicker than the vena cava and this may account for those results.

SILBERT, Boston I just want to sound a note of caution. I suspect that the radioactively labeled heparin that you are using is made by tritium gas exchange. Raby's is S^{35} but the other was tritiated. Is that correct, Dr. Hiebert? This procedure results in a lot of degradation and changes in the molecule. I think one has to be very cautious in interreting what it's really doing and that it is really heparin as we know heparin. It may have very subtle changes, very subtle differences. I think that the experiments do have to be confirmed by chemical measurement of the heparin as well as the radioactive label.

UVNÄS, Stockholm I just wanted to say a few words, to defend the mast cells. If I understand Dr. Padawer correctly, he thinks that the mast cell is some kind of garbage can that we go around with our whole life. It gets more and more filled with things which the body doesn't like to have running around or waste products of various kinds. Now, even if that is an interesting thought, you should not forget that the mast cell has very effective secreting machinery. The mast cell is a glandular cell and many people have studied the mechanism by which the active response of a mast cell occurs. The release of histamine, the degranulation, requires the same factors (calcium, energy, etc.) which the release of transmitters at the nerve terminal requires. The mast cell has effective secretory machinery. It synthesizes biologically active substances like histamine. If the cell synthesizes heparin, I can't see from a teleological point of view, such a cell which makes these biologically active substances and has secretory machinery to get rid of them, that this doesn't correspond to some kind of a function. I don't know if this is a valid assumption but I don't like the idea that it should be only a garbage can.

PADAWER, New York I don't think that Dr. Uvnäs has to defind the mast cells because I'm one of its defenders. As a matter of fact, I think I'm as much a proponent as he is. It is not a garbage can, it is not collecting things that the body doesn't want. In fact, it is keeping track of things that are key in our well-being and it is, in effect, keeping a file of those things that might really do us in, if somehow we were not ready to cope with them. It's rather selective in what it picks up. (By the way, I should say that both Selye and Michaels who wrote two of the best known reviews on mast cells, concluded that mast cells are not phagocytic, but we shouldn't fault the earlier workers because they defined the reticulo endothelial system mainly by using two compounds, tryphan blue and colloidal carbon, unfortunately the mast cell does not pick up either.) We have here a cell that does pick up material, which is certainly not garbage, it is possibly IgE bound to antigenic complexes. For the body to know what these things are and to take appropriate measures to defind us against them is a very worthwhile function. As far as the various secretory machinery that you mentioned, calcium, energy, etc., one could mention others, but I'm very impressed with the fact that those very same things are involved with virtually everything that cells do. One cell uses calcium to contract, another cell uses it to absorb, another cell uses it to secrete. These are rather basic mechanisms that cells use and the body, being very conservative, uses these particular mechanisms for whatever function desired. The system can work in either direction and I am not so convinced that when you force a cell to somehow lose its granules, this doesn't reverse a normal process. So I don't know that we can really take these changes in either calcium or energy as really evidence of what is going on, just as likely the ionic changes will then affect the microtubule, micro-filament system and this perse will result in changes in ATP which, in effect, leads back to the energy mechanisms you're talking about.

HIGGINBOTHAM, Louisville Noxious substances and detrimental things that mast cells can take care of are readily taken care of by the macrophage and macrophages are, in many people's minds, good cells for processing substances and distribution to an informational system, the immune system. If one compares the mast cells of a normal animal and one that has secreted its granules during an immune type of response, e.g., IgE fixation, the things that should be noted experimentally are that the granules are swollen, as has been discussed before and are readily penetrable by various cations from the extracellular medium. Also, they are now highly metachromatic which suggests that they are binding much more dye than they would in the normal. The dye can be readily eluted by the so-called histamine releasers, there are many of them, and since it's a cationic dye we have a cation exchange process going on. Since heparin can bind certain of these histamine releasers such as compound 48/80, polymyxin, Russell's viper venom, etc., and neutralize their toxicity, some of these complexes are ingested by adjacent macrophages. We have a system that appears as a protective mechanism in which mast cells facilitate transfer to the mononuclear phagocyte.

CLINICAL APPLICATION

HEPARIN THERAPY IN VENOUS THROMBOSIS AND PULMONARY EMBOLISM: CLINICAL AND EXPERIMENTAL OBSERVATIONS

J. Hirsh, W.G. van Aken, and H. Chiu

Department of Pathology, McMaster University

Heparin is considered to be the drug of choice in the treatment of venous thromboembolism. The aim of heparin treatment is to prevent local extension of venous thrombosis and subsequent recurrent pulmonary embolism without causing bleeding. The reported frequency of recurrent pulmonary embolism and bleeding during heparin treatment of patients with venous thromboembolism has varied considerably (1).

A number of recent publications have compared the effectiveness of heparin given by continuous intravenous infusion with intermittent four hourly IV injection and have demonstrated that, although both methods are effective in preventing recurrent thromboembolism, there is considerably less bleeding when heparin is given by continuous infusion in a dose that maintains laboratory tests within a defined range (2,3).

The response to a standard dose of heparin assessed by laboratory tests differs considerably among patients with venous thromboembolism (4). In this chapter, it is proposed to review the results of clinical and experimental studies that were performed to explore 1) the reasons for the variation in individual response to a standard dose of heparin in patients with venous thromboembolism, and 2) the relationship between the response to heparin as measured by laboratory tests of blood coagulation and the antithrombotic effect of heparin.

I. VARIATIONS IN RESPONSE TO HEPARIN

A. Clinical Studies

The response to a standard dose of heparin was investigated in 20 patients with proven venous thromboembolism. An initial dose of 70 units/kg of aqueous sodium heparin was given by bolus intravenous injection. After 90 min a maintenance dose of 400 units/kg/24 hr was given by continuous intravenous infusion using a precision syringe pump. The dose of heparin was adjusted on the basis of results of the activated partial thromboplastin time (APTT), measured 6-15 hr after starting heparin, the aim being to maintain the APTT in the range of 60-80 sec (control 40 sec).

ISBN 0-12-484850-8

The APTT was performed before heparin was given and at 15, 45, and 90 min after the bolus injection and then 6-15 hr after the maintenance infusion was started. Heparin activity, measured using the heparin protamine titration test (5), was performed on all of the post heparin injection samples. In addition, an *in vitro* heparin tolerance test was performed by measuring the APTT response of pretreatment plasma to varying concentrations of heparin over a range of 0.05-0.4 units/ml of plasma. The relationship between the heparin activity and the corresponding APTT was calculated by subtracting the pretreatment APTT from the APTT obtained on samples drawn after heparin infusion and dividing the result (the ΔAPTT) by the heparin activity in the samples. This was referred to as the heparin effect index (HEI).

The APTT values and the heparin levels in response to the intravenous bolus dose of heparin and to the maintenance heparin infusion varied considerably from patient to patient (4). There was a relatively poor correlation between the *in vivo* heparin activity and the ΔAPTT for individual patients at 15, 45, and 90 min after bolus injection; the correlation coefficient being $r=0.48$. This was because there was considerable interindividual variation in the ΔAPTT response at each plasma heparin activity measured *in vivo*. In contrast, the correlation between the APTT and the heparin activity for each individual patient on blood samples taken at 15, 45, and 90 min after heparin injection was very good with a correlation coefficient of between 0.82 and 1.00.

The *in vitro* HEI obtained by adding heparin to pretreatment plasma showed a strong correlation ($r=0.87$) with the HEI observed after heparin administration, a finding that suggested that the factors responsible for modifying *in vivo* APTT response in any particular patient was present in the patient's plasma before heparin treatment. The reason for the variation between individuals in the anticoagulant response to heparin (HEI) is not entirely clear but could be due in part to differences in the levels of coagulation factors in these patients that are known to influence the APTT response to heparin. Such an effect was produced *in vitro* by adding cryoprecipitate to plasma and demonstrating that this markedly influences the APTT response to heparin without affecting the heparin activity determined by the protamine sulphate titration method. The half-life of heparin in these patients, and in four additional patients with pulmonary emboli, was calculated using the heparin activity assay.

The mean heparin half-life was significantly shorter for patients with pulmonary embolism than for those with venous thrombosis ($p<0.005$ (Fig. 1). The mechanism for this difference in heparin half-life between patients with pulmonary embolism and venous thrombosis was not clear and

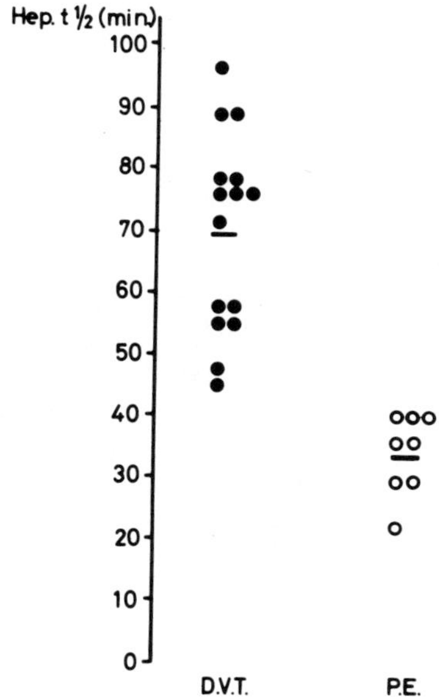

Fig. 1. Heparin half-life (min) in 15 patients with deep venous thrombosis (DVT) and in 8 patients with pulmonary embolism (PE) following the intravenous injection of 70 U/kg heparin. The difference between these two groups is statistically significant ($p<0.005$).

further studies were carried out using an experimental model of venous thrombosis and pulmonary embolism in rabbits.

B. Experimental Studies

Previous investigations by Thomas and associates (6) demonstrated that experimental pulmonary emboli become rapidly covered with a layer of platelets, whereas the thrombi from which these emboli were derived were relatively free of platelets. This raised the possibility that the observed differences in heparin clearance in venous thrombosis and pulmonary embolism could be due to release of antiheparin activity from platelets. Investigations of heparin clearance were therefore performed in rabbits with venous thrombosis or pulmonary embolism to determine whether heparin clearance is increased in experimental pulmonary embolism and to explore the possible contribution of platelets to the heparin clearance in acute pulmonary embolism (7).

In these investigations, plasma heparin concentration was measured in two ways; by protamine sulphate titration and by ^{35}S radioactivity measurements following the injection of ^{35}S heparin mixed with commercial heparin. It was initially demonstrated that the heparin clearance measured by the radioactivity was significantly faster than the clearance using heparin activity for calculation. Gel filtration studies with unlabeled heparin and ^{35}S heparin showed that the molecular size distribution of the latter was consistently in a relatively lower range. Therefore, both heparins were fractionated by gel filtration on a Sephadex G 200 column to obtain samples in the same molecular size range. This fractionated ^{35}S heparin gave a similar heparin clearance to unlabeled heparin in normal rabbits.

Heparin clearance was measured from serial blood samples at 1.5 min after heparin injection, at 5 min and then at 5 min intervals for 30 min. An average of six to eight blood samples were collected after heparin injection and the heparin $t\frac{1}{2}$ was calculated from the samples taken between 5 and 30 min after heparin injection.

Experimental venous thrombi and pulmonary emboli were produced in anesthetized rabbits. Venous thrombi were produced in internal and external jugular veins using a stasis hypercoagulability method. The induced thrombus was held in place by a proximal stenotic suture that narrowed the lumen to approximately 30% but did not completely occlude blood flow. Experimental pulmonary emboli were produced in rabbits by removing the stenotic suture from the jugular vein and gently squeezing the thrombus manually in the direction of the heart. Three thrombi were produced and all of these were embolized. The presence of pulmonary embolism was confirmed at autopsy.

In order to study the effects of platelets on the increased heparin clearance, investigations were performed in thrombocytopenic animals. Thrombocytopenia was produced by exposing animals to whole body irradiation from a cesium source (930 rads). The necks of the animals were protected by a lead shield to prevent radiation damage to the jugular veins. Seven days later, the rabbits received an intravenous injection of 0.3 ml antirabbit platelet serum. In some animals, heparin clearance was measured after the introduction of polyether urethane coated glass emboli. In these animals, jugular veins were exposed, blood flow in one of the jugular veins was temporarily occluded, and a small incision was made in the vessel through which the pellet was introduced. After squeezing the vessel, the pellets embolized. Eighty percent of these pellets were recovered in the pulmonary arteries.

The heparin $t\frac{1}{2}$ in normal animals was 21 ± 3.2 min using heparin activity and 18 ± 2 min using ^{35}S radioactivity. The heparin $t\frac{1}{2}$ in rabbits with PE was 13.5 ± 1.2 min using heparin activity and 12.3 ± 2 min using ^{35}S radioactivity. The results in PE were significantly different than in normal controls. The experiments were then repeated using the heparin activity assay only. When 50 units/kg of heparin was injected into each of three groups of 15 rabbits following the formation of PE, VT, or after sham operation, the heparin $t\frac{1}{2}$ in rabbits with PE was 12.0 ± 3 min in rabbits with VT was 18.2 ± 3.3 min and in sham operated rabbits was 20.2 ± 3.5 min. The heparin $t\frac{1}{2}$ was significantly shorter in animals with PE when compared with VT or control animals, while the differences between VT and control animals were not significant. On the other hand, when 200 units/kg of heparin was injected following PE, VT, or sham operation, the heparin $t\frac{1}{2}$ was 19.4 ± 5 min in PE, 22.7 ± 9 min in VT and 19.3 ± 3 min in sham operated animals. These values were not significantly different from each other.

The experiments were repeated using emboli derived from aged thrombi to exclude the possibility that the shortened heparin $t\frac{1}{2}$ in PE was due to injected thrombin that was used to induce the venous thrombi. In these animals, the heaprin $t\frac{1}{2}$ was again significantly shorter in the PE than in the VT or control animals.

Venous thrombi and pulmonary emboli were removed at autopsy and investigated by light electron microscopy. Whereas the venous thrombi consisted mainly of densely packed red cells with leukocytes, fibrin and platelet aggregates distributed at random between the cells, the pulmonary emboli, which were of identical age to the venous thrombi, were coated with a rim of platelets of variable thickness. Electron microscopy demonstrated that most of these platelets had undergone degranulation.

The organ distribution of ^{35}S was measured in PE and in control animals and was not found to be significantly different. In addition, the pulmonary emboli removed 60 min after heparin injection had less than 0.01% of the injected ^{35}S radioactivity.

The effect of thrombocytopenia on heparin clearance in animals with induced venous thrombi and pulmonary emboli was investigated in animals 24 hr after injection of antiplatelet serum when the platelet count was less than 20,000/cu mm. Thrombocytopenic animals with PE had a heparin $t\frac{1}{2}$ that was significantly shorter than in rabbits with VT or sham operation, and the heparin $t\frac{1}{2}$ in thrombocytopenic rabbits with pulmonary emboli, which was 12.8 ± 3.2 min was not significantly different than the heparin $t\frac{1}{2}$ in rabbits with pulmonary emboli with normal platelet counts (12.5 ± 3 min).

Heparin $t\frac{1}{2}$ in rabbits with coated glass emboli was not any different than in sham operated animals.

The results of these studies, therefore, showed that heparin $t\frac{1}{2}$ is shorter in rabbits with experimental pulmonary embolism than in animals with either VT or control animals and therefore confirms the observations obtained in patients with thromboembolic disease. It is of interest that the heparin $t\frac{1}{2}$ was not reduced in animals with PE that were treated with 200 units/kg of heparin. It is possible that the higher dose of heparin masked an increased rate of clearance of a portion of the heparin dose. Alternatively, it is possible that the increase in heparin clearance in experimental pulmonary embolism is mediated by humoral or other factors that are generated as a consequence of PE but whose production or effect is inhibited by larger doses of heparin. The fact that heparin clerance is not increased when polyether urethane glass coated pellets were embolized suggested that the increased heparin clearance depends on the nature of the embolic material. The finding of increased heparin clearance in animals with pulmonary embolism that were made thrombocytopenic indicates that shortened heparin $t\frac{1}{2}$ in PE is not due to platelet factor 4 released from platelets that aggregated on the surface of the embolus. Thus, these findings confirm the more limited studies in man and raise the possibility that in order to counteract the effects of increased heparin clearance, larger initial doses of heparin should be used in the treatment of acute pulmonary embolism.

II. RELATIONSHIP BETWEEN THE ANTICOAGULANT AND ANTI-THROMBOTIC EFFECTS OF HEPARIN

As shown in the clinical study, the relationship between the level of circulating heparin activity and its effect on coagulation varies considerably from patient to patient and it is currently uncertain which of these measurements reflects the antithrombotic effect of heparin more accurately. A model of experimental venous thrombosis was developed in rabbits that provided a means of accurately quantifying fibrinogen accretion onto an existing thrombus (8). This model was used to explore the relationship between the antithrombotic effect of heparin and its anticoagulant effect, the latter being measured both by heparin assay with protamine sulphate titration and by the activated partial thromboplastin time (APTT).

Venous thrombi were produced in the jugular veins as described above. After the thrombus was produced, the animals were infused with ^{125}I-fibrinogen. The amount of fibrinogen accreted onto thrombi was calculated by relating the ^{125}I activity of the washed thrombi to the integrated mean specific activity of plasma fibrinogen during the experiment. Each experiment lasted 10 hr and during this time the rabbits were infused either with saline or with various concentrations of heparin delivered as a continuous infusion using a precision pump.

The amount of fibrinogen accreted in 20 animals infused with 0.9% sodium chloride was 122.5 ± 52 mg, which represented an increase of fibrinogen content of the thrombus over the 10 hr period of 56.5%. The relationship between the antithrombotic and anticoagulant effect of heparin given by continuous infusion indicated that there was a sharp reduction in fibrinogen accretion with increasing anticoagulant effect measured either by the APTT, the APTT ratio $\frac{\text{(post heparin APTT)}}{\text{(pre heparin APTT)}}$ or heparin activity (8).

The relationship between heparin activity and APTT showed a highly significant correlation, r=0.92 and p<0.001. By comparison with these results in rabbits, the patients with venous thrombosis, who were studied as part of the clinical investigation, showed a much more variable anticoagulant response to heparin when this was measured either by protamine sulphate titration or by APTT and the correlation between these two tests was poor. Porcine cryoprecipitate was therefore infused into rabbits in an attempt to dissociate the results of the APTT response and the results of heparin assay. Pretreatment of the animals with cryoprecipitate altered the slope of the regression line between heparin activity and APTT values so that there was a considerably smaller increase in APTT for any given level of heparin activity. In addition, the pretreatment APTT in animals treated with cryoprecipitate was significantly less than in control animals. After treating the animals with cryoprecipitate, the experiments with heparin and saline were repeated and the relationship between inhibition of fibrinogen accretion and anticoagulant effect of heparin in normal and cryoprecipitate-treated animals was obtained by comparing the APTT and heparin levels required to decrease accretion to 15 mg, which represented approximately a 90% reduction in fibrinogen accretion. In normal animals this reduction was achieved with an APTT of 48 sec a $\frac{\text{posttreatment}}{\text{pretreatment}}$ APTT ratio of 1.5 and a heparin level of 0.17 units/ml. In contrast, a similar reduction was produced in the cryoprecipitate-treated animals with an APTT value of 29.7 sec that was significantly less than the level required in normal animals but with a similar APTT ratio (1.4) and a similar heparin level (0.21) units/ml.

The results of this study therefore showed that estimations of plasma heparin activity and APTT are equally sensitive in predicting the antithrombotic effect of heparin in rabbits with experimental venous thrombosis, and that these tests are highly correlated with each other. Fibrinogen accretion was markedly inhibited at a similar heparin level in both the cryoprecipitate-treated and normal animals, but this level of inhibition of fibrinogen accretion was obtained with a significantly lower APTT value in the cryoprecipitate-treated animals than in the normal animals. Cryoprecipitate was used to dissociate the APTT response to heparin since it had been shown that elevated levels of Factor VIII may mask the APTT response in patients treated with heparin (9). Thus, in the experimental model used, the minimum dose of heparin required to produce a marked antithrombotic effect was more accurately predicted by the heparin assay than by the APTT.

The clinical significance of these findings is uncertain. In patients with venous thromboembolism, the incidence of clinical recurrence and of bleeding is low when heparin is given by continuous infusion in a dose that increases the APTT to 1½-2½ times the normal control level. Nevertheless, there are clinical situations, such as the development of venous thromboembolism in the early post-operative period, in which it would be desirable to avoid bleeding by using the minimum effective dose of heparin. In some of these patients, the pretreatment APTT is short and large doses of heparin may be required to increase the APTT to twice the normal control value. The experimental findings described above raise the possibility that in these patients it might be safer to monitor heparin treatment by using the heparin assay or by relating the degree of prolongation of the APTT to the pretreatment test result rather than to increase the APTT to twice the normal control value.

ACKNOWLEDGEMENTS

This work was supported in part by the Province of Ontario, the Canadian Heart Foundation, and the Medical Research Council. Dr. van Aken was a Visiting Research Fellow of the Ontario Heart Foundation and was supported by a grant from the Ontario Heart Foundation of Canada and by a Travel Grant from the Nils Stensen Foundation, Amsterdam.

REFERENCES

1. Gallus, A.S., and Hirsh, J., Sem. Thromb. Haemost. *2*, 291 (1976).
2. Salzman, E.W., Deykin, D., Shapiro, R.M., and Rosenberg, R., N. Engl. J. Med. *292*, 1046 (1975).
3. Glazier, R.L., and Crowell, E.B., JAMA *236*, 1365 (1976).
4. Hirsh, J., van Aken, W.G., Gallus, A.S., Dollery, C.T., Cade, J.F., and Yung, W., Circulation *53*, 691 (1976).
5. Refn, I., and Vestergaard, L., Scand. J. Clin. Lab. Invest. *6*, 284 (1954).
6. Thomas, D.P., Gurevich, V., and Ashford, T.P., N. Engl. J. Med. *274*, 953 (1966).
7. Chiu, H.M., van Aken, W.G., Hirsh, J., Regoeczi, E., and Horner, A.A., J. Lab. Clin. Med. (in press) (1977).
8. Chiu, H.M., Hirsh, J., Yung, W.L., Regoeczi, E., and Gent, M., Blood *49*, 171 (1977).
9. Edson, J.R., Drivit, W., and White, J., J. Lab. Clin. Med. *70*, 463 (1967).

HEPARIN BY INHALATION

L.W. Kavanagh and J. Mahadoo

Department of Physiology
University of Saskatchewan

Since heparin must be given by injection, possible alternatives such as oral or pulmonary administration have been attempted. Windsor and Freeman (1) observed no anticoagulant effect when 230 to 286 units/kg of heparin was sprayed into tracheostomy tubes of dogs. Rosner (2) observed a mild anticoagulant effect following inhalation of heparin aerosol in humans. Koh and Barucha (3) found an anticoagulant effect after the tracheal instillation of amino acid-heparinic acid complexes into dogs. This laboratory found a marked anticoagulant effect after tracheal instillation of sodium heparin into dogs (4). Further, in 1973, Molino and Belluardo (5) reported that administration of heparin by aerosol was effective in preventing thrombotic incidents in selected patients. Sunderland and Klein (6) reported hemorrhagic symptoms after 2.4 million units of heparin were added to pulmonary lavage. These studies, therefore, established that heparin is absorbed by the lung, and further studies were designed to investigate the type of response. These studies gave interesting unexpected results and also provided a useful research model for further investigations.

I. ANTICOAGULANT EFFECT WITH PULMONARY HEPARIN IN DOGS

In our initial study the anticoagulant effect, its magnitude and duration, and the dose response relationship were examined. Mongrel dogs were anesthetized, an endotracheal tube inserted, and a fine polyethylene tube pushed down into the trachea. Heparin at doses from 8 to 20 mg/kg in 2 ml of distilled water was then delivered through the tubing.

ISBN 0-12-484850-8

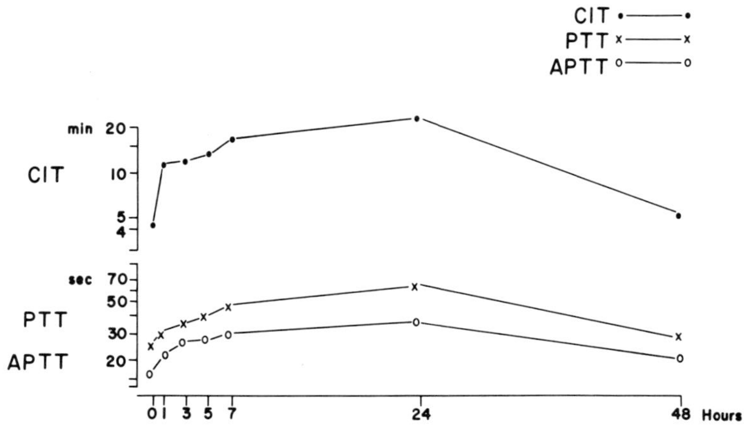

Fig. 1. Coagulation test values after intrapulmonary instillation of heparin in one dog at a dose of 15 mg/kg at 0 time. ●—● CI.T = Lee and White whole blood coagulation time; X——X PTT = partial thromboplastin time; o———o APTT = activated partial thromboplastin time. (Reproduced by permission from (4).)

Figure 1 shows the type of anticoagulant response obtained, in this case at a dose of 15 mg/kg. The heparin used was approximately 150 μ/mg. What was striking was that the response to pulmonary heparin was markedly different from that observed with intravenous heparin. Pulmonary heparin produced a very prolonged moderate anticoagulant state without wide fluctuations in values. The effect began within 1 hr and lasted 48 hr or more. The clotting time did not reach the incoagulable range seen with intermittent intravenous therapy, but the effect was prolonged beyond the 2 or 3 hr effect of intravenous heparin. The response of different doses was studied, and the effective dose in dogs was between 8 and 15 mg/kg or 1200 to 2250 μ/kg. Doses below 8 mg/kg did not give a significant anticoagulant effect as measured by clotting time or partial thromboplastin times and doses at 20 mg/kg or higher yielded incoagulable blood with hematoma formation at the site of venipuncture. This was the only hemorrhagic problem, no hematuria or other signs of bleeding were noted.

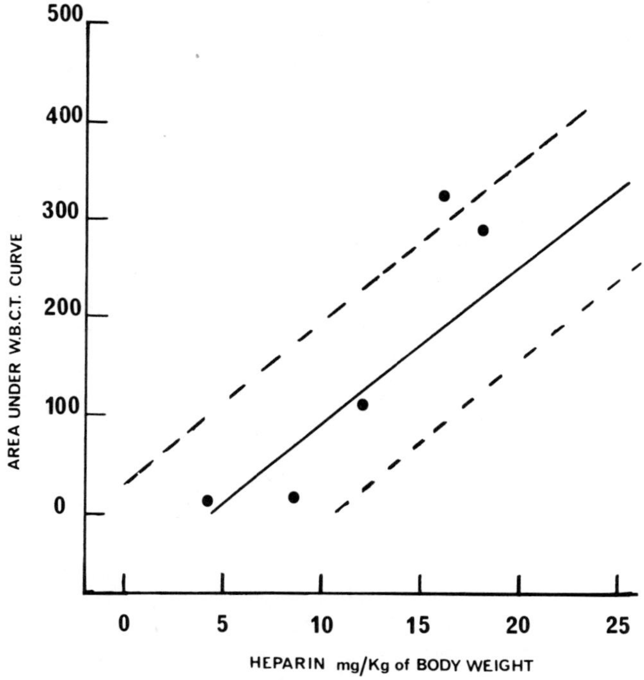

Fig. 2. Dose-response to intrapulmonary heparin. Regression line between response (area under the W.B.C.T. curve) and dosage for 18 positive responses in dogs. Dotted lines show 2 x standard error of estimate (95% of data). ● = values obtained for intrapulmonary administration with human volunteers. Area by planimeter in square inches. (Reproduced by permission from (7).)

To obtain an indication of the reproducibility of the response, five doses of heparin, 8, 10, 12, 15, and 20 mg/kg, were repeated three to five times in five dogs. Some variation in anticoagulant effect, that is in maximum clotting time reached and its duration, were seen for each dosage, but in general a greater effect was seen with increasing dose. In order to express the total response more fully and quantitatively, the area under the dose-response curve was calculated for each trial. The area values were found to correlated significantly with the dosage as shown in Fig. 2. There is scatter in the area values for any one dose, but this is also seen with intravenous heparin administration in dogs. The heparin may have been instilled into different levels of the pulmonary system, which could alter the rate of absorption. Also area values are only a crude measure of the total response since the clotting times were measured infrequently in order to reduce blood loss to the dogs. However, a positive correlation between dose and the area under the whole blood clotting time curve was found.

II. ANTICOAGULANT EFFECT OF HEPARIN AEROSOL

This study has shown that heparin is absorbed from the lung and the response was longer and milder than when given intravenously. Since this prolonged hypocoagulant state could be of possible clinical use, the response to heparin in aerosol form was studied in mice and humans as described by Jaques *et al.* (7). Mice were exposed to a heparin aerosol for 10 to 30 min from a *Vaponefrin* nebulizer in a glass chamber. The dosage was regulated by the amount of heparin solution nebulized. Human volunteers inhaled a heparin aerosol from a DeVilbiss ultrasonic nebulizer containing the appropriate volume of heparin in a 10-12 mg/ml solution to give the required dose. The inhalation procedure required about 1 hr for effective doses. The coagulation parameters measured were whole blood clotting time, and in some trials Factor Xa inhibition by the method of Yin *et al.* (8). Sodium heparin of pig intestinal mucosa was used for most studies, and ^{3}H-labeled heparin was used in some of the mouse trials.

Figure 3 shows the changes in whole blood clotting times obtained. In humans, after inhaling 12 to 18 mg/kg doses, or a total of 100,000 to 190,000 units, a moderate degree of anticoagulation resulted which lasted 8 to 16 days. The percentage increase in clotting time is not as great in humans as in the dog but lasts considerably longer. This increase in clotting time was significant with a P value of < 0.01. The response was intermediate in mice, lasting about six days.

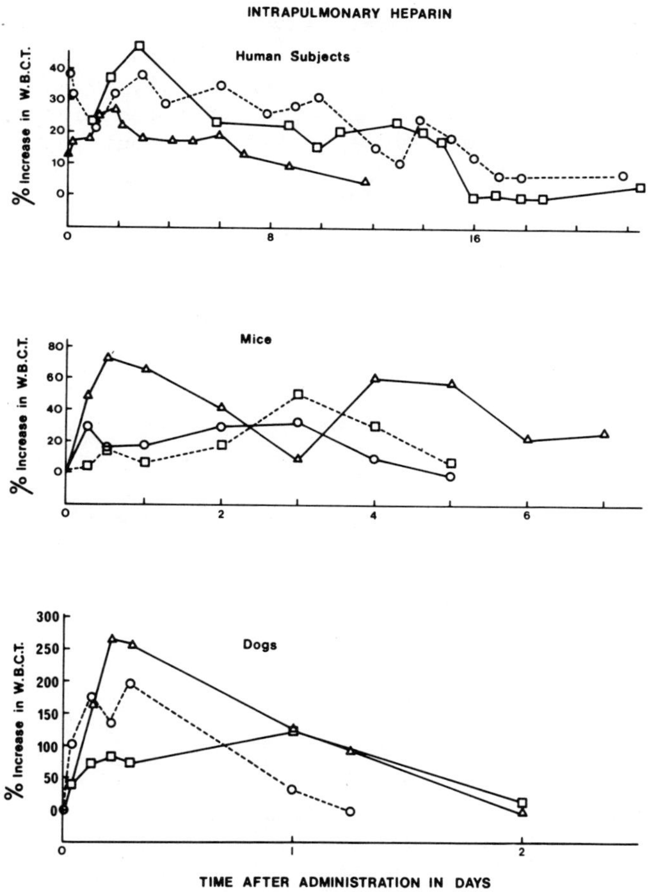

Fig. 3. Effect of intrapulmonary heparin on whole-blood clotting time (W.B.C.T.). Three human volunteers inhaling 12 (△), 16 (□), 18.7 (O) mg heparin/kg body-weight. Mice inhaling 4.4 (O), 6.6 (□), 10.1 (△) ppm heparin (mins). Each point on the curve represents a mean of 3 W.B.C.T. values obtained from three mice. Three dogs receiving heparin by instillation after intubation, 10 (O), 12 (□), 15 (△) mg heparin/kg. (Reproduced by permission from (7).)

III. PHARMACOKINETICS OF RESPONSE TO INTRAPULMONARY, INTRAVENOUS AND SUBCUTANEOUS HEPARIN

It is apparent that the effect of heparin depends on the route of administration. Intrapulmonary heparin requires a large initial dose and gives a prolonged mild effect; intravenous heparin gives an almost immediate high clotting time with a short half-life of about 1.5 hr. The effect of subcutaneous heparin is intermediate between these two effects. What is the explanation for the extended effect of inhaled heparin? The prolonged mild effect of intrapulmonary heparin could be explained by a variety of hypotheses, but it is the final product of the rate of absorption, storage within the body, rate of metabolism, and rate of excretion of the undegraded drug.

TABLE I Distribution of Radioactivity After Tracheal Instillation of ^{3}H-Heparin in Rats

	% of radioactivity administered		
Tissue/excreta	*1.5 hr*	*24 hr*	*7 days*
Lungs	*60.9*	*9.8*	*6.3*
Plasma	*3.3*	*1.3*	*0.6*
Red blood-cells	*3.3*	*1.1*	*0.5*
Platelets	*0.1*	*0.07*	*0.03*
Urine	--	*14.8*	*23.2*
Feces	--	*0*	*19.1*
Other tissues	*53.8*	--	--
Total	*121.4*	*27.07*	*49.73*

Each value is an average of data from three rats.

Amount of heparin administered per rat was 39 to 110 units (4.3-12.2 x 10^{6} cpm).

Values under the 7-day column are for the 7th day sample of plasma, red cells, platelets, and lungs and for total collected from day 1 to 7 for urine and feces.

Weight of rat = 250 g.

To study absorption and distribution, ^{3}H-heparin was instilled via the trachea into rats which were then killed and examined at various times. Table I shows the approximate distribution of radioactivity in various organs. 98.9% of the radioactivity was recovered from the lung immediately after instillation. At 1.5 hr 60.9% was recovered from the lung,

6.7% from the blood, and the remainder from other tissues (muscle 39%, liver 3.6%, and kidney 3.26%). After 24 hr only 10% of the radioactivity was left in the lungs. Approximately 42% had been excreted in 7 days. Thus the prolonged effect does not depend on slow absorption from the lung. The total recovery of radioactivity was found to be more than the amount administered mainly because the muscle and other organs were not exsanguinated before the determination of radioactive counts. This resulted in some duplication of radioactivity in the final analysis.

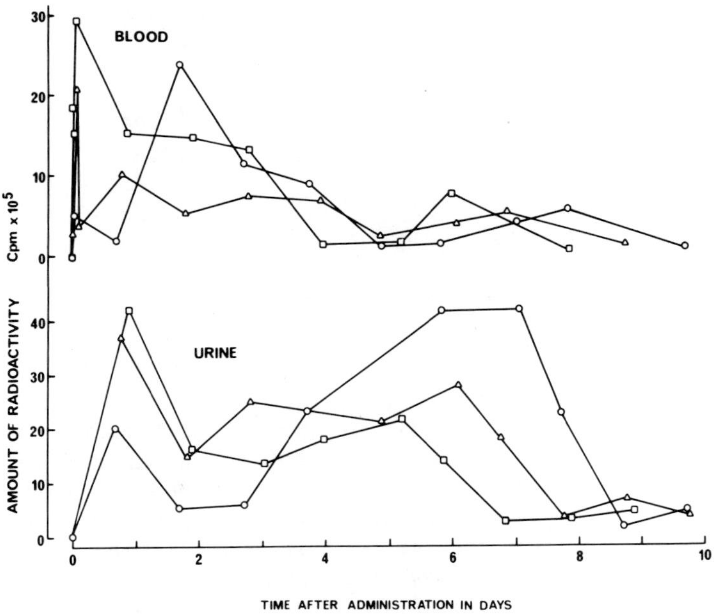

Fig. 4. Radioactivity in rat blood and urine after instillation of tritium-labeled heparin. 300-500 units heparin/kg body-weight. □ 17.5 μCi, O and Δ, 25 μCi, of ^{3}H-heparin. Each curve is plotted from values obtained from a single rat. (Reproduced by permission from (7)).

Figure 4 shows the radioactivity in blood and urine in rats following tracheal instillation of ^{3}H-heparin. The highest blood levels appear on the first day and gradually decreased over the next four to seven days. Peak values occur in the urine on the first day and rise slightly again on the fifth to seventh days. These patterns are similar to the increase in clotting times shown in Fig. 3.

Plasma levels in rats 1.5 hr after heparin administration as measured by inhibition of activated Factor X were essentially the same at all dose levels tested as shown in Table II. When tritiated heparin was used, the radioactivity in plasma corresponded to about 1 unit of heparin. Thus it appears the plasma levels do not depend directly on the dosage. These data suggest that heparin is rapidly cleared from the lung and

TABLE II Heparin Levels in Rat Plasma (Yin et al.) 1.5 hr After Tracheal Insufflation

Dose of heparin (units/kg)	*Plasma-heparin (units/ml)*
0	0
550	1.25
1000	0.6
10.000	1.65
10.000	2.55
10.000	1.25
20.000[a]	1.35

Weight of rats 350-785 g.
[a] *^{3}H-heparin.*

stored within an unknown pool, a process which then allows gradual release and appears to protect the heparin from rapid metabolism and excretion. As indicated by Mahadoo in this publication, heparin appears to be taken up by macrophages, which then may slowly release heparin into plasma. Our initial studies on dogs showed the presence of metachromatic granules in many cells found in lung smears, not present in control animals. The identity of the cells was not clear, but these cells were different in appearance to mast cells. Oh *et al.* (9) have shown that mouse peritoneal macrophages take up and hold heparin in granules without degradation until disintegration of the macrophage releases the heparin. Since heparin is a highly charged molecule it is not expected to pass through biological membranes readily. The large surface area of the lung with an abundance of phagocytic cells may explain how this fairly large molecule with a strong negative charge enters the body. The heparin appears to be engulfed within a vesicle. How these phagocytes transport the heparin into the blood stream is not yet clear. It would appear that the heparin enters the blood stream continuously at a gradual rate. In one dog, anticoagulated at 7 hr after tracheal heparin instillation, protamine titration of the blood indicated a heparin concentration of about 0.5/ml. An appropriate amount of protamine was then administered and the clotting time decreased to 4 min. However, after 24 hr, the clotting time had again risen to 50 min indicating additional heparin had entered the blood stream. The same phenomenon was observed by Sunderland and Klein (6) who performed pulmonary lavage on a patient with alveolar proteinosis with a solution containing 2.4 million units of heparin, which can be recalculated to a dose of approximately 200 mg/kg. Symptoms of abdominal hemorrhage were noted on the first day. Protamine neutralization was carried, but hemorrhagic symptoms appeared again the following day. This is not at all surprising when one observes the completely different pattern of response to intrapulmonary heparin.

IV. COMPARISON OF RESPONSES TO PULMONARY HEPARIN IN DOGS AND MAN

Comparison of clotting time values in dogs following tracheal instillation and in man following inhalation shows that the hypocoagulation in man is not as marked as that in the dog. However, the effect lasts for up to 16 days in man, as compared to 2-3 days in dogs. Blood levels of heparin were also determined by the inhibition of Factor Xa procedure (8), which may be more sensitive to the effects of low levels of heparin. Values thus obtained confirmed these findings.

To compare the response in the two species the areas under the curve were recalculated using the percentage increase in clotting time times the duration. Figure 2 shows the linear relationship found in the 18 trials in dogs. The solid dots indicate the responses found with the five trials in man indicating a similarity in total response between the two species, although the extent is less and the duration longer in man.

V. COMPARISON OF DOSAGES

The effective dose of pulmonary heparin that gave a measurable anticoagulant response in man was between 12 to 18 mg/kg. Converting a 15 mg/kg dose into units for comparison with other regimes, this amounts to 1050 mg for a 70 kg man. Each milligram of heparin had an activity of approximately 150 units so the total units inhaled were 157,500 units for a treatment that appeared to last two weeks. For an intravenous dosage of 500 units every 4 hr or 30,000 units per day, 157,500 units is about five days of treatment. For a subcutaneous treatment regime of 5000 units twice a day this represents 15 days of treatment. Thus in man about the same overall response is obtained when giving heparin by either the subcutaneous or pulmonary route, but inhalation requires a very large loading dose and infrequent administration.

VI. TOXICITY

Possible toxic effects to be considered are hemorrhagic effects, effects attributable to the pulmonary route of administration, and those associated with long term heparin therapy, such as effects on platelets, fibrinolysis, and bone. Much of this knowledge is incomplete at this time. It is quite possible that effects on these systems may vary with the route of administration.

Dog lungs were examined carefully for any sign of pathological change showing long term toxicity, and mice were examined shortly after inhalation for immediate toxicity. In the dog lung no difference in cellular infiltration, alteration in alveolar size or wall thickness, or change in number of mast cells present was found between experimental and control animals. No sign of previous hemorrhage was found. All animals were observed and no sign of hemorrhage were noted during the therapeutic period at the lower doses (8-16 mg/kg). At 20 mg/kg doses hematoma formation at the site of venipuncture was found if local pressure was not adequately applied. No hematuria, hemoptysis, or other signs of bleeding were noted.

No signs of toxicity were noted in tissue sections of mice that had inhaled heparin. However, in the rats prepared for tracheal instillation of heparin by a tracheostomy, it was noted that the surgical site that had been previously dry began to ooze blood in as little as 15 min following intrapulmonary instillation of high doses of heparin, and at times these animals died from blood loss. This was at very high doses of 60 to 120 mg/kg. This would indicate a very rapid absorption of at least a portion of the heparin from the lungs. The four male and two female human volunteers were examined thoroughly before and after heparin inhalation and no signs of toxicity or bleeding were noted. No change in chest x-ray was noted. Hemorrhagic symptoms can appear with higher doses. Sunderland and Klein administered 2.4 million units of heparin in a pulmonary lavage (approximately ten times the dosage used in our study), and noted epistaxis, hematuria, lower abdominal pain and an incoagulable blood picture. The hemorrhagic symptoms disappeared with protamine treatment but were present again the following day and were gradually improved. There was no evidence of residual lung damage a year later (10). The effect of long term inhalation of heparin on humans has not been studied as yet.

VII. USE OF HEPARIN INHALATION

Can we expect to use heparin by inhalation in the future? It is only when one realizes the pharmacological effect of heparin by this route that one can initiate a rational plan for its use. As with all drug therapy there should be a firm indication that the benefits of the drug will be greater than the hazard created. The positive aspects of this method include the avoidance of injection and the fact that the effect is prolonged and mild. This may be a method that provides good prolonged antithrombotic activity without creating the hazard of bleeding present with indirect anticoagulants. There is thus no need for frequent monitoring of heparin concentration in blood.

What are the disadvantages of this method? As yet the human response has only been studied in a small number, and variation in response has not been widely assessed. We would not recommend this method for treatment of actual thrombotic episodes as one would likely undertreat the patient. As with the subcutaneous heparin regimes this form of treatment seems best suited for prophylactic use in patients with high risk of thrombosis. However heparin therapy by inhalation should not be lumped together with the current evaluation of the value of subcutaneous administration of heparin as a prophylactic measure to reduce post surgical pulmonary emboli. This would not be recommended at this time as the necessary trials have not been performed. The prolonged effect, the normal variation in response to heparin in each individual could increase the danger of bleeding either at surgery or shortly afterwards. The important point is that if bleeding did occur the mild anticoagulant effect would be expected to persist for 8 to 16 days. This could require frequent protamine neutralizations, a procedure that is not without some risk and that has not been studied as yet to my knowledge, after heparin inhalation.

The benefits of heparin inhalation are likely to be greatest in patients with high risk of venous thrombosis where heparin therapy has shown some benefit. These conditions include hospitalized elderly nonsurgical patients, those with repeated episodes of deep venous thrombosis, pulmonary emboli, arterial embolism, and cerebral embolism. Other high risk categories such as hyperviscosity and neoplastic states, rheumatic valve disease with or without atrial fibrillation, and artificial valve grafts are high risk groups and would likely benefit from long term heparin therapy. In such groups heparin by aerosol would be convenient and nonhemorrhagic and provide prolonged antithrombotic protection, and we would recommend clinical trials in this type of patient.

However the effects of heparin when administered by different routes on antithrombin III levels, platelet function, and fibrinolysis are not clear, and future use will depend on all these effects. Thonnard-Neuman (11) has been using heparin by aerosol for prophylactic reduction in migraine headaches and reports a favorable effect. The basis of improvement may be due to alterations in blood antithrombin levels. Various others have used heparin aerosol for a variety of reasons. Sunderland and Klein had added heparin to a pulmonary lavage as a mucolytic agent for alveolar proteinosis. Molino and Belluardo have used 100 mg of heparin by aerosol twice daily for five months on a group of 86 *Thrombophilic* patients. In these patients, inhalation of heparin raised clotting time values to the normal range and was associated with no incidence of thrombosis or embolism. No evidence of toxicity was noted. Youngchaiyud (12) has reported some increase in airway conductance following heparin aerosol therapy in patients with chronic obstructive pulmonary disease. This method of heparin therapy could also be of considerable value as a research tool. Heparin can be administered repeatedly and painlessly to experimental animals and human volunteers for studies on toxicity, senility, enzyme activation, and a number of biological actions that have been attributed to heparin.

Clearly, heparin is absorbed by inhalation to give a prolonged mild anticoagulant effect without hemorrhagic effects. While this route is not recommended yet as a prophylaxis for post-surgical thrombosis, inhalation may prove to be of significant value in preventing thrombosis in other high risk groups, with greater convenience to the patient.

ACKNOWLEDGEMENT

Supported by grants-in-aid from the Saskatchewan Heart Foundation, Canada Packers Ltd., Toronto, Ontario, and the Medical Research Council of Canada.

REFERENCES

1. Windsor, E., and Freeman, L., Am. J. Med. *37*, 408 (1959).
2. Rosner, S.E., Vasc. Dis. *2*, 131 (1965).
3. Koh, T.Y., and Bharucha, K.R., U.S. Patent #3, Vol. 577, p. 543, Continuation-in-part of U.S. Patent #3, Vol. 506, p. 506 (1971).

21. Crafoord, C., Acta Chir. Scand. *79*, 407 (1937).
22. Cramer, R., Moore, R., and Amplatz, K., Radiology *109*, 585 (1975).
23. Elias, G., Shukla, S.K., and Mink, I.B., Cancer *36*, 129 (1975).
24. Falb, R.D., Leininger, R.I., Grode, G., and Crowley, J., Adv. Exp. Med. Biol. *52*, 365 (1975).
25. Follath, F., "Antikoagulantien bei künstlichen herz-klappen" *in* "Blutgerinnung und Antikoagulation," (K. Neuhaus and F. Duckert, eds.), p. 11. F.K. Schattauer Stuttgart-New York, 1976.
26. Francken, I.V., Johansson, L., Olsson, P., and Zetterquist, E., Lancet *70* (1963/I).
27. Frick, P.G., Acta Haemat. *16*, 11 (1956).
28. Friesen, R.H., and Clement, A.J., J. Thorac. Cardiovasc. Surg. *72*, 875 (1976).
29. Fujimoto, K., and Ueno, R., Z. Orthop. *111*, 310 (1973).
30. Fye, K.H., Hancock, D., Moutsopoulos, H., Humes, H.D., and Arieff, A.I., Arch. Intern. Med. *136*, 995 (1976).
31. Gastpar, H., and Goossens, N., "Untersuchungen über die Dosisabhangigkeit der ausgeschiendenen Heparinmengen in den Urin des Menschens, "Proc. 8th Congr. Europ. Soc. Haematol., II, 437. S. Karger, Basel-New York, 1962.
32. Gastpar, H., "Nebenwirkungen der Heparinoide," Proc. 3rd Intern. Congr. Chemother., II, 1798. G. Thieme, Stuttgart, 1964.
33. Gastpar, H., "Physiologische Bedeutung und pharmako-logische Wirkungen des Heparins," F.K. Schattauer, Stuttgart, 1965.
34. Gastpar, H., Thrombos. Diathes. Haemorrh. Suppl. 42, 291 (1970).
35. Gastpar, H., Hemat. Rev. *3*, 1 (1972).
36. Gastpar, H., "Heparin und Heparinoide" *in* "Klinik und Theeapie der Nebenwirkungen" (H.P. Kuemmerle, and N. Goossens, eds.), 2. Aufl., p. 399. G. Thieme, Stuttgart, 1973).
37. Gastpar, H., Med. Welt *27* (N.F.), 1737 (1976).
38. Gastpar, H., ed. "Onkohaemostaseologie" F.K. Schattauer, Stuttgart-New York, 1976.
39. Gastpar, H., "Platelet Cancer Cell Interaction in Metastasis Formation," J. Med. (in press).
40. Gatot, D., Smith, P.J., and Eckert, H., Aust. Paediat. J. *12*, 53 (1976).
41. Gentry, P.W., and Alexander, B., Biochem. Biophys. Res. Comm. *50*, 500 (1973).
42. Goossens, N., Gastpar, H., and Seitz, W., Klin. Wschr. *36*, 524 (1958).

43. Gordon, L.A., Richards, V., and Perkins, H.A., N. Engl. J. Med *255*, 1025 (1956).
44. Gott, V.L., Adv. Exp. Med. Biol. *52*, 351 (1975).
45. Graeff, H., Kuhn, W., and Zander, J., "Endotoxin Shock in Obstetrics" *in* "Gram-Negative Bacterial Infections," (B. Urbaschek, R. Ubaschek, and E. Neter, eds.), p. 446. Springer, Vienna-New York, 1975.
46. Greiling, H., and Kaneko, M., Drug Res. *23*, 593 (1973).
47. Grode, G.A., Anderson, S.J., Grotta, H.M., and Falb, R.D., Trans. Amer. Soc. Artef. Int. Organs *15*, 1 (1969).
48. Gross, R., Nieth, H., and Mammen, E., Klin. Wschr. *36*, 107 (1958).
49. Hagmar, B., Path. Europ. *4*, 283 (1969).
50. Hagmar, B., and Norby, K., Intern. J. Cancer *5*, 72 (1970).
51. Hagmar, B., Acta Path. Microbiol. Scand. *80*, 357 (1972).
52. Harker, L.A., and Slichter, S.J., N. Engl. J. Med. *283*, 1302 (1970).
53. Heene, D.H., Schöndorf, T., and Matthias, F.R., Proc. 20th Symp. Blutgerinnung, Hamburg, 1977. F.K. Schattauer, Stuttgart-New York (in press).
54. Hiebert, L.M., "Heparin and Endothelium," Proc. Intern. Heparin Symp., Saskatoon, July 6,7,8, 1977. (N.M. McDuffie, ed.) Academic Press, New York, 289.
55. Husemann, E., Pfannemüller, B., and Hertlein, W., Experientia (Basel) *9*, 379 (1953).
56. Jones, F.E., Black, P.J., Cameron, J.S., Chantler, C., Gill, D., Maisey, M.N., Ogg, C.S., and Saxton, H., Brit. Med. J. *547* (1975).
57. Kalmar, Pokar, H., and Tilsner, V., "Antikoagulantien und extrakorporaler Kreislauf," Proc. 20th Symp. Blutgerinnung, Hamburg, 1977. F.K. Schattauer, Stuttgart-New York (in press).
58. Kaulla, K.N. v., and Husemann, E., Experientia (Basel) *2*, 222 (1946).
59. Kaulla, K.N. v., "Klinische Fortschritte auf dem Gebiet der Blutgerinnung," Med. Klin. (Monographie H. 7) 1949.
60. Kaulla, K.N. v., "Coagulation Problems in Transplanted Organs" (K.N. v. Kaulla, ed.), C.C. Thomas, Springfield, Ill., 1972.
61. Kaulla, K.N. v., "Discussion Comment" *in* "Onkohaemostaseologie", p. 152. (H. Gastpar, ed.). F.K. Schattauer, Stuttgart-New York, 1976.
62. Kavanagh, L.W., and Mahadoo, J., "Heparin by Inhalation," Proc. Intern. Heparin Symp., Saskatoon, July 6,7,8, 1977. (N.M. McDuffie, ed.). Academic Press, New York, 333.
63. Khanh, B.T., Bathema, D., Vasquez, M., and Luke, R.G., Nephron *66*, 292 (1976).

64. Kincaid-Smith, P., Saker, B.M., and Fairley, K.P., Lancet, *1360* (1968/II).
65. Kincaid-Smith, P., Kidney Int. *7*, 242 (1975).
66. Kiricuta, I., Todorutio, C., Muresian, T., and Risca, R., Cancer *31*, 1392 (1973).
67. Koike, A., Cancer *17*, 450 (1964).
68. Kojima, K., and Sakai, I., Cancer Res. *24*, 1887 (1964).
69. Kolff, A.J., Effler, D.B., Gross, L.K., Peerboom, G., and Moraca, P.P., Clevel. Clin. Quart. *23*, 69 (1956).
70. Kuhn, W., and Graeff, H., *in* "Septischer Abort und bakterieller Schock" (J. Zander, ed.), p. 74. J. Springer, Berlin-New York, 1968.
71. Kuhn, W., and Neuhof, H., Personal Communication (unpublished).
72. Laki, K., J. Med. *5*, 32 (1974).
73. Lasch, H.G., and Heene, D.L., Thrombos. Diathes. Haemorrh. *33*, 105 (1974).
74. Leval, M.R., Hill, J.D., Mielke, C.H., Jr., and Macur, M.F., J. Thorac. Cardiovasc. Surg. *69*, 144 (1975).
75. Little, J.R., J. Amer. Med. Ass. *169*, 36 (1959).
76. Ludwig, H., and Ries, J., "Zur Indikation einer Parallelbehandlung tumorkranker Frauen mit Antikoagulantien" *in* "Strhlen, Blutgerinnung und Haemostase," (R. Marx, and H.A. Thies, eds.), p. 219. F.K. Schattauer, Stuttgart-New York, 1974.
77. Ludwig, H., Gynaekologe *7*, 204 (1974).
78. Lüscher, E.F., and Käser-Glanzmann, R., Thrombos. Diathes. Haemorrh. *33*, 113 (1974).
79. Luke, R.G., N. Engl. J. Med. *294*, 396 (1976).
80. Marx, F.J., Carl, P., and Schramm, W., Verhdl. ber. Dtsch. Ges. Urol. *26*, 223 (1975).
81. Marx, F.J., Staehler, G., Faul, P., and Schramm, W., Urologe *A14*, 127 (1975).
82. Marx, F.J., "Klinische Anwendung Klassischer Antikoagulantien in der Urologie", Proc. 20th Symp. Blutgerinnung, Hamburg, 1977. F.K. Schattauer, Stuttgart-New York (in press).
83. Marx, R., and Vath, A., Aerztl. Forsch. *3*, 131 (1950).
84. Marx, R., "Wichtige klinisch-haematologische Phaenomene bei Malignomen" *in* "Onkohaemostaseologie", (H. Gastpar, ed.), p. 3. F.K. Schattauer, Stuttgart-New York, 1976.
85. Merskey, C., Johnson, A.J., Part, J.H., and Wohl, H., Blood *24*, 701 (1964).
86. Merskey, C., Johnson, A.J., Kleiner, G.J., and Wohl, H., Brit. J. Haematol. *24*, 701 (1967).
87. Merskey, C., "Defibrination Syndrome" *in* "Human Blood Coagulation, Haemostasis and Thrombosis", (R. Biggs, ed.), 2nd Ed., P. 492. Blackwell, Oxford, 1976.

88. Messmer, B.J., Okies, J.E., Hallman, G.L., and Colley, D.A., Surgery *72*, 772 (1972).
89. Mielke, Ch., Jr., J. Thorac. Cardiovasc. Surg. *66*, 854 (1973).
90. Millar, R.C., and Ketcham, A.S., J. Med. *5*, 23 (1974).
91. Minna, J.O., Robboy, S.J., and Colman, R.W., "Dis-semminated Intravascular Coagulation in Man," C.C. Thomas, Springfield, Ill., 1974.
92. Mobin-Uddin, K., Utley, R.J., Bryant, L.R., Dillon, M., and Weiss, D.L., Ann. Thorac. Surg. *17*, 351 (1974).
93. Monkhouse, F.C., Gyanecologia *138*, 103 (1954).
94. Nuutinen, L.S., and Mononen, P., J. Thorac. Cardiovasc. Surg. *70*, 707 (1975).
95. Nyman, D., Thurnherr, N., and Duckert, F., Thrombos. Diathes. Haemorhh. *23*, 102 (1974).
96. Ødegard, O.R., Lie, M., and Abildgaard, U., Thrombos. Res. *6*, 287 (1975).
97. Paeschke, K.D., and Anger, H., Dtsch. Krebskongr., München, 1974.
98. Piper, J., Acta Physiol. Scand. *9*, 28 (1945).
99. Pollak, V.E., Ann. Intern Med. *73*, 334 (1973).
100. Popov, S., Kalinke, H., Etzel, F., Baymann, E., and Egli, H., "Coagulation Changes During and After Liver Transplantation in Man" *in* "Coagulation Problems in Transplanted Organs (K.N. v. Kaulla, ed.), p. 31. C.C. Thomas, Springfield, Ill., 1972.
101. Popov-Cenić, S., "Die Antikoagulantienbehandlung bei Gefässoperationen" (unpublished investigations).
102. Proesman, W., and Eeckels, R., Clin. Nephrol. *2*, 169 (1974).
103. Pulver, R., Chemotherapia *3*, 1 (1961).
104. Quellhorst, E., Reichel, W., Fernandez-Redo, E., and Scheller, F., Med. Klin. *72*, 981 (1977).
105. Regelson, W., Hemat. Rev. *1*, 193 (1968).
106. Regelson, W., Adv. Cancer Res. *11*, 223 (1968).
107. Regelson, W., Adv. Chemother. *3*, 303 (1968).
108. Regelson, W., Interferon *6*, 353 (1970).
109. Regelson, W., Annul. Rep. Med. Chem. *8*, 160 (1973).
110. Regelson, W., J. Med. *5*, 50 (1974).
111. Rent, R., Myhrman, R., Fiedel, and Gewurz, H., Clin Exp. Immunol. *23*, 264 (1976).
112. Reo, W.J., Whitley, D., and Eberle, J.W., Trans. Amer. Soc. Artif. Int. Organs *18*, 360 (1972).
113. Saliba, J.J., and Saliba, R.J., Thrombos. Diathes. Haemorrh. *33*, 113 (1974).
114. Salzman, E.W., Merrill, E.W., Binder, A., Wolf, C.F.W., Ashford, T.P., and Austen, W.G., J. Biomed. Mater. Res. *3*, 69 (1969).

115. Shires, D., Holcomb, H., and Cade, J., Clin. Res. *14*, 387 (1966).
116. Simon, G., and Chatelanat, F., Path. Microbiol. (Basel) *26*, 191 (1963).
117. Staehler, G., Carl, P., and Marx, F.J., Med. Welt *26* (N.F.), 990 (1975).
118. Stamm, H., Thrombos. Diathes. Haemorrh. Suppl. *15*, 9, 43, 51 (1965).
119. Strauli, P., Thrombos. Diathes. Haemorrh. Suppl. *20*, 147 (1966).
120. Strunk, R., and Colten, H.R., Clin. Immunol. Immunopath. *6*, 248 (1976).
121. Studdiford, W.E., and Douglas, G.W., Amer. J. Obstet. Gynec. *71*, 842 (1956).
122. Styk, B., and Kociskowa, D., J. Hyg. Epidemiol. Microbiol. Immunol. (Praha) , 483 (1964).
123. Suemasu, K., and Ishikawa, S., Gann *61*, 125 (1970).
124. Sullivan, J.M., Harker, D.E., and Gorlin, R., N. Engl. J. Med. *284*, 1391 (1971).
125. Thaler, E., and Schmer, G., Abstr. 73, 20th Ann. Meet. Soc. Artif. Int. Organs, 1974.
126. Vitacco, M., Avalos, J.S., and Gianantonio, C.A., J. Pediatr. *83*, 271 (1973).
127. Vogel, G.E., and Kopp, K.F., Med. Klin. *71*, 116 (1976).
128. Vogel, G.E., Hansen, W., and Goldmann, F.L., "Die Heparinisierung der chronischen Dialysepatienten." Med. Klin. (in press).
129. Walton, K.W., Brit. J. Pharmacol. *7*, 370 (1952).
130. Wardle, E.N., and Uldall, P.R., Brit. Med. J. *135*, (1972/II).
131. Weily, H.S., Steele, P.P., Davies, H., Pappas, G., and Genton, E., N. Engl. J. Med. *290*, 534 (1974).
132. Wessler, S., Adv. Exp. Med. Biol. *52*, 309 (1975).
133. Wood, S., Jr., Holyoke, E.D., and Yardley, J.H., Proc. 4th Canad. Cancer Conf., p. 167. Academic Press, New York, 1961.
134. Zimmermann, S.W., and Bergin, J.J., Nephron *12*, 219 (1974).

Friday, July 8, 1977, afternoon session

CARD, Saskatoon Dr. Kavanagh, how close are we to clinical application? Should we start using this next Monday or do you think one year or ten years?

KAVANAGH, Saskatoon The appropriate clinical studies to characterize the response haven't been done yet, but we anticipate this will soon be underway.

KRAEMER, Los Alamos Professor Jaques, in his recent paper (Jaques *et al.*, Lancet, 1, 411-413, 1977), which I thought was extremely interesting, provoked the following question: is there a relationship between the species differences in basophils and the species differences in mast cells, pariticularly in regard to whether they have any heparin in them or evidence that they make heparin?

JAQUES, Saskatoon There has only been an adequate examination of basophilic leukocytes from the standpoint of mucopolysaccharides in man and rabbit. This is because the percentage of basophilic leukocytes is so limited on other mammalian species. The rabbit is the experimental animal of choice because its basophilic leukocytes can be as high as 10% of the total. Certainly Tak Sue has shown that the basophilic leukocytes in the rabbit contain only chondroitin sulfates and this has been shown for man as far back as 1952. There are about four papers in the literature, all with the same results. The surprising thing is really how relatively little we do know about the basophilic leukocytes. On the other hand there is the query which is made by Michaels in his review and it had been in the literature before that, well over 40 years ago now, the surprising thing is that when one goes through the different mammalian species those animals that have large numbers of mast cells in tissues have relatively few basophilic leukocytes in the blood. That's why the rabbit is again the experimental animal of choice. It has a high basophilic leukocyte count and very few mast cells in tissues.

CUNNINGHAM, Saskatoon I wonder whether Dr. Jaques or perhaps any of the earlier contributors might offer some guidance for the pathologist on the significance that he ought to attribute to the accumulations of mast cells. I don't mean neoplastic accumulation but accumulations of mast cells where they are reactive in some manner, for example, finding them in relation to lymphoid centers in marrow or lymph nodes. The issue of

ISBN 0-12-484850-8

Ginsberg's work (Ginsberg and Lagunoff, J. Cell Biol., Vol. *35*, 685, 1967) on the possible derivation of mast cells from T cells I think is very provocative to me, in this regard.

PADAWER, New York That's quite a question and let me give it a stab. First, I think, recently its been shown similar results obtain, without the presence of fibroblasts, so that it is possible that these lymphocytes, and I hesitate to think of them as only T cells, could end up in that way. Second, there is a good deal of evidence that mast cells are affected by some tumors and by some autoimmune disease. You recall Burnett had found what he called clones of mast cells in the thymus of NZB mice that had developed Coomb's sensitivity. So there is some relationship to the immune system which I think, at this point, is inescapable, even though what it means is a very hard one to follow. Again, Burnett has suggested that the mast cell might be an end cell of the T lymphocyte, very similar to the plasmocyte, being the end cell of the B series. The difficulty with that is that nude mice that are congenitally athymic have perhaps more mast cells than average. They cannot reject foreign grafts but, on the other hand, they do not seem to come down with more cancer normally than other mice, suggesting that their surveillance system is still quite operative so we have a lot to develop in terms of the mast cell. I think the statement that the mast cell accumulation represents a certain experience towards antigen, is probably correct in some way, although I would like to leave it rather undefined because I find it difficult to define it at the moment. I would like to take this opportunity to say that, in my mind, there isn't as much difference between Dr. Uvnäs' viewpoint and my own, as might appear at first sight, and similarly, Dr. Higginbotham's viewpoints are part of one and the same thing. First I should announce my debt to Dr. Higginbotham for some of the ideas that I have presented. I might say, I'm a little like whoever it was that said that he reached so high because he stood on the shoulders of giants. Bob Higginbotham was the first one, I think, to come up with the idea that the mast cell was acting as an ion exchange resin, and I merely said its been happening outside the cell. It's happening inside the cell and I have suggested that some enzymes are tacked onto it but basically it's the same concept. I think what is happening is that Dr. Uvnäs has been looking at a system which has been pushed to the extreme, where it is so pushed that it's actually falling apart, whereas I have been looking at the same system from the opposite end where it has been functioning at a low level of activity that it can cope with. Normally the mast cell does all of these things without degranulating unless you push it so hard that it no longer can cope. I think that in some way we are really all working in the same area and Dr. Jaques, I don't know that there's any need to apologize for the word *garbage* in this content because I am very aware that one man's garbage is another's fertilizer, and New York City is spending millions of dollars trying to get rid of its garbage while Milwaukee has the garbage that made Milwaukee famous. These concepts are really very similar and I think perhaps from the pathological point of view, if there is one thing I might suggest to pathologists, and this on the basis of our own pathologists who think that they can tell mast cells without special stain, is that if you really want to look at mast cells I think you ought to go to stains that are much more specific than Hemotoxylin and Eosin and decrease the bravado that pathologists have by saying *this* is a mast cell.

CUNNINGHAM, Saskatoon I would have to agree with you on that because certainly Hemotoxylin and Eosin is the best way of making mast cells invisible that I know of. This issue about the nude mice, we have looked at this in a thymoplastic subject who had very, very minimal lymphocytes in the circulation. The autopsy report showed lots of mast cells, so that in the human situation the absence of lymphocytes didn't preclude the histogenesis of mast cells.

CONCLUDING REMARKS

40 YEARS OF HEPARIN RESEARCH - PAST AND FUTURE

L.B. Jaques

University of Saskatchewan

On a similar occasion the late Sir Lionel Whitby compared himself to the final batsman in a cricket match who had the responsibility of bringing in badly needed runs. Equally applicable is the analogy of the final batter in the lower half of the ninth inning in baseball with the winning runs on base. Both these situations have been described in verse but whereas Newbolt (1) concluded with the stirring exhoration *"Play up, Play up and Play the game!";* as you know, Casey struck out (2), which indicates that the position may result in an anticlimax.

I asked that my talk be listed as *40 years of Heparin Research - Past and Future* to indicate that I would attempt both to do some summing up and also some projection into the future. I believe one should only attempt to see the future in science from the records of the past. Like all outstanding fairy stories, the Water-Babies by Charles Kingsley (3), is a philosophical work, in this case an allegory of science and its procedures. In the story, Tom, the Water-Baby, to become a man is starting out for the Other-Side-of-Nowhere. He starts out and is immediately lost. The mythical figure, Mother Carey instructs Tom that what he must do is swim backwards holding on and looking into the eyes of his dog, and in this way will reach his goal. This is the analogy for the scientific process. By continually going over the past records and making sure that we do not miss the important parts of the record, we can project something of what the future has in store for us.

We have listened and participated for three days in a mind-stretching exercise. To me what has been tremendously appealing is the interelationships of all aspects of this topic. The discussion of chemistry and chemical problems is of vital importance to the clinical use of heparin. On the other hand the clinical problems presented give practical significance for many aspects of the chemical problems. The discussion with regard to the cellular aspects of heparin and related compounds is closely related with both, since on the one hand it is the cellular aspect that provides the complex chemistry, and on the other hand is vital to understanding how heparin does exert its effects clinically. In the process,

ISBN 0-12-484850-8

certain assumptions which have been widely held, and in fact have been the working background for all of us have not only been challenged at this conference, but successfully *refuted*. In this presentation I propose then not only to try and summarize the conclusions of the talks of these three days, but also to identify assumptions and from there point out that with the refuting of generally held assumptions, we now have a responsibility to expand our knowledge so as to replace the old principles with new principles that will serve for another forty years.

I. THE CHEMICAL NATURE OF HEPARIN

The discussions of the chemical nature of heparin demonstrated that commercial heparin is a mixture of at least 22 different chains all having the same main chemical structure being polymers of a hexasaccharide containing in 1,4α-linkage, 2,6-disulfoglucosamine, 2-sulfoiduronic acid, and glucuronic acid. Dimers of all the chains lengths are found in pig intestinal mucosa heparin. Only some of these chain lengths are active anticoagulant and the activities differs with respect to different stages of the coagulation cascade. This has been documented by the demonstration in many tests that only a third of commercial heparin is active and that this varies with the test. When the examination is extended to the heparin present in the rat skin, rat peritoneal mast cells, monkey skin by Horner and Lindahl, further complexities are found. The native heparin present is frequently in much larger molecular aggregates, as large as 75,000 - 1,000,000 daltons. Degradation of these larger aggregates can be achieved by ascorbic acid demonstrating side to side linkages of chains by a nonglycosidic bond. Alan Horner has proposed that *macromolecular heparin* be used for all ascorbic acid degradable heparins, which of course will include the dimer in the commerical pig intestinal mucosal heparin. Also, evident in these macromolecular heparins and to a lesser degree in commercial heparins is a carbohydrate core and xylose-serine which attached heparin to protein in its synthesis.

The first assumption that has been refuted is that heparin represents a single principle and all that has been necesary is the further purification to obtain the active principle. It is now evident that this assumption is not true.

II. CHEMISTRY OF MUCOPOLYSACCHARIDES VERSUS PROTEINS AND NUCLEIC ACIDS

I think one can also see further consequences from the

results reported. The elucidation of this complex situation has not been obtained by any one particular technique but a battery of techniques that have been used in combination. These are specific bacterial enzymes, nuclear magnetic resonance, chromatographic techniques of greater sophistication, electrophoresis in a variety of gels and with different buffers, electrofocusing, and with many of these the utilization of the principle of critical electrolyte concentration formulated by J.E. Scott. These techniques are not only clarifying the chemistry of heparin but also of the related sulfated mucopolysaccharides. In so doing, I think that they demonstrate that another assumption on which we have been operating is not valid. This is that the techniques that by themselves have been so satisfactory for elucidating the chemistry of polysaccharides, of nucleic acids, of proteins, can be effective in elucidating the chemistry of the mucopolysaccharides. Granted, we would not have been able to achieve the results that have been reported and discussed in the last several days if there has not been the development of these techniques in connection with proteins and nucleic acids. The fact that the elucidation of the problems of the mucopolysaccharides has required the combination of a number of techniques seems to me to indicate that the common assumption that these compounds have a general similarity to proteins and nucleic acids is not valid. These compounds are anionic polyelectrolytes. A similar group of compounds have been developed in industrial chemistry and have wide application. They are used to increase the production of oil wells, to clean floors, etc. They have very many applications and we all encounter them every day without being aware of it. Anionic polyelectrolytes (and the corresponding cationic polyelectrolytes) have rather unique properties. First, I remind you that in distinction to proteins and nucleic acids, these polyelectrolytes are not ampholytes and do not possess isoelectric points and, therefore, do not possess certain characteristic properties of proteins and nucleic acids. As shown by Dr. Stone and others, heparin (and other mucopolysaccharides) can have a helical structure. However, in solution the shell of negative charges surrounding the molecule results in marked extension of the chains. This results in very remarkable chemical properties, in terms of modifying the behavior of other ions in solution and even to the extent of *catalytic* activities. This is why the approach of Dr. Stivala and others in examining the polyelectrolyte behaviour of these compounds along the lines of Scatchard and others is so important. There is considerable overlap in this with Dr. Davis' approach in terms of colloid theory.

III. NOMENCLATURE REFORM

I have used the term mucopolysaccharide rather than glycosaminoglycan. Dr. Gastpar, Dr. Bianchini, and Dr. Kakkar have discussed representatives of an important group of these compounds, the heparinoids. These have identical properties and I'm sure still have an important medical future, yet many of them do not contain amino sugar as a part of their skeleton. This indicates then the amino sugar is not an important component. I suggest that as the word mucopolysaccharide has been defined in various ways in the past, it should now be redefined as covering those compounds that are anionic polyelectrolytes of biological and medical interest.

In appealing to reform nomenclature, I should point out that we do need to improve the nomenclature with regard to sulfate in these compounds. There is increasing use of the term *polysulfate* in the literature. A polysulfate refers to a compound with a sulfate radical containing more than one sulfur atom, analogous to polyphosphates, but with even higher energy bonds. Since PAPS is involved in the synthesis of the sulfated mucopolysaccharides and heparin as shown by Silbert, it is not unlikely that when people start to look for polysulfate compounds as with polyphosphates, these will be found to occur biologically. For compounds such as heparin that have more than one sulfate per sugar unit, *multisulfated* is satisfactory. Further it has the advantage of indicating the sulfate groups are of different types, which of course they must be when substituted in different positions in the sugar. The use of sulfate with chondroitin and heparitin can only be confusing or misleading to anyone outside of our own field of specialty. Is there any point in continuing this perpetuation of an early error?

IV. STANDARDIZATION OF HEPARIN

The demonstration that heparin is not a single principle but a mixture of a number of chains only some of which inhibit a given coagulation step and not the same for different steps challenges the assumptions on which standardization of heparin is based and even the assumption on which pharmacopeias are written. This is that a single test can be prescribed for a drug to constitute a legal qualification. It is not widely appreciated that the science of biological standardization and assay was developed in connection with insulin. This was necessary because, for this first time, a drug was to be used clinically that was first known by its specific biological activity and that required a narrow range of dosage control (too little, the diabetes was not under control, a little too much, and the patient could go into convulsions). Now the chemists (in Toronto and Stockholm) were fresh from developing the standardization of insulin. It was natural then that they used the same approach and definitions as for insulin. However, the discussions of the last three days have demonstrated that heparin and insulin are antiethical in chemistry, biological activity, clinical use, and control. Heparin is not one drug principle but many. No single biological test describes the activities present in the mixed mucopolysaccharides, and a completely different approach is required for standardization of the drug for clinical use. It would appear that it is necessary to set this up in physicochemical terms. The methods are now available for identifying chemically the carbohydrate skeleton and the various chains present. It would therefore appear that the next step is to identify which of the chains are of clinical importance. In this connection it is essential not to limit the examination to one particular property such as the ability to combine with antithrombin. Nor is it possible to limit the investigation to *in vitro* tests since Dr. Horner demonstrated that an ^{35}S-commercial heparin introduced into the body appeared in a higher molecular weight fraction, i.e., conversion of inactive commercial chains to active chains can occur in the circulation after injection of heparin. We now realize that this is the explanation of the observation made by Levy in this laboratory 25 years ago (4). He injected heparin in rabbits, dogs, and man, took blood samples, separated the heparin, and measured the antithrombin activity and toluidine blue combining activity. After the initial peak, the antithrombin value was always considerably greater than the toluidine blue value. Now, we realize he was observing the conversion proposed by Alan Horner of conversion of inactive chains to antithrombin active chains.

For the standardization of heparin, it may well be that for clinical use, heparin will be found most suitable which is a mixture of a number of chain lengths. This should offer no problem since it is possible to determine the size and chain distribution of a number of commercial heparins that are satisfactory clinically. Then the pharmacopeia can adopt specifications in terms of the range of the desirable components.

V. HEPARIN AND MAST CELLS

The identification of heparin and mast cells has been discussed in many ways at this conference. I believe there has been a considerable clarification of and disposal of certain assumptions. The first of these is that heparin and mast cells are more or less synonymous terms. Other sulfated mucopolysaccharides are present in mast cells. In fact this was first pointed out by Professor Jorpes with the Fuchsin-sulfurous acid reaction (5). Further, the heparin found in the mast cell is not identical with commercial heparin. Those cases already examined (from rat skin and rat peritoneal mast cells) appear to consist of chiefly high molecular weight heparins of the order of 750,000 to a million. It does appear, however, that high molecular weight heparins are still essentially polysaccharides containing a polysaccharide core with the heparin chains attached to the core.

We have heard various proposals regarding mast cells and their functions. We have made progress in the amount of information about mast cells that indicate that this is not an identical cell wherever it is found. One characteristic of mast cells is the presence of granules in very large numbers that have a high affinity for toluidine blue and show a metachromatic staining of this dye. The staining is due to the presence of high concentrations of sulfated mucopolysaccharides. What this tells us is that the mast cells are characterized by their accumulating sulfated mucopolysaccharides synthesized in the cell. Radioisotope-labeling has demonstrated that synthesis of histamine and heparin is very active within mast cells, but uptake of these compounds by mast cells is slow. What causes the cell to accumulate the histamine and heparin it synthesizes and thus become a mast cell? Ginsberg (6) showed in an *in vitro* system where lymphocytes were grown in tissue culture on a fibroblast monolayer, a mass differentiation of mast cells followed exposure to the specific antigens. That is, the accumulation of the large amounts of SMPs in lymphocytes to the point of being recognized as mast cells is a response that occurs in association with fibroblasts. Does the presence of a large number of mast cells constitute evidence of previous series of exposures to sensitizing agents? If so we must include metals as stimuli, since the development of large mast cells occurs as response to metals after prior treatment with a sensitizing agent (7). If mast cells are a record of previous challenge by foreign substances, how can the mast cell be a secreting cell as proposed by Dr. Uvnäs or as a cell controlling the composition of tissue fluid as presented by Dr. Padawar. Are we talking about the same cells or is it simply that they all look the same but these are different cells with these different functions? Alternatively, normal tissue (as in gnotobiotic animals) contains a few mast cells that carry out normal physiological functions. Exposure to foreign agents results in the transformation of large number of lymphocytes to mast cells that develop to the wellbeing of the tissue concerned. I think we must conclude that we have not as yet resolved these questions. On the other hand the development of methods described at this sympsoium should provide means for experiments to answer to some of these questions.

The close association of mast cells with blood vessels has led most people to assume that heparin is secreted from the mast cells and goes directly into the blood vessel lumen. Dr. Padawer pointed out on his slide that the mast cells, even when related to blood vessels, are at a significant distance from the vessel. Further, as Dr. Davis pointed out to me, the flow of fluid is from the vessel to the lymph. All of this points to heparin from mast cells being released as granules into the connective tissue spaces and then engulfed by macrophages, etc., locally. Only with extreme anaphylaxis in the dog is much heparin and histamine released and dissociated in the tissue fluid to be transported to the general circulation.

VI. HEPARIN AND OTHER CELLS

Discussions of the relation of different mucopolysaccharides to other cells has demonstrated that possibly recognition of cells depends on mucopolysaccharides in or associated with the cell membrane. Since only a small number of heparin chains have anticoagulant activities and yet 22 chains occur naturally, this would suggest that heparins have a much wider biological function than the one rather limited anticoagulant role, important though this may be to clinical medicine. Anionic polyelectrolytes represent the obvious chemical complementary form to biogenic amines. As such one must think of them as the most likely candidates for receptor structures. As demonstrated by Dr. Uvnäs, in the mast cell, heparin appears to be attached to proteins by the sulfate groups and attached to histamine by carboxyl groups. This opens up another angle for investigation with regard to these compounds.

The identification of the cellular pool in the reticuloendothelium system for heparin administered as a drug disposes of a number of assumptions long current. The first of these, of course, is that heparin is simply mixed with the blood in circulation. It is now evident that by any route of administration the plasma levels are a reflection of the effect of the cellular pool. This explains the observation reported particularly by Refn *et al.* (8) at the 1954 Thrombosis-Embolism Conference that intermuscular and subcutaneous injection of heparin actually gave blood levels much like continuous intravenous injections. Low plasma heparin levels of heparin can be the consequence of administration of heparin intermuscularly, subcutaneously, or intrapulmonary. These methods of administration introduce considerable amounts of heparin into the cellular pool for later release to the circulation. The successful clinical results for thrombo-embolism with *low-dose* heparin has demonstrated the clinical effectiveness of low plasma concentrations of heparin. However, *low-dose* is relative to large doses of heparin given previously subcutaneously. It would appear better now to describe this procedure (irrespective of route) as maintenance of *low plasma levels of heparin*. Particular routes will then be selected as most suitable to the patient.

The demonstration of the cellular pool for heparin is accompanied by the failure to find any significant effect on the mast cell. This is in agreement with the finding that the heparin in the RES cells is simply stored and later released and enters the circulation again. On the other hand, mast cell granules when they discharge from the mast cell, as indicated by Dr. Higginbottom, appear to be taken up by macrophages and destroyed. This represents a significant difference. Is it due to the inflammatory response elicited by the accompanying histamine of the granule, or by activation of macrophages, or is it due to enzymes accompanying the histamine and heparin in the granule? It should be pointed out in this regard that when rat peritoneal mast cells are caused to release their granules by 48/80, the granules are reformed in a few hours, but when the granules are released by distilled water, the mast cells are destroyed and do not reappear for many months (9).

VII. NONMAST CELL HISTAMINE AND HEPARIN

The demonstration of nonmast cell histamine has resulted in many recent papers on important physiological roles for histamine including that of transmitter function. It would seem logical then to look for nonmast cell heparin. Engleberg (10) drew attention to tissues that contain considerable heparin and few mast cells. If nonmast cell heparin and histamine are in other cells, then presumably in these cells the heparin and related sulfated mucopolysaccharides are stored in a form that does not stain with toluidine blue to give typical granules. Such nonmast cell heparin, however, might very well be (like nonmast cell histamine) in a form much more readily utilized for purposes of secretion. As shown by S. Wice & A. Wollin in their exhibit, in the small intestine of the rat, the synthetic mechanisms for these are adaptive to increased fat load, as previously characterized by Schayer for nonmast cell histamine in other locations.

VIII. CLINICAL USES OF HEPARIN

It has been generally assumed that the clinical use of heparin is simply an extension of the early laboratory use, i.e., that the anticoagulant effects of heparin *in vivo* are identical with that of mixing heparin with blood *in vitro*. Of course, the appearance of lipoprotein lipases and diamine oxidase demonstrates differences. Actually, Solandt and Best (11) in the initial paper on heparin in an extracorporeal loop also showed a difference for the clinically desirable action of heparin. After the injection of heparin in dogs, the clotting time reached infinity immediately, as with the addition of comparable amounts of heparin to the blood outside of the body. However, formation of thrombi in a glass cell in the loop was not prevented until 20 to 60 min after the injection. Two to six hours later the clotting time again became measurable but thrombus formation did not occur. In other words, there was a dissociation of the effects on coagulation time and on blocking thrombus formation.

With the demonstration that heparin is a mixture of principles it is necessary to identify the various components of the mixture with regard to their clinical action. The demonstration that only one-third of commercial heparin is active in a given coagulation test carries with it the conclusion that monitoring heparin by a coagulation test means monitoring only one-third of the heparin that is being administered. This, of course, immediately explains discrepancies that have been reported from time to time between different coagulation tests used to monitor heparin. It does suggest that on the whole, nothing is to be gained by trying to decide which test is better because all of them are measuring a part of the heparin. The problem remains. Is the heparin not giving a positive indication in the test for monitoring, contributing to the clinical effectiveness of the therapy? Sharnoff (12) made the point that the considerable variation between commercial heparins demonstrated by coagulation tests *in vitro* has not been the experience of clinicians in using different heparin preparations from different manufacturers or from different batches from the same manufacturers. This tends to suggest that total mixtures have equal clinical therapeutic effectiveness.

The observation that administered heparin enters into biocellular pools for later release to the circulation is probably a factor in the remarkable clinical success of heparin and also in the lack of extremes of variation of hypocoagulable activity. This is probably a factor in the success of heparin, adding an additional safety factor of which we have been unaware. It would appear that continuous intravenous, repeated intravenous injections, subcutaneous injections, intrapulmonary administration of heparin differ only in the amount of heparin that is introduced into the cellular stores and total number of cells storing heparin. These can then be used as alternatives as most suitable for the given patient.

Heparin has two major clinical uses. The first is for cardiovascular surgery, cardiac diagnostics, external circulations (lung, artificial kidney, etc.). This is the consumer in hospitals of the largest amount of heparin. Second is its use of heparin in treatment and prevention of thromboembolism. I emphasize that there are many other uses of heparin and Dr. Gastpar has reviewed some of these. It is evident that these two main uses of heparin differ considerably in requirements. In the arterial system much more heparin is required for protection. Associated with this is the fact that in the uses cited there is much more tissue damage, the blood is exposed to much more foreign surface, etc. The importance of this was demonstrated in the initial experiment leading to these two uses of heparin. For the second use in treatment and prevention of venous thromboembolism, it was also shown that the quantity of heparin required for protection also depended on the degree of tissue damage (endothelium, shift in the coagulation balance). Hence, low dose heparin (maintenance of low plasma levels) is effective only when started with reasonably normal endothelium and hemostatic balance. With these deranged, more heparin is required.

To sum up, the baffling chemical complexity of heparin matches the complexity of the thrombotic process. The overall negative charge of these polyanions is of higher density than of any other biological substance. This is responsible for the special features of cellular storage and inability of sodium salts to pass membranes. These properties are the basis of the long success that this drug has had clinically.

IX. CONCLUSION

In concluding this rather rambling survey of some of the results of this three day conference and of what the future has in store for further heparin research, I recall that at the Josiah Macey Conference on Blood Clotting and Allied Problems in 1950, the late Professor Knisely closed the conference with a recitation of the children's poem *"The Blind Men of Hindustan"*. The point of this poem is - seven blind men examined an elephant. Each came up with a different theory about the nature of the elephant on the basis of the part that he took hold of as judged by his sense perceptions.

I would like to refer to another literary elephant. C.S. Lewis (13) identified a great defect of academics. C.S. Lewis referred to people who claimed to be able to see fern-seeds when they were unable to see an elephant 10 yards away in broad daylight. In this presentation, I have referred directly or indirectly to 25 assumptions that we have held for the past 40 years and that are no longer tenable. I hope for the next 40 years of heparin research, less and less time will be spent examining nonexistent fern-seeds and as much time as possible be spent examining the visible elephants.

REFERENCES

1. Newbolt, H., "Vitai Lampada" *in* "Poems of Today. An. Anthology," p. 115. Sidgwick & Jackson Ltd., London, 1916.
2. Thayer, E.L., "Casey at the Bat" *in* "Innocent Merriment. An. Anthology of Light Verse," (selected by Franklin P. Adams) p. 487. Whittlesey House Division of McGraw-Hill, New York, 1942.
3. Kingsley, C. "The Water-Babies. 1863." J.M. Dent & Sons Ltd., London; Dutton, New York, 1957.
4. Levy, S.W., M.Sc. thesis. University of Saskatchewan, Saskatoon, Sask., Canada, 1951.
5. Jorpes, E., Werner, B. and Aberg, B., Jour. Biol. Chem. *176*, 277, 1948.
6. Ginsburg, H., Ann. N.Y. Acad. Sci. *103*, 20, 1963.
7. Selye, H., "Calciphylaxis." University of Chicago Press, Chicago, 1962.
8. Refn, I., Raasch, F. and Vestergaard, L., 1st International Conference on Thrombosis and Embolism, Basel p. 758, 1954. B. Schwake, Basel, 1955.
9. Keller, R., Arch. Intl. Pharmacodyn.Therap. *110*, 300, 1957.
10. Engelberg, H., "Heparin: Metabolism Physiology and Clinical Application." C.C. Thomas, Springfield, 1964.
11. Solandt, D.Y. and Best, C.H., The Lancet *i*, 1042, 1940.
12. Sharnoff, J.G., The Lancet *i*, 258, 1973.
13. Lewis, C.S., "Fern-seed and Elephants," (Walter Hooper ed.) p. 111. Fontona - Collins, Glasgow, 1975.

INDEX

I

L

M

N

P

T

U

W